For modesty's sake?

Rijksmuseum voor Volkenkunde Leiden

For modesty's sake?

ISBN: 90 5613 017 X

Publishers and printers: Barjesteh, Meeuwes & Co / Syntax Publishers in co-operation with Haveka B.V.
Lay-out: Manten Grafische Communicatie & Advies, Rotterdam

G.M. Vogelsang-Eastwood

For modesty's sake?

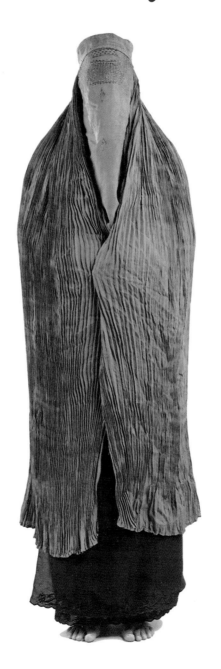

 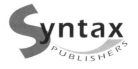

Barjesteh, Meeuwes & Co | Syntax Publishers Tilburg

Two women from Western China (courtesy of K. de Vries).

Table of contents

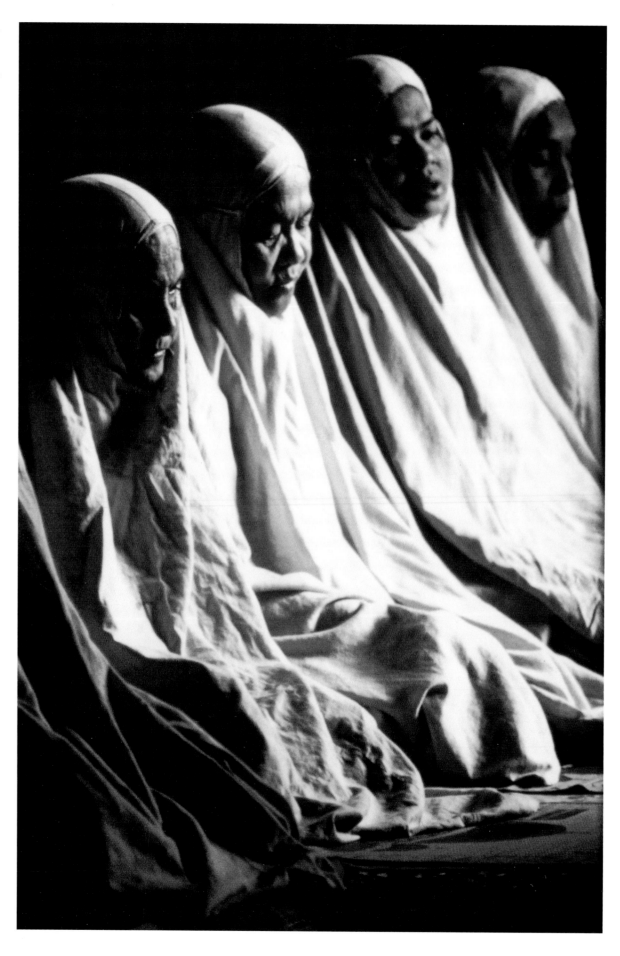

Preface

This book is intended to be an overview of the history and development of veiling. It was written in order to accompany an exhibition (*Sluiers*), held at the National Museum of Ethnology, Leiden between October 1996 and March 1997.

The origins of the book and the exhibition lie in the discovery of three face-veils at the medieval site of Quseir al-Qadim, on the Red Sea coast of Egypt. The site was being excavated by D. Whitcamb and J. Johnson, The Oriental Institute, Chicago and in 1982 I was working there as the textile and clothing specialist. I became intrigued by the idea and history of veiling at that time and gradually the subject of veiling became a mini-obsession. However, it was not until I was appraoched by the Natinal Museum of Ethnology, Leiden, to create an exhibition about veiling that I had the chance to make a more detailed study of the subject. The research involved in writing the book and preparing the exhibition has opened the way to many ideas, as well as doors which I never suspected existed.

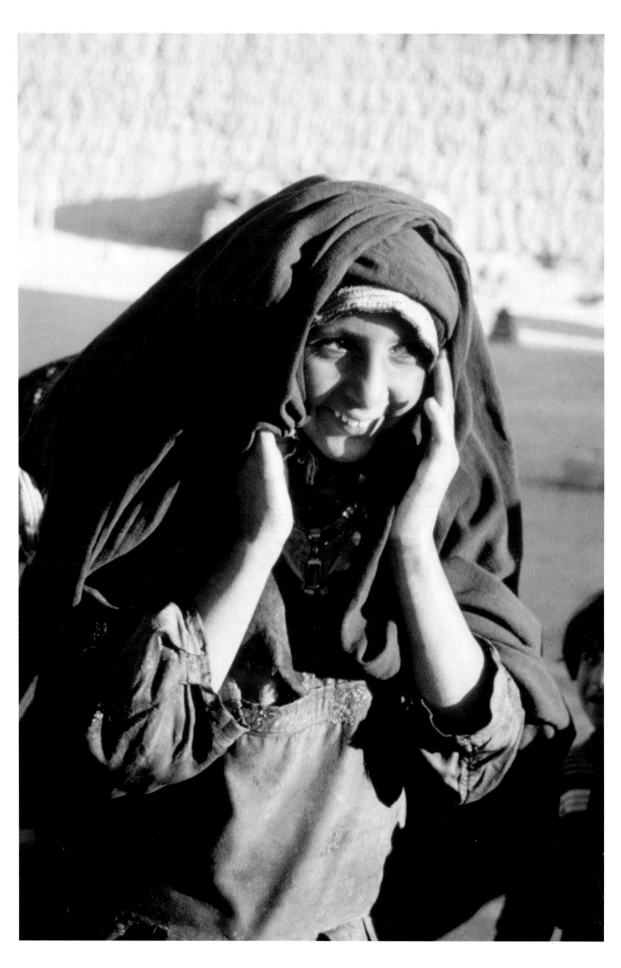

Woman from a village near Saada, Yemen (courtesy of K. de Vries).

Acknowledgements

I should like to thank various people for their help during the preperation of this book and the exhibition, including, at the National Museum of Ethnology, Leiden, the director S. Engelsman, A. v.d. Sande, R. Bedaux, R. Munneke, H. de Boer, F. Scholte and J. Groenendijk. M. Lemann and J. Daas should be acknowledged for their on conserving the textiles and preparing the stands. Without their experience (especially that of Maria's) the attractive nature in which the objects were displayed would never have been achieved. L. Helm should also be thanked for putting many ideas into practise (he also makes a wonderful chauffeur!).

In addition, J. van Haarst should be thanked for just being there with the cups of tea. While it was the secetaries of the museum (while enjoying trying on various veils), who helped me to understand just how interested people would be in my 'obsession'.

Within Leiden University, I should like to thank Prof. R. Kruk form the Department of Islamic Art, for her advise and help throughout the preparation of the exhibtion. The staff of the Near Eastern Library, for their interest and help with advise and the Hotz photographs. A special word of thanks should go to B. Grieshaven for his work on many of the photographs in this book. Mention should also be made of Arzu who was our model and who made all the garments look extremely attractive. In addition, K. de Vries, R.E. Kon and N. Monastra shoud be thanked for allowing me to use their photographs.

The kindness of staff from the Tropen Museum, Amsterdam and the Museum of Ethnology, Rotterdam, also need a special mention. Their generosity of time and spirit was greatly appreciated.

In Egypt, I should like to thank the staff of The Netherlands Institute for Arabic and Archaeological Studies, Cairo, especially, F. Leonar, H. de Heijer, T. Mulde. In addition, Lyla and Somya should not be forgotten for their help with the various shopping trips to the Khan al-Khali.

In Yemen help was provided by Ursula Dreibholz and Sadek Noha of the American Institute for their help with providing suitable Yemen garments. A word of thanks also needs to go Kefah Abduwani (fashion designer), Muscat, Oman, for her patience and kindness with regards her wonderful garments.

A word of thanks should go to the Egyptian Ambassador, His Excellency Ambassador Badawi and Mrs. Badawi, for their support and enthusiasm from the initial stages of both the book and the exhibition. Finally, I should also like to thank the the staff members of the Oman Embassy, The Hague, especially the Ambassador, His Highness Jaifer Salim Al-Said, the Second Secretary and the Ambassador's secretary for their continous help in this project.

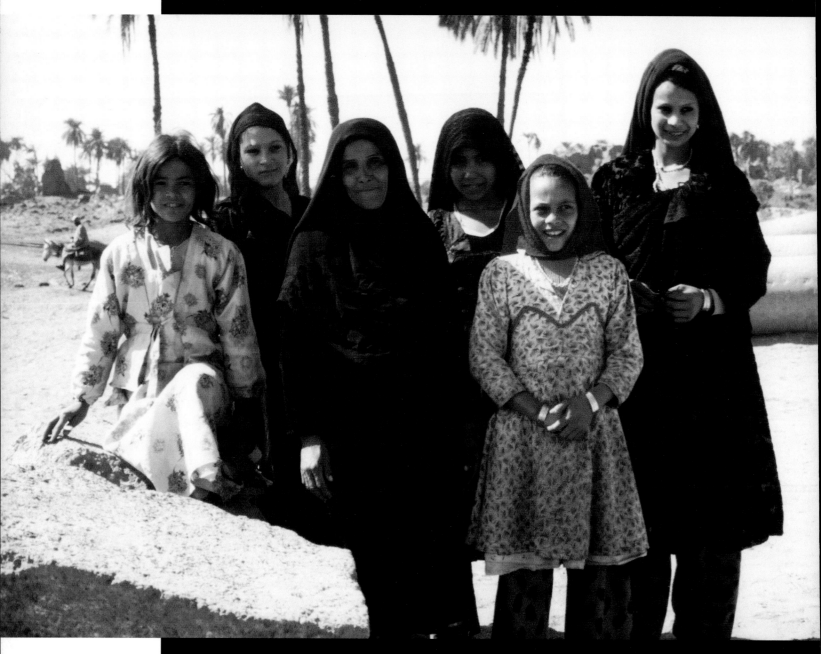

Group of women from Middle Egypt.
Included in the photgraph is a young girl
(no head covering), a pubescent girl
(colourful headscarf), a young married woman
(black headscarf) and a mature woman
(enveloping headcovering).

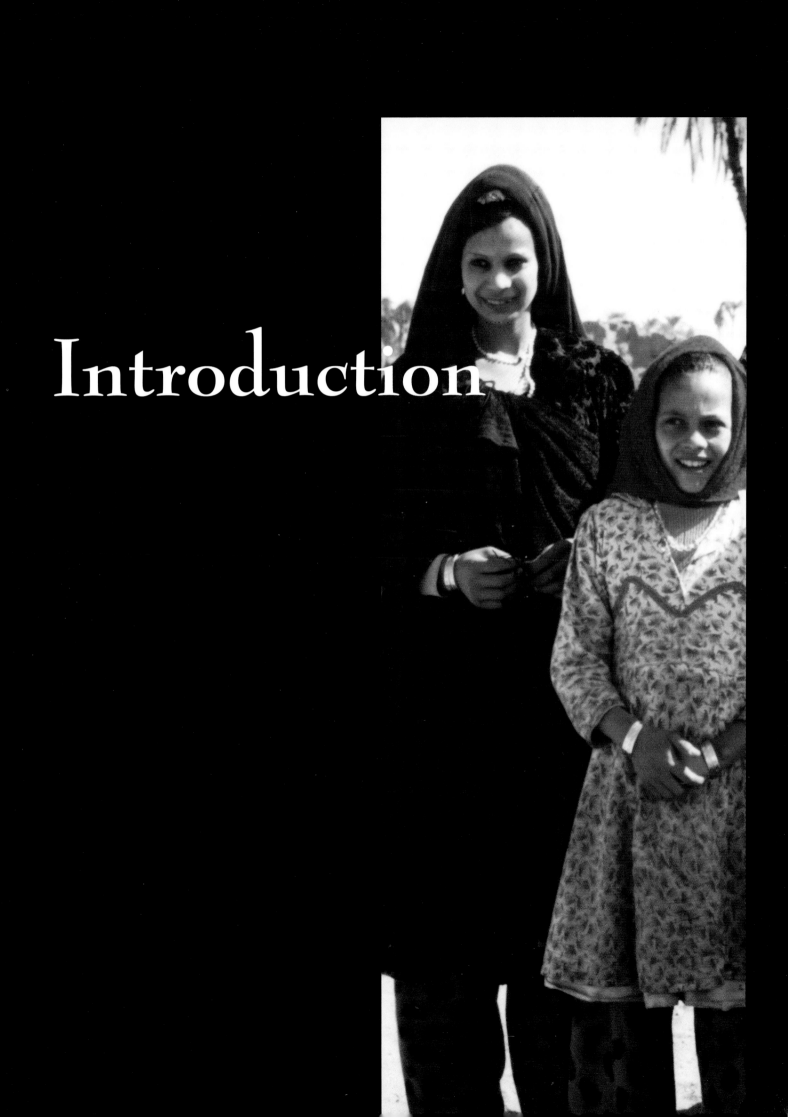

Introduction

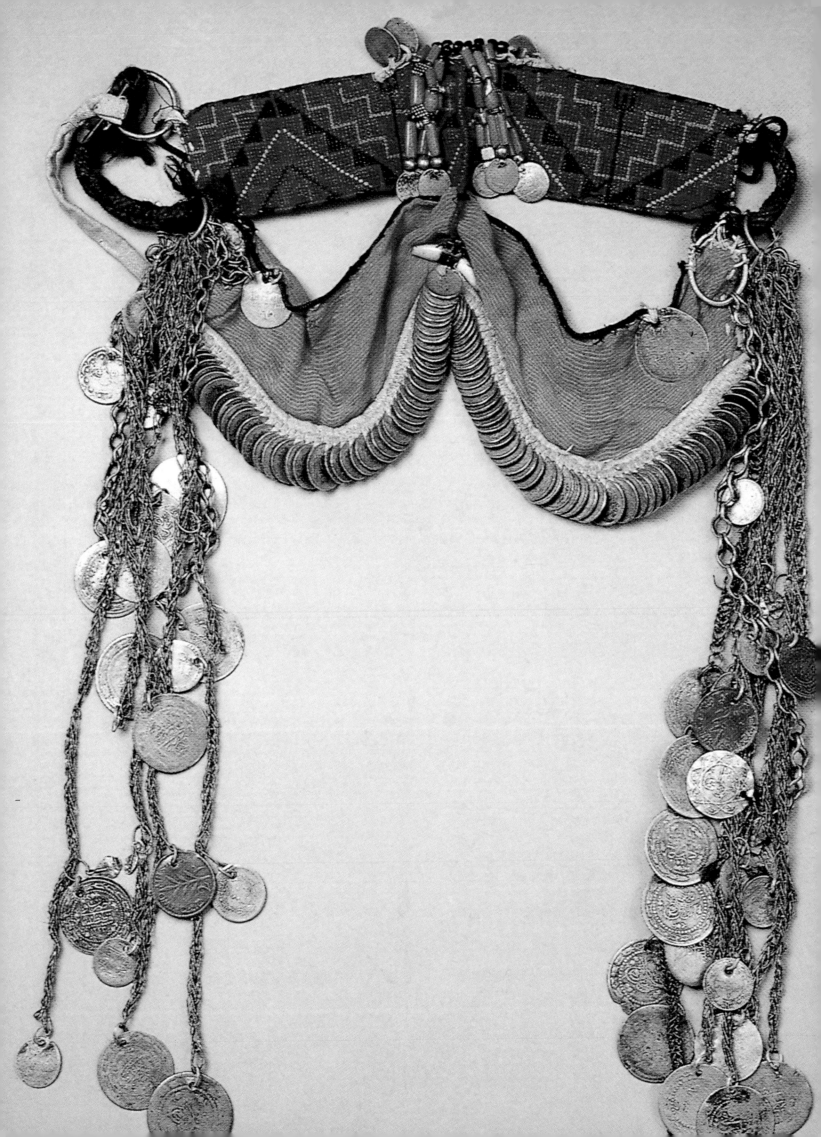

Chapter 1

The image of veils

The wearing of veils is currently one of the most emotive subjects within costume history. This applies to both the participants and the observers. Newspapers and magazines frequently carry articles about the dreaded "headscarf" and how "unfortunate" girls are made to wear this garment as a token of their (or their parents') religious beliefs. But the situation is not so simple. This study is intended to show that veiling is not a new development, but one which has ancient and diverse antecedents.

This book will concentrate on the various sorts of headscarves and veils worn in Southwest Asia and North Africa (Map 1). This region has been picked for two reasons. Firstly, many women in these areas of the world wear such garments as part of their day-to-day public and private costume. Secondly, as noted above, considerable emphasis has been placed in the media on the wearing of headscarves and what this 'means'. This is not to say that headscarves and veils from other parts of the world will be neglected. They form important comparative material for placing veils and veiling in a wider context and as such these parallels will be referred to constantly.

The book is divided into four sections. Firstly, there is a general history of veiling from the second millennium BC onwards. Next there is a description of the main types of veils (head, face and body) worn in Southwest Asia and North Africa. This is followed by a discussion of the various reasons, real and alleged, for the wearing of veils. Finally, there is a short section about the

way in which the West has perceived veiling and the 'oriental' woman.

Definitions of Veils and Veiling

But what is a veil? Basically it is a length of material which is tied around the head in some manner. It is intended to cover the hair and in some cases to screen the wearer (normally female) from the outside world. The veils discussed here are all lengths of material which are normally wound around the head in some form. Usually it is regarded as important that most if not all of the person's hair is covered. This means that, in general, hats and caps which are a shaped headcovering can be excluded from this study. The various types of 'veils' which are discussed in this book are:

Kerchiefs, scarves and headveils: kerchiefs are lengths of material which are worn over the head and cover most or all of the hair. They are worn around the head only. A scarf is a relatively small square of cloth which is worn over the head and hair and fastened around the neck in some manner. In contrast, a headveil is a long length of material which again covers the head and hair, but which is worn around the shoulders. It can also be draped as far as the waist. Various forms of kerchiefs, scarves and hair veils are worn by men and women throughout the world.

Face veils: face veils are separate garments which cover all or part of the face. The use of face veils is found in

Figure 1. Coin face veil (burqa`) of the type worn by Bedouin women.

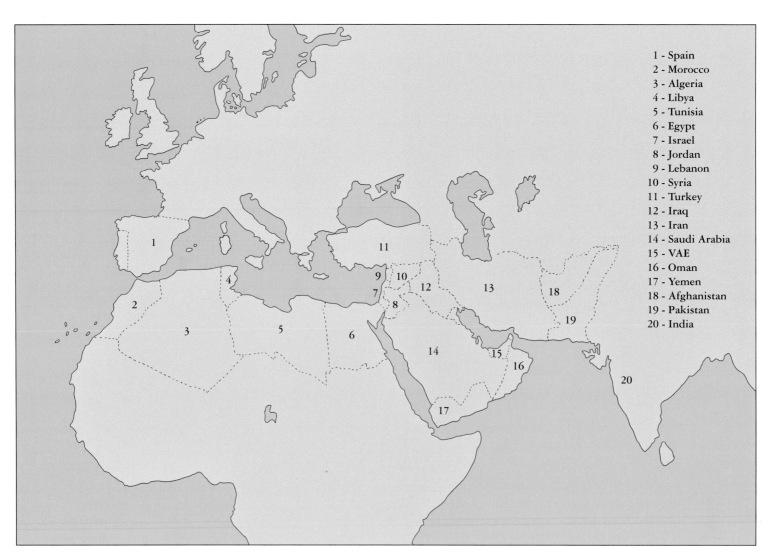

| 1 - Spain |
| 2 - Morocco |
| 3 - Algeria |
| 4 - Libya |
| 5 - Tunisia |
| 6 - Egypt |
| 7 - Israel |
| 8 - Jordan |
| 9 - Lebanon |
| 10 - Syria |
| 11 - Turkey |
| 12 - Iraq |
| 13 - Iran |
| 14 - Saudi Arabia |
| 15 - VAE |
| 16 - Oman |
| 17 - Yemen |
| 18 - Afghanistan |
| 19 - Pakistan |
| 20 - India |

Map 1. Map showing the main regions of the world where women traditionally wear veils.

regions as far apart as Algeria, Turkey, and Oman. The Turkish *yashmak* is perhaps one of the best known examples of the face veil.

Mantles, outerwraps, body covers and garment veils: the word mantle is generally used for a length of material loosely draped over the head (leaving the face uncovered) and which also covers the rest of the body, usually down to the ankles. The traditional Spanish *mantilla* is a suitable example of this type of garment. The Iranian *chador*, on the other hand, is very similar to the mantle, but it is worn closely wrapped around the body. Such a garment is often called an outerwrap. A body covering, on the other hand, is a tailored garment which covers the head and body completely. It usually reaches down to the ankles. Such garments are worn in Afghanistan and north-western Pakistan. Finally, in some regions of the world coat-like garments are frequently worn over the head to act as an enveloping veil. This type of garment can be seen in Arabia where the *abaya* or sleeveless coat is worn as a veil.

One of the problems encountered while preparing this study was to define when a veil or scarf should be called a mask. It was decided that when a head or facial covering is only used during a ritual or religious function, rather than on a daily basis, and when it is worn to represent another person, deity or character, then it should be regarded as a mask, and as such it is not included in this work.

Problems of Terminology

One of the problems encountered in this study is that of local terminology. Sometimes the same word is used for different garments in various regions. A good example of the confusion that may arise with local names is the term *burqa*. There are references to the use of this word dating back from the tenth century AD. According to the Arabic Geography, the *Hudud al-'Alam*, Bailakan, the ancient capital of Arran (a region near the Caspian Sea), was famous for its production of: "striped textiles *(burd-ha)* in great numbers, horse-rugs *(jul)*, veils *(burqa)* and natif-sweets" (Minorsky 1937:144). Unfortunately, the account does not specify what sort of veil was being referred to.

Nowadays a garment locally called a *burqa* is worn by married nomadic women in various parts of Palestine and Egypt (figs. 1 and 2). This type of veil is usually made from a forehead band and two bands covered in coins and beads of various types which flow down the lower half of the face. This *burqa* is not a face veil which is used to cover all or part of the face, but a facial ornament which enhances certain areas of the face such as the eyes. On the other hand, some Western writers talk about the *burqa`* of Afghanistan. This is a very different garment from the Palestinian garment, in that it is made up of a small cap to which lengths of pleated material are sewn (fig. 3; Doubleday 1988:3). The cloth normally reaches to just above the ankles. The wearer can only see the world through a small mesh. In this case the *burqa`* should be seen as a body covering intended to disguise rather than enhance a woman's body. The *burqa`* of Afghanistan is also described by some Western and Eastern writers as a *chadri*, which comes from the same root as the Iranian word *chador*.[1]

Wherever possible, therefore, the local or regional term for a particular garment has been given.

Sources of Information

With respect to veiling, the range of potential information is considerable. There are numerous representations from all over the world, including sculptures, paintings, and reliefs which depict veiled figures. There are written accounts including lists of dowries and receipts for objects which record the presence and use of veils. There are also laws dating back to the second millennium BC in Mesopotamia, which forbid certain groups of women to go out of their houses without being veiled. There are very similar prescriptions now in place in lands such as Iran. In addition, literature, both fictitious and factual, provides a rich source of information about veils. Tales as well as biographies and autobiographies play their roles in understanding the role

of veiling. Finally, however, and this is the most important source of information, we have the garments themselves. The combination of all of these sources help to provide an insight into this fascinating subject.

Some Western Problems with Veiling

Clothing has long been used as a symbol of political or religious affiliations. During the twentieth century the fascist "Black Shirts" and "Brown Shirts", and Mao's blue suits for Communist China, represent suitable examples of the political use of clothing. Similarly, Islamic clothing, especially the headscarf worn by women, is being seen and used as a symbol of the growing rise of militant Islam and its opposition to the West.

To date, most Western preconceptions about veiling seem to come into two categories. Firstly, that of "Orientalism", whereby the veil is seen as an important element of the Oriental myth of mystery, seduction and harems. Secondly, the alleged negative role that *hijab* or Islamic clothing, plays in modern society, for instance in the supposed subjugation of women and the growing rise of fundamentalism within Islam. Both of these subjects will be discussed in greater detail in later chapters. Nevertheless, it is worth highlighting several aspects of *hijab*, which have recently come to the public's attention.

Over the last ten years there have been numerous items in the international press about the growing interest in and use of *hijab*. Part of this interest developed after the fall of the Berlin Wall. The fear of the "Red under the Bed" was replaced by the 'threat' of Islam. All too often attention is focused on one element of Islam,

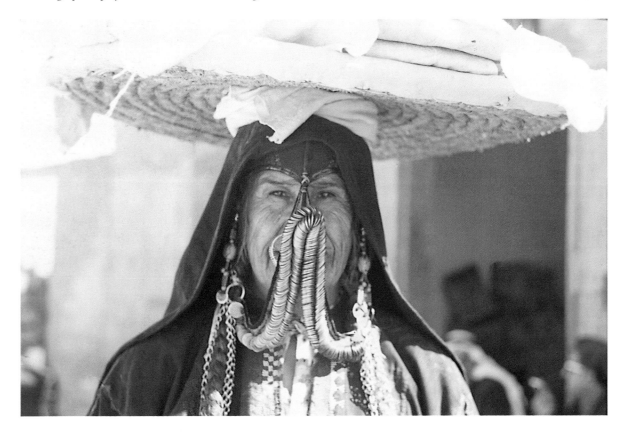

*Figure 2. Coin face veil (*burqa`*) worn by a Bedouin woman (courtesy of Shelagh Weir).*

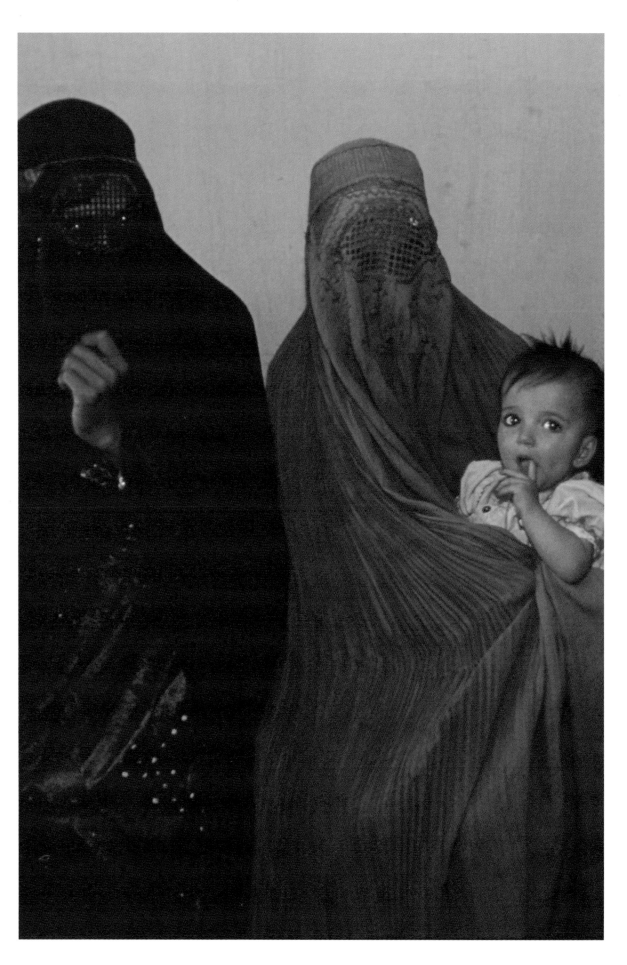

namely the type of clothing worn, and in particular the headscarf. One reason for this, almost obsessive, attention on scarves is that it is a very visual aspect of the clothing form, whose presence can be seen in most if not all of the major European cities. A second reason is related to what is often regarded as a soft target, namely, the role and position of women. In some cases, there is a strong degree of patronisation in the various reports. The writers try to protect the "ladies", while there is a presumption of either a woman's lack of intelligence or free will in agreeing to wear what seems to be such an obvious badge of subjugation.

In several European countries, including France, Belgium, Britain and The Netherlands, authorities have tried to ban the wearing of headscarves in schools. In the autumn of 1994, for example, nearly seventy Muslim girls in French schools were sent home from school for wearing headscarves. This action was the result of a circular sent around French schools whereby the Education Minister, François Bayrou, ordered schoolheads to ban Islamic headscarves and other obviously religious symbols. The order went against a 1992 ruling by the State Council that said that the banning of headscarves was a restriction on civil liberties. However, the minister said that he was against any sign which separated pupils or which were considered to be linked with proselytism. This argument has been used by the government since the time of the French Revolution. Since then the state has tried to keep a neutral position when it comes to religion and religious symbols. Priests, for example, have to hang up their cassocks on a coat hook before giving lessons at a university. Nevertheless, it should be noted that the proscriptions on discreet outward signs such as small crucifixes and the *kippa* or skull cap worn by Jewish boys were not included in the ban.

In The Netherlands the movement against headscarves came to the fore in 1985 when Prof. J. Brugman, an Arabist, advised the mayor and council of Alphen-aan-den-Rijn that girls should not be allowed to wear headscarves in schools. As recently as November 1994 two girls of Turkish origin living in Vlaardingen were sent home from school for wearing such scarves.

One of the reasons officially given for the ban on headscarves is that they present a danger for girls while having gym or sport lessons, as it is possible for the scarf to catch in the sport equipment. Girls (no matter what their religion) with long hair are normally recommended (not forced) to wear their hair tied back while in gyms for the same reason. Various suggestions have been put forward to solve the problem. For example, that gym lessons should operate on a single sex basis, or that Muslim girls should wear swimming caps. However, the aim of the scarf is to cover the hair and the neck, the areas of the female body which have to be hidden according to Islamic tradition. Wearing a swimming cap would cover the hair, but it would leave the neck bare. As may be expected, the latter suggestion was not taken very seriously. The current compromise is that Muslim girls wear a thin, high collared jumper to cover their necks, while over their hair they wear a headscarf tied at the back of the head.

More recently, there has been a series of items on Dutch television and in the press about the question whether a woman can be fired from her job if she is wearing a headscarf. This situation developed because a cleaning firm forbid the wearing of headscarves by its female Muslim workers. The question of the firm's right to ban headscarves was taken up by the *Algemene Commissie Gelijke Behandeling* (General Commission for Equal Treatment; CGB). They decided that on the grounds of the *Algemene Wet Gelijke Behandeling* (General Law on Equal Treatment; AWGB) that such a ban constituted discrimination because it made a difference between people on the grounds of religion.

The decision by the Commission also has consequences for the question of whether schoolgirls should be allowed to wear headscarves or not. Under the ruling it becomes illegal for state schools to ban the wearing of headscarves (by Muslim girls). It should be noted, however, that this ruling does not apply to special schools such as those which are specifically Catholic or Protestant.

Notes:

1   Dupree 1973:246; Scarce 1975; Scarce 1987:181.

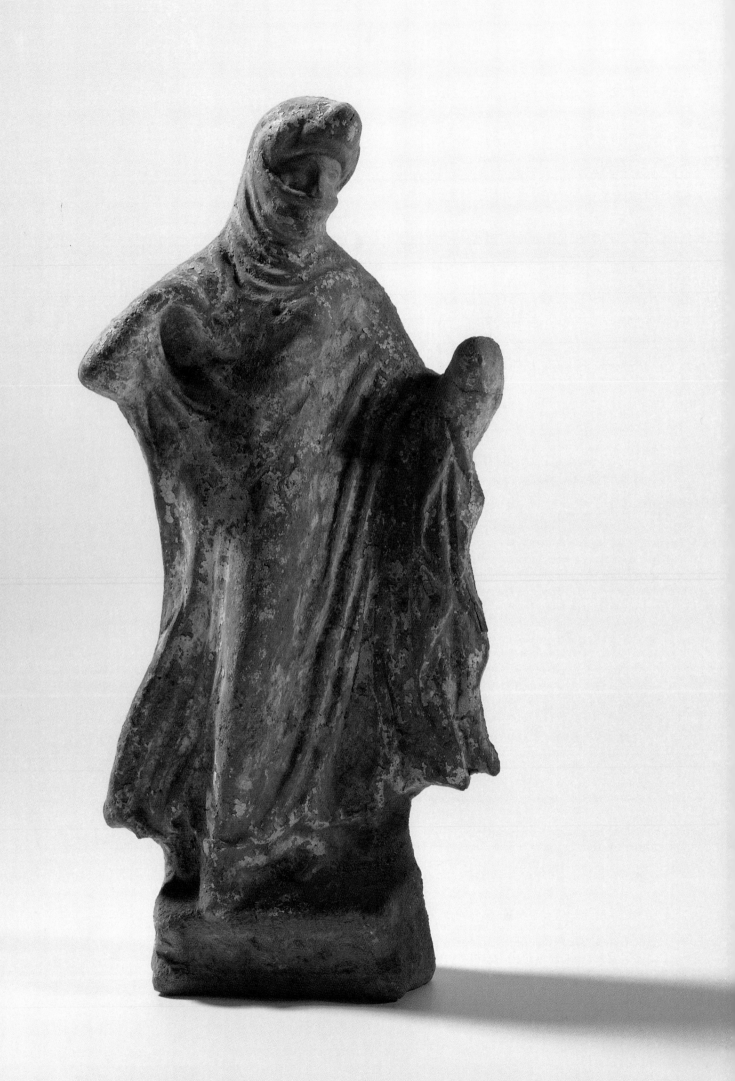

Chapter 2

Figure 14. An Hellenistic figure of a woman, possibly from Boetia in mainland Greece, c. 4-3th c. BC (no. OC(ant) 6-39; courtesy of the Gemeentemuseum, The Hague).

The early history of veiling

One of the questions posed in this chapter, is when did 'true' veiling develop? And who was the first to use a 'true face veil', namely, a separate piece of material across the face, as opposed to a large piece of cloth that covers head, face and part of the body? As may be expected, it is not possible to provide an easy answer to these questions, basically because the origins of the veil, in all its forms, date back to ancient times and relevant information is difficult to find. Nevertheless, it would appear from written as well as visual sources, that mantles and outerwraps represent the oldest form of veiling. It was only by the late first millennium BC that a separate garment, the face veil, developed. In order to look further at this question the history of veiling in North Africa, the Mediterranean and Southwest Asia until about the fifth century AD needs to be considered.

Mantles and Outerwraps

Although the basic concept of the mantle and outerwrap is the same, namely, a square or rectangle of material used as an outer covering, there are a number of different forms. As will be seen the types of mantles and outerwraps used in the eastern Mediterranean regions differ from those in the North Africa.

Mesopotamia

The use of a mantle or length of cloth for covering all or part of the body has a very long tradition, especially in

the Mediterranean and Middle East. It can be traced back to at least ancient Mesopotamia in the second millennium BC, although it is probably much older.

There is very little visual evidence that women wore mantle-type veils before the beginning of the second millennium BC. But this may be deceptive as there are so few depictions of women in general, and most of these figures are shown indoors within a palace or house. The only example of a woman wearing even a short piece of material over her head dates from the fourth millennium BC and comes from the site of Warka in modern Iraq. The representation in question is of a queen or a goddess on an alabaster vase (fig. 4; Griebewegen-Frankfort 1951:150-2). She appears to be wearing a short length of material under a crown. In general, figures of ordinary women from this period tend to show them with their hair uncovered or tied back with a single head band. Similarly, during the Early Dynastic period in Mesopotamia (c. 3000-2340 BC), there are a few depictions of women, but these are rare. It would appear that again, women had long hair which was bound around their head and kept in place with several bands, one of which went over the forehead.

By about 1800 BC, however, there is written evidence from this region indicating that women were covered in some manner. It would also appear that 'respectable' women, namely wives and concubines, were covered, while slave women went bare headed. This information is derived from a collection of royal letters dating to period

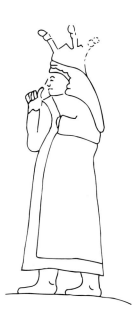

Figure 4. Queen from the Warka vase (based on Frankfort 1963, fig. 10).

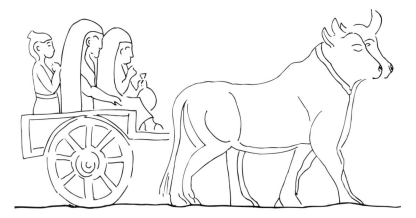

between 1790 and 1745 BC from the site of Mari on what is today the Iraq-Syrian border.

Various letters have been found at Mari from its then king, Zimri-Lim, to one of his wives in which he gives orders concerning the fate of some female captives[2]:

"Choose from the 30 female-weavers - or however many who are choice (and) attractive, who from the toenails to the hair of the heads have no blemish (?) - and assign them to Wara-ilisu. And Wara-ilisu is to give them the Subarean veil"

In a later letter to his wife, the king noted:

"There will be more (booty) available for my disposition ... I will myself select from this booty which I will get, the girls for the veil and will dispatch them to you".

By the time of the Assyrians (c. 1350-612 BC), the garments to be worn by women when outside of the house had been codified (fig. 5). There are surviving written accounts from this period which give some of the earliest descriptions of women being compelled to wear some form of covering over their heads and possibly their faces when in public. These accounts come in a Middle Assyrian law (c. 1450-1250 BC) in which it is stated that married women, Assyrian women and "ladies by birth" had to be veiled when in public.[3] Similarly, concubines and "captive" maids also had to be veiled when accompanied by their mistresses. On the other hand, the wearing of veils in public by prostitutes and female slaves was a punishable offence. The text then goes on to state that prostitutes who were caught wearing these garments were to be punished by being beaten fifty times with a rod and then pitch being poured on their heads. Slaves were similarly beaten, but instead of pitch being poured over them, their clothes were taken away from them and their ears were cut off:

"Who(ever) sees a veiled harlot shall arrest her; he shall produce witnesses (and) bring her into the residency. Her ornaments shall not be taken (from her, but) the man who arrests her shall take her

clothing; she shall be beaten 50 blows with rods (and) pitch shall be poured on her head.

And if a man sees a veiled harlot and lets (her) go (and) has not brought her into the residency, that man ... he shall be beaten 50 blows with rods; the informer [?] against him shall take his clothing; his ears shall be pierced (and) a cord shall be passed (through them) (and) be tied behind him ... he shall do labour for the kind for one full month."

"Who(ever) sees a veiled slave-girl shall arrest her (and) bring her into the residency. Her ears shall be cut off, (and) the man who arrests her shall take her clothes. A veiled slave girl - if a man sees her and lets (her) go (and) has not arrested her (and) has not brought her into the residency, (and) charge (and) proof have been brought against him, he shall be beaten 50 blows with rods, the informer [?] against him shall take his clothing; his ears shall be pierced (and) a cord shall be passed (through them) (and) be tied behind him ... he shall do labour for the kind for one full month."

"Women, whether married or (widows) or (Assyrians) who go out into the (public) street (must not have) their heads (uncovered). Ladies by birth must be veiled. A concubine with her mistress must be veiled. A hierodules [captive] whom a husband has married must be veiled. One who is not married must have her head uncovered in public."

"If a man will veil his concubine (?) he shall summon 5 (or) 6 of his neighbours to be present (and) veil her before them (and) shall speak saying: "She (is) my wife, she (thus) becomes his wife.""[4]

There is a also warning to the high-born ladies of Babylon in the Old Testament (mid-first millennium BC). Here it is stated that following the Lord's vengeance upon Babylon, the Babylonian women would be compelled to perform menial tasks, remove their veils, strip their trains and uncover their legs:

"Come down and sit in the dust, O virgin daughter of Babylon;
sit on the ground without a throne,
O daughter of the Chalde'ans!
For you shall no more be called tender and delicate
Take the millstones and grind meal, put off your veil,
strip off your robe, uncover your legs" (Isaiah 47, 1-2)

The type of veiling referred to above can be seen in two bas-reliefs from Mesopotamia now in the British Museum, London (figs. 6 and 7). In the first representation a group of women and their daughters are shown leaving the stricken city of Lachish (c. 704-681; BM 124989). In the second relief, a group of women are depicted talking with each other (c. 704-681 BC; BM 124786). In both reliefs the women are wearing long mantles, loosely placed over their heads with their foreheads showing. The mantles worn by the second group are fringed and it would appear that these women are wearing some form of kerchief under the mantle.

During the fourth century BC, Xenophon described the appearance of the wife of Abradatus of Susa when she was taken captive by Cyrus, the king of the Achaemenids:

> "... And when we went into her tent, upon my word, we did not at first distinguish her from the rest; for she sat upon the ground and all her handmaids sat around her. And she was dressed withal just like her servants; but when we looked round upon them all in our desire to make out which one was the mistress, at once her superiority to all the rest was evident, even though she sat veiled, with her head bowed to the earth ... she was conspicuous among them both for her stature and for her nobility and her grace, even though she stood there in lowly garb" (Xenophon, *Cyropaedia*, V.i.4).

The Greek word used to describe her veil is *kalumma*, which can be translated as headcovering, hood or veil. These descriptions are vague and it would be possible to interpret the clothing worn by the queen as meaning either a mantle or a face veil. However, a little further on in the text, Xenophon wrote that when the queen was given to Cyrus she:

> "... rent her outer garment from top to bottom and wept aloud; and her servants also cried aloud with her. And then we had vision of most of her face and vision of her neck and arms" (Xenophon, *Cyropaedia*, V.1.6).

This second description indicates that Xenophon was indeed referring to a garment which covered the queen's head, neck and shoulders, rather than a face veil.

The type of mantle which the queen was probably wearing is shown worn by a group of Ackaemenid women depicted on a carpet found in a Barrow 5, High Altai at Pazyryk in Siberia not far from the Chinese border (Rudenko 1970:168, 296-7, pl. 177). The carpet dates to the fifth century BC and is perhaps Persian in origin. The women are shown wearing long gowns with crown-like headdress over which are long mantles which reach nearly to the ground (fig. 8).

The Eastern Mediterranean

The Eastern Mediterranean is a general term to cover lands stretching from the Greek mainland, west and south Turkey, down to the Levant (Syria, Israel, Palestine), and Egypt. Strictly speaking Rome should not be included. However, as this chapter also briefly discusses the use of mantles in the Roman Empire, especially that of the eastern parts, it was found appropriate to discuss the Roman use of mantles in this section.

Ancient Anatolia

The first region to be looked at is Anatolia, in what is now Turkey. In particular, attention is focused on the mantles worn by women during the Hittite Period (1400-1200 BC) and afterwards.

One form of this mantle can be seen at Yazilikaya, where Pudehepa, the wife of Hatusili III (c. thirteenth century BC), is shown wearing a mantle over her head (no headdress is indicated; fig. 9; Lloyd 1967:67, fig. 65). The mantle reaches down to her ankles. Later depictions of Hittite women show them wearing a tall headdress (nowadays often called a *polos*), with a long mantle. These garments can be seen on a procession of priestesses from the so-called Herald's Wall at the site of Carchemish (Lloyd 1967:97, figs. 95-6). All of the women are wearing the high headdress, which is covered with a long mantle reaching down to their ankles.

There are also a number of Neo-Hittite stelae which depict veiled women, for example, an eighth-seventh century BC basalt stele (fig. 11; Adama Museum, acc. no. 1756). In this relief a seated lady is shown spinning. She is wearing a long, fringed mantle which covers her from head to ankles.

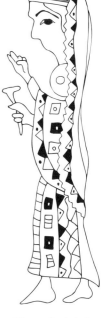

Figure 8. A lady from the so-called Pazyryk carpet (5th c. BC; based on Rudenko 1970, pl. 177).

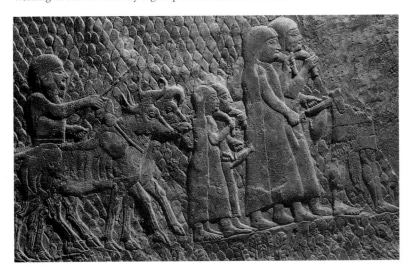

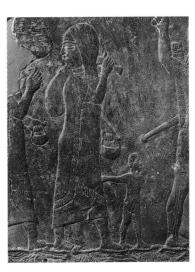

Figure 6. A group of women and their daughters leaving the city of Lachish (c. 704-681 BC; BM 124989; courtesy of the British Museum, London).

Figure 7. A group of women talking to each other (c. 704-681 BC; BM 123786; courtesy of the British Museum, London).

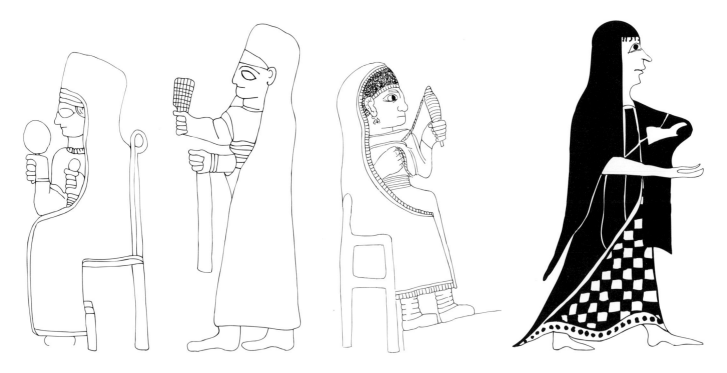

Figure 9. A Hittite lady wearing a long mantle, from Yazilikaya in modern Turkey (c. 13th c. BC; based on Lloyd 1967, fig. 65).

Figure 10. A Hittite priestess wearing a long mantle, from the site of Carchemish (after Lloyd 1967, fig. 95-6).

Figure 11. Neo-Hittite relief showing a seated woman wearing a long mantle (based on an 8th c. BC stele, Adama Museum, Turkey, acc. no. 1756).

Figure 12. An archaic Greek woman wearing a long mantle over her head (c. 630 BC; from a 'Melian' vase, National Museum, Athens no. 3961).

The Greek World

During the Archaic Period (about 630-480 BC) Greek women tended to wear a long dress with a loose mantle slung diagonally across the upper part of the body with the end of the material in folds across the legs (fig. 12). The head and hair was not normally covered in statues from this period, although occasionally depictions of women with mantles over their heads can be found on pottery.

In the late sixth century BC, however, a major change took place in the way women were dressed and after that date they are frequently shown totally wrapped in a large outerwrap which covered the head, hair and all of the body. At this time Greek architecture and decorative arts in general, in addition to clothing, were influenced by the Ionic style which derived from the eastern Greek colonies of Ionia in what is now western Turkey.[5]

Examples of Hellenistic statuettes of both veiled and unveiled women have been found at various sites in Turkey, for example, at Troy and Myrina (on the west coast of Turkey).[6] The statuettes date from the third century BC to the first century AD. In some cases the mantles are simply draped over the head, but in other examples the garments are closely wrapped around the body of the wearer. In respect to the garments worn in this region it is worth noting a reference to the use of an outerwrap cum veil worn by the women of the Ionic city of Chalcedon which lies opposite what is now Istanbul. The reference comes from the first century AD work *Quaestiones Graecae* by Plutarch:

> "... Why have the women of Chalkedon the custom, when they meet strangers and particularly magistrates, to veil the other cheek?"

The answer given was that following a battle, eight thousand men of the city were killed and some of the women were 'reduced' to marrying slaves or freed men. Their more virtuous and noble sisters who remained unmarried started to wear a veil across their face when forced to deal (as there were no male members of their own families), with magistrates and other officials. As a result, those who had married, "out of shame", adopted the same custom (Halliday 1928:194-6; Question 49). It is apparent from the above description that Plutarch is referring to the use of a mantle which was pulled across part of the face, rather than a true face veil which would have remained in place all the time when in public.

One of the earliest depictions of closely wrapped women can be found on a fifth-century BC krater in the collection of Mount Holyoke College (Galt 1931:374, fig. 1). There is a group of six women, five of which are dancing while the sixth is playing a double flute (fig. 13). All of the dancers have their outerwraps drawn over their heads and in front of their faces so that only their eyes and the foreheads are visible.

In the Gemeentemuseum, The Hague, there is a small figurine of a veiled woman, which is reputed to be from Boetia in mainland Greece (fig. 14).[7] Again her whole body is covered, with only her eyes and part of her nose visible.[8] The manner in which The Hague figure is depicted is very similar to a description by Herakleides, a Greek writer who was writing in about 250 BC. He noted that women living in Thebes in Boetia wore an enveloping outerwrap:

> "The way they wrap their heads in their himatia is such that the garment seems to cover the whole face like a little mask; the eyes alone peep out; all the

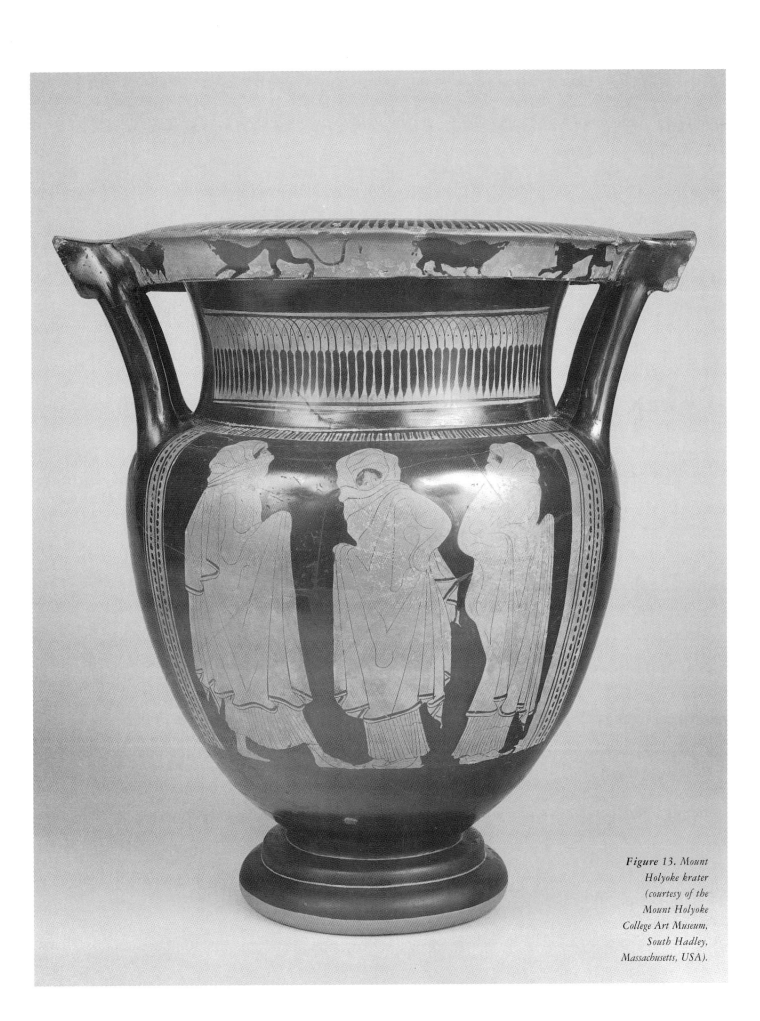

Figure 13. Mount Holyoke krater (courtesy of the Mount Holyoke College Art Museum, South Hadley, Massachusetts, USA).

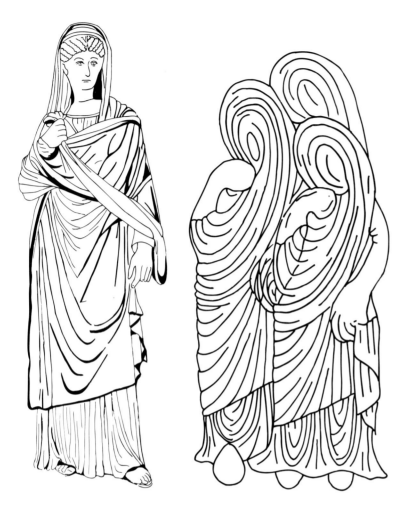

Figure 15.
Drawing of a Roman
lady, based on a
statue of the Empress
Faustina the elder
(105-41; Palazzo
de Conservatori,
Rome Galleria, inv.
no. 57).

Figure 16.
A group of women
from the city of
Palmyra, Syria,
c. AD 250 (based
on Seyrig 1934,
pl. XIX).

other parts of the face are covered by the mantles. They all wear these pure white. Their hair is yellow and fastened upon the crown of the head" (Herakleides, *Diakaiarchos* I, 18ff).

As can be seen, there is a very strong link between the description of the garments worn by Theben women given above and that of the clothing on the figure.[9] The figure has been dated to the fourth century BC.

The Roman World

Women during the early Republican period generally did not wear head veils. This can be seen on numerous statues and busts of ladies from this period. However, by the time of Augustus (63 BC - AD 14) the use of veiling was added to a woman's clothing repertoire. A few centuries later it was quite normal for a Roman lady to be depicted with a head veil or long mantle of some kind (fig. 15). Thus, by the first half of the first millennium AD head veils and mantles were in widespread use throughout North Africa and the Eastern Mediterranean.

During the Roman period, North Africa was noted for what was regarded as its distinctive style of dress. Classical sources seem to have considered the peoples (including the Berbers) of this region to be barbarians because they wore animal skins draped over their shoulders.[10] For Roman

writers one of the most striking features of North African clothing was the flowing unbelted tunic.[11]

Another feature of pre-Islamic clothing from the region described by Greek and Roman writers, was the large wrapping cloth used as an outer garment by both men and women. Although it should be noted that even at this stage the outerwrap was worn in different ways by men and women. In later centuries, this outerwrap is known by various names including Arabic *ha'ik, kisa'* and *barrakan* (see page 67), and in Berber as *a'aban, akhusi, afaggu* and *tahaykt*.[12]

There is more information, both written and visual, about the garments worn in the eastern parts of the Roman Empire. One of the most detailed sources of information about the appearance of costume of this region comes from the caravan city of Palmyra in what is now Syria. Numerous funerary statues and busts have survived from this site, and these intricately sculptured representations present a detailed picture of what was being worn by both men and women. It is quite clear from these sources that women were veiled, and in some cases quite heavily.

In most cases the head coverings worn by women are simply drawn over the hair and left hanging on either side. However, in a bas-relief from the same city there is a depiction of a procession in which a camel and horse are flanked on either side by two groups of women (fig. 16; Seyrig 1934, pl. XIX). The women to the right of the relief are depicted with swirls of cloth coming from under the right arm over the left shoulder and head. The women's faces are not clearly shown. But it would seem acceptable to suggest that the garments constituted long overwraps which went over their heads and which were then pulled across their faces using their right hands.

There have been various arguments about these women, whether they represent worshippers of baal, Christians, Jews or Nabateans, or even some other group. But what is clear is that by the third century AD, the sight of totally covered women was not unknown within the eastern parts of the Roman Empire.

The Palmyrian reliefs, however, are not the earliest evidence for veiling in the Levant. There are, for example, in the Bible various references to women who have covered their hair and faces. Most of these references, however, seem to be linked to the use of mantles and outerwraps of some kind, rather than face veils.

One of the earliest references is to be found in the Old Testament, the Song of Songs:

"Behold, you are beautiful, my love,
behold, you are beautiful!
Your eyes are doves
behind your veil
....
Your cheeks are like halves of a pomegranate
behind your veil (The Song of Songs, 4:1,3).

It would also appear that during the first millennium BC young girls were unveiled as the unmarried Rebekah was described without a veil:

"The maiden was very fair to look upon, a virgin, whom no man had known" (Genesis 24:16).

Married women on the other hand were normally veiled in public, as can be deduced from a later account of Rebekah after she had been married:

Rebekah lifted up her eyes, and when she saw Isaac, she alighted from the camel, and said to the servant, "Who is the man yonder, walking in the field to meet us?" The servant said, "It is my master". So she took her veil and covered herself' (Gen. xxiv, 66).

Widows had a special set of clothing which marked them as such, and these probably did not include a face cover. Yet prostitutes were expected to be veiled even while working, as the story of Tamar relates:

"She put off her widow's garments, and put on a veil, wrapping herself up, and sat at the entrance to Enaim, which is on the road to Timnah; for she saw that Shelah was grown up, and she had not been given to him in marriage. When Judah saw her, he thought her to be a harlot, for she had covered her face" (Gen. xxxviii, 14).

Judah slept with Tamar without realising that she was his daughter-in-law, so apparently she never removed her veil.

Another story about veiled women dates from the Hellenistic period and refers to the life of Susanna, daughter of Helkias and wife of Joakim the Judge (Charles 1913:638-651). Two elders had heard about the beauty of Susanna and concealed themselves in her garden (v.7) where they spied upon her unveiled form (apparently she was about to enter a bath). They went up to her and made an 'indecent proposition'. Susanna rebuffed them and so they brought an accusation against her in court accusing her of having propositioned them. According to one version, Susanna appeared discreetly dressed in court "and these wicked men commanded her to be unveiled (for she was veiled) that they might be filled with her beauty" (v. 32). Susanna was about to be condemned when the Lord heard her cries of innocence and sent Daniel to declare her unsullied character. As a result, she was allowed to go home, while the two elders were punished by death for bearing false witness.

In addition to the Bible references given above, there is also a representation of a Jewish woman from the Syrian city of Dura-Europos which was destroyed in AD 257. The depiction comes from the synagogue and shows women wearing long tunics with simple lengths of cloth covering there hair (fig. 174).[13] Unfortunately, although these women are wearing outerwraps of some kind, the exact nature of the garments is not clear.

There is also a passage in the Talmud which refers to the veiling of urban women in Palestine in the third century AD. The passage contains a discussion on the Mishna regulations regarding Sabbath observance (TB Shabbath 80a; Goldschmidt 1930:672). The discussion concerns the question what could or could not be carried on the Sabbath from an enclosed area to an unenclosed area, and vice versa. The Mishna states that a quantity of eye-paint sufficient for the adornment of one eye must be carried on the Sabbath before the penalty could be applied (TB Shabbath 8,3). In an early Jewish commentary on the Talmud called the Gemara this statement was subjected to the dialectical process, whereby it was asked if a quantity of eye paint sufficient for one eye only could serve a practical purpose (Goldschmidt 1930:672). According to (rabbi) Rabh Huna modest women adorn only one eye with eye paint because only one eye was exposed. The discussion was continued by Hillel, the son of Rabbi Shemuel bar Nahmani, who stated that women in villages did not cover themselves, while those in the towns did.

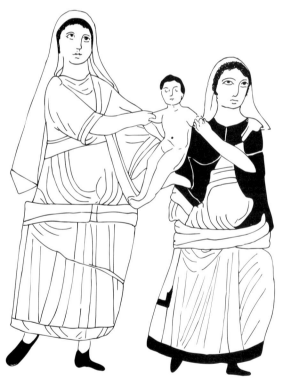

Figure 17. *Two women from the synagogue at Dura-Europos, Syria, before AD 257 (based on Goldman 1994, fig. 10.18).*

There are similar comments in early Christian literature about the 'fact' that women should be covered. Perhaps one of the most famous is by St. Paul in I Corinthians (11:2-16):

But I want you to understand that the head of every man is Christ, the head of a woman is her husband, and the head of Christ is God. Any man who prays or prophesies with his head covered dishonours his head, but any woman who prays or prophesies with her head unveiled dishonours her head - it is the same as

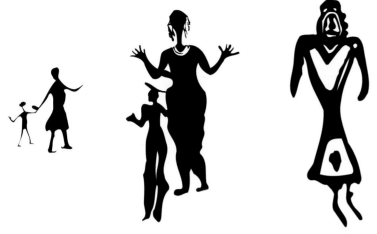

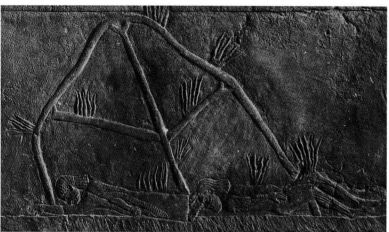

if her head were shaven. For if a woman will not veil herself, then she should cut off her hair; but if it is disgraceful for a woman to be shorn or shaven, let her wear a veil. For a man ought not to cover his head, since this is the image and glory of God; but woman is the glory of man ... That is why a woman ought to have a veil on her head, because of the angels."

Other comments about veiling can be found in St. Jerome's letters to Eustochium (*Letters* XXII). This group of epistles was written in Rome during the spring of AD 384 and one, no. XXII, was intended for Christian women who were planning a religious life:

"Go not out from home, nor wish to behold the daughters of a strange country ... You will be wounded, you will be stripped, and you will say, lamenting: The keepers that go about the city found me, struck me, wounded me; they took away my veil from me ... Jesus is jealous. He does not wish your face to be seen by others. You may make excuses and plead: "I have drawn my veil, I have covered my face, I have sought thee".

The concept of being covered and veiled within the framework of Christianity continues to this day in the form of the headcovering worn by traditional nuns.

Veiling in the Arabian Peninsula

There is very little known about the early clothing of Arabic women and what is known has to be put together from various sources of information.

Some of the earliest evidence comes from prehistoric rock carvings from Arabia which date to the second and first millennia BC. It would seem that even at this early date women wore a long garment of some kind (fig. 18; Anati 1968:195). There is also a bas-relief from the period of Ashurbanipal (668-627 BC), which depicts a dead Arab woman and man sprawled on the ground near a burning tent (fig. 19; BM 124927; Albenda 1983:84). The woman is wearing a long gown over which was a fringed mantle. Her hair was left uncovered and it would appear that this was done as an artistic device to highlight the fact that she died through violence.

There are a number of written records of veiled Arabian women dating from the first millennium AD. The third century AD writer Tertullian, for example, noted that Arabian women appeared in public totally enveloped with only one eye showing:

"2. Iudicabunt nos Arabiae feminae ethnicae quae non caput, sed faciem quoque ita totam tegunt ut uno oculo liberato contentae sint dimidiam frui lucem quam totam faciem prostituere. 3. Mauult femina uidere quam uideri" (Tertullian De *Virginibus Velandis*, XVII).

"2. The women of Arabic origin, who cover not only their heads, but also their faces, would condemn us, because they prefer to enjoy the light with one eye, rather than show their whole face. It is better for a woman to see, than be seen."

There is also a reference in the Mishnah to the wearing of veils, of some kind, by women in Arabia: "... They may go out with the *sela* (a silver coin) ... women of Arabia may go out veiled and the women of Media with their cloaks looped up over their shoulders ..." (Shabbath 6⁶).

The evidence for the early use of veiling in the Arabian peninsula can also be traced in several pre-Islamic Arabic poems from the sixth century AD, which refer to veiled women. In some cases, the dropping of the veil is desired in order to see the beauty underneath.

"She drips with saffron and with ambergris. She has let fall her striped head-scarf because of her beauty".14

In such cases the emphasis is usually placed on the neck and eyes which were regarded as erotic regions:

"She turned her head - and you were enslaved by her smooth white throat like that of a gazelle with its graceful neck. And by those bright eyes (a sleepy glance, you might think) of a beauty ready to brim with tears" (Beeston *et al.* 1983:58-9).

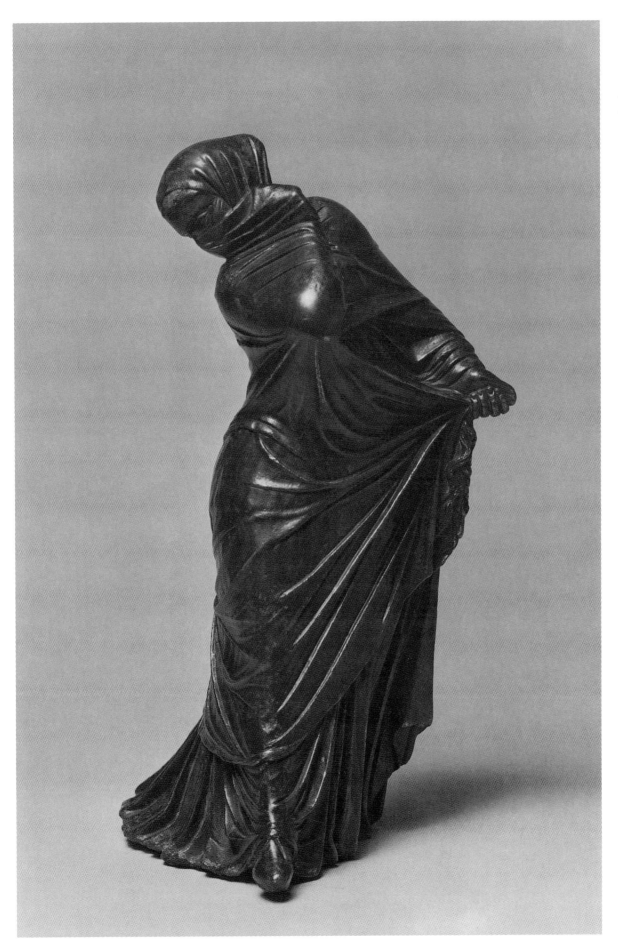

Figure 20.
A Hellenistic figure
of a veiled woman
("The Baker
Dancer"; c. 220 BC;
MMA #1972.118.95;
courtesy of the
Metropolitan
Museum of Art,
New York).

In other examples of pre-Islamic Arabic poetry, the modest movements of a woman were being praised:

> "She won me when as, shamefaced, no maid to let fall her veil. No wanton to glance behind as she walked with steady tread.
> Her eyes seek the ground, as though she had looked for a thing lost there; Straight forward she goes; if you speak to her, few are her words and low.
> Not one is Umaymah for gossip to bring to her husband shame. When mention is made of women, pure and unstained is she".[15]

Women in early Islamic times normally covered their head and faces with various types of veils when in public. One of the most important garments was an outerwrap called a *djilbaab*. According to contemporary descriptions this wrap totally enveloped the body, leaving only one eye free (Stillman 1986:735). There are also references to a form of headveil called *mandiil* being worn during this period, but its nature is not exactly clear.[16]

In conclusion, it is likely that both the nomadic and the settled people of Arabia maintained a fairly conservative and constant style of dressing. For women this included the use of a large and enveloping outerwrap when in public. The use of such garments in this region seems to date from at least the second millennium BC.

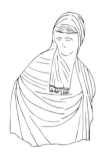

Figure 21. Figure of a woman wearing a face veil (based on Adriani 1948, pl. III, i).

Some Early Examples of the Use of Face Veils

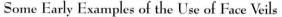

It is often presumed that the face veil is the product of Islam because it is with this cultural group that face veiling is now most commonly associated. However, as can be seen from the Assyrian laws quoted above, the concept of veiling in general can be traced to pre-Islamic times. Nevertheless, there is no direct evidence that these laws are referring to separate pieces of material drawn across the face, the 'real' face veils. Similarly, all the veils and references to veils discussed so far in this chapter exclude any direct evidence, they could be mantles and outerwraps that covered the body.

Surprisingly, the earliest actual evidence for face veils comes from Greek sources. During the third and second centuries BC a series of statuettes were made which are now called the "Mantle Dancers". These figurines depict dancing women who are totally enveloped in a long wrap. In one example now called the Baker Dancer, now housed in the Metropolitan Museum, New York, the woman is clearly wearing a face veil whose upper edge is shown just below her hair line (fig. 20; c. 220 BC; MMA #1972.118.95).[17]

The face veil she is wearing belongs to the type of veil which is now called a *niqab* (see page 57). Face veils of this type are still worn in the eastern Mediterranean and the Arabian Peninsula. The veil is made from a length of material fastened around the forehead and allowed to drape over the face. Eyeslits are cut out of the material in order to allow freedom of vision.

A second type of face veil (face panel) is depicted on

Figure 22. Figure of a woman from the Turkish site of Myrina, c. 3rd c. BC (Louvre 1163 0.09; courtesy of the Louvre Museum, Paris).

an Hellenistic statuette which is now in the Graeco-Roman Museum in Alexandria (fig. 21; Adriani, 1948, pl. III, 1). The woman wears a face screen which hangs from her forehead down to her chest (see page 50). The garment is fringed along the lower edges. Presumably the material was fairly sheer as no eye holes have been cut out of the material. In this respect it resembles the Yemeni veils described in the following chapter.

There are other examples of this type of face veil, but in these cases the veil has been thrown back over the head. One such example can be seen in a statuette of a standing woman from Tanagra in mainland Greece.[18] The figure dates to about 250-230 BC (Higgins nd, 132, pl. 159). In an article on some Graeco-Roman reliefs, the Italian historian, A. Adriani, noted two other examples (Adriani 1948). One of these was a statuette in the hands of an antiquities dealer in Cairo (first century BC), while the other was in the British Museum, London (first century AD). In both cases the women are wearing fringed veils similar to the one depicted on the Alexandrian statuette and again the veils have been flung back over the women's heads.

A third type of veil, which is made from a length of cloth wrapped around the lower face covering the lower part of the nose, mouth and chin can be seen on a statuette now in the Louvre Museum (fig. 22; Louvre Myrina 1163 0.09; Mollard-Besques 1963, pl. 130). The figure comes from the site of Myrina on the west coast of Turkey and dates to the third century BC. This type of veil is now called a *lithma*, and is still worn in a large part of the Islamic world, from North Africa to Yemen.

These representations of veiled women mean that the history of face veiling can be traced back to at least the third century BC. It would also appear that by this period the use of face veils by Greek ladies had spread to Alexandria in Egypt. The question remains, however, where did the Greeks obtain the idea of face veils?

Earlier in this chapter reference was made to the changing use of women's outer garments in Greece during the sixth and fifth centuries BC. This was the period when the Greek towns maintained close contacts with more eastern kingdoms, namely that of the Lydians in west Turkey. Eastern influences upon the Ionian Greeks have been suggested for many fields, including literature, architecture and art.[19] The Ionians, in their turn, passed on many cultural elements to the mainland Greeks. Costume may well have been one of the traits transferred. This apparently was the case with the outerwrap. Whether or not the same situation can also be applied to the face veil is a moot point.

In conclusion, it would appear that there were two lines which need to be followed in this discussion. Firstly, there is the ancient Mesopotamian/Persian concept of veiling. Secondly, there is the spread of these ideas, via eastern Greek colonies, into the Greek and Roman worlds.

What is certain is that by the first millennium AD the concept of face veiling was well established within the Eastern Mediterranean and Southwest Asia. Not only that, but the three forms of face veiling which have been identified, namely, the *niqab, lithma* and face-panel, are currently in use in North Africa and the eastern Mediterranean.

Notes:

2   Batto, 1974:24-25; Lerner 1986:70-71.
3   Driver and Miles 1935, no. 40; Jastrow 1921:209-239.
4   A similar set of regulations concerning the use of veils by married women is described in a twelfth to eleventh century BC Assyrian text (Weider 1954-6:257-293, no. 21).
5   Burns 1971:100-3; Boardman 1989:61-2.
6   Thompson 1951; Mollard-Besques 1963.
7   Leyenaar-Plaisier 1986, no. 27, inv. OC(ant) 6-39.
8   Two similar, veiled dancing women are now in the Museum of Fine Arts, Boston. Both are believed to be from Corinth (01.7923 and 01.7924).
9   A similar passage concerning the garments worn by Theban women can be found in Dicaearchi's *Messenii* 59:17-18. For another classical reference to veiled women, see Plutarch *Moralia* 232.
10 It has been suggested by W. Björkman that a prehistoric rock carving from Moghrar-Tashtani in the Sahara may represent an early example of a veiled woman (Björkman 1986:769). In the representation, however, the figure is shown with no mouth or nose, only the eyes are depicted (Frobenius and Obermaier 1925:49, pl. 80). It is more likely that the lack of the mouth and nose is an artistic device rather than representing a particular type of garment.
11 See for example, Virgil *Aeneid*, viii, 724; Livy 35:11.7; Plautus, *Poen* 5.2,48; Sil. 3, 235; Juv. 8.120 and Corippus *Johannidos*, ii, 130-1.
12 The sixth century AD writer, Corippus, described this garment as a: *horrida substrictus dependens stragula membris. Ex umeris demissa iacet* (*Johannidos*, ii, 134ff). The medieval Arabic Historian, Ibn Khaldun, noted that most Berbers wrapped themselves with a *kisa'* thrown over the shoulders. Later European travellers also described this garment (see Marçais 1930:25-30).
13 Kraeling 1956, pls. LII-LIII; Goldman 1994:186, figs. 11.5-6
14 Lyall 1921, I, 52-3, no. VIII; trans., 16-20, verses 3-4.
15 Lyall, 1921, I, 200, no. XX, verses 6-7; trans. 69-70. Beeston *et al*, 1983:59.
16 The word *mandiil* can also mean a small hand cloth or handkerchief. This word may also be the origin of the Latin word *mantellum* (cloak ?) and the later Spanish word *mantilla* (see page 33; Rosenthal 1971).
17 A similar veil can be seen in Perdrizet 1921, pl. CXVII, 517. See also Louvre Myrina 1325, Mollard-Bosques 1963:211:f.
18 BM acc. no. 1875.3-9.4. Higgins 1967:102, pl. 44c.
19 Richter 1987:56-9; Broadman 1985:62.

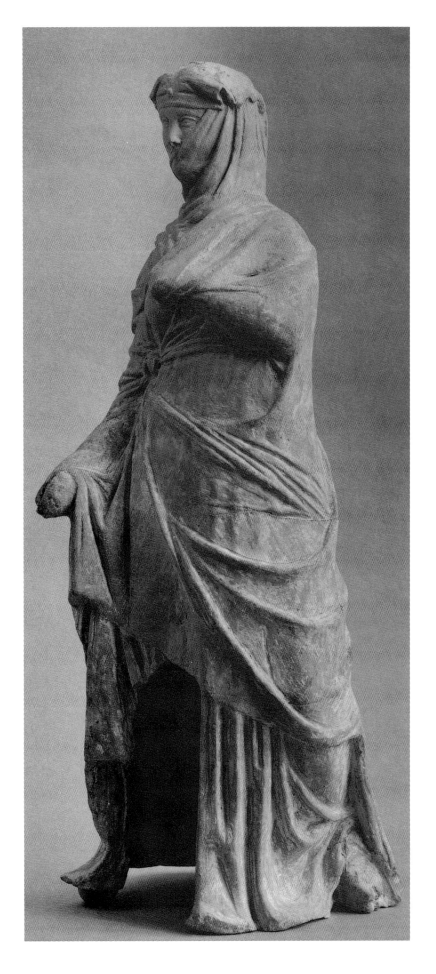

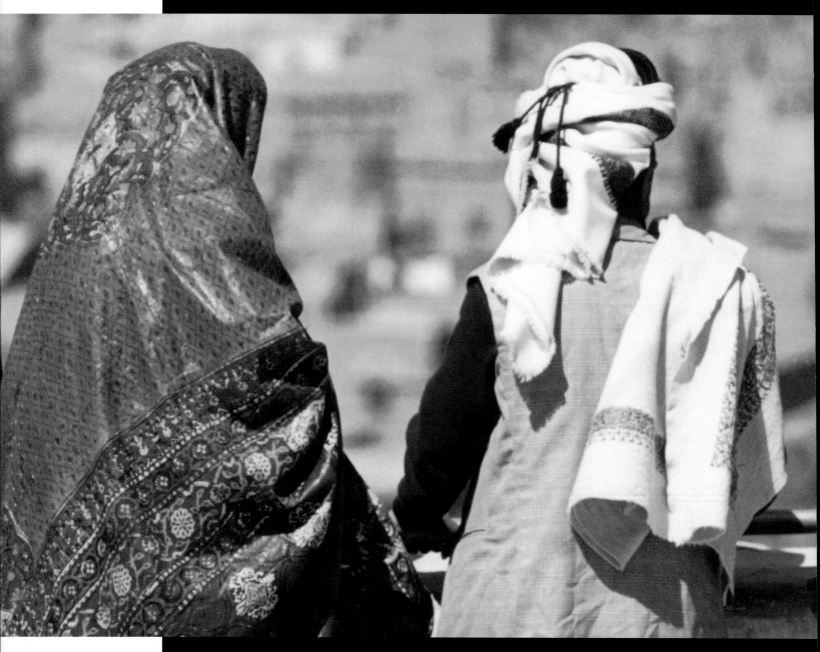

*Women from the San`a region of Yemen
(copyright R.E. Kon).*

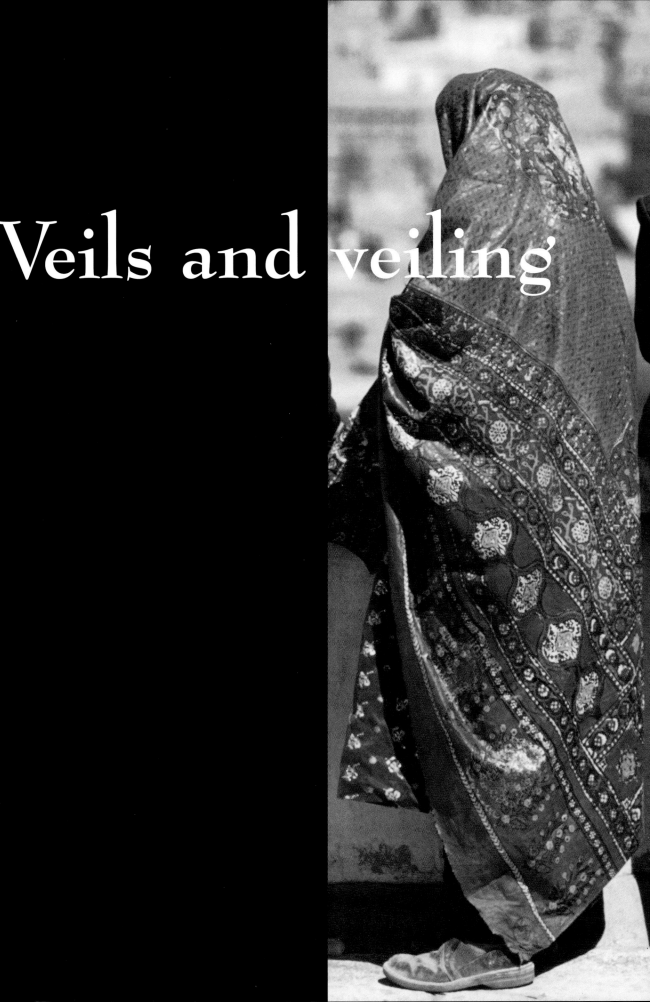

Veils and veiling

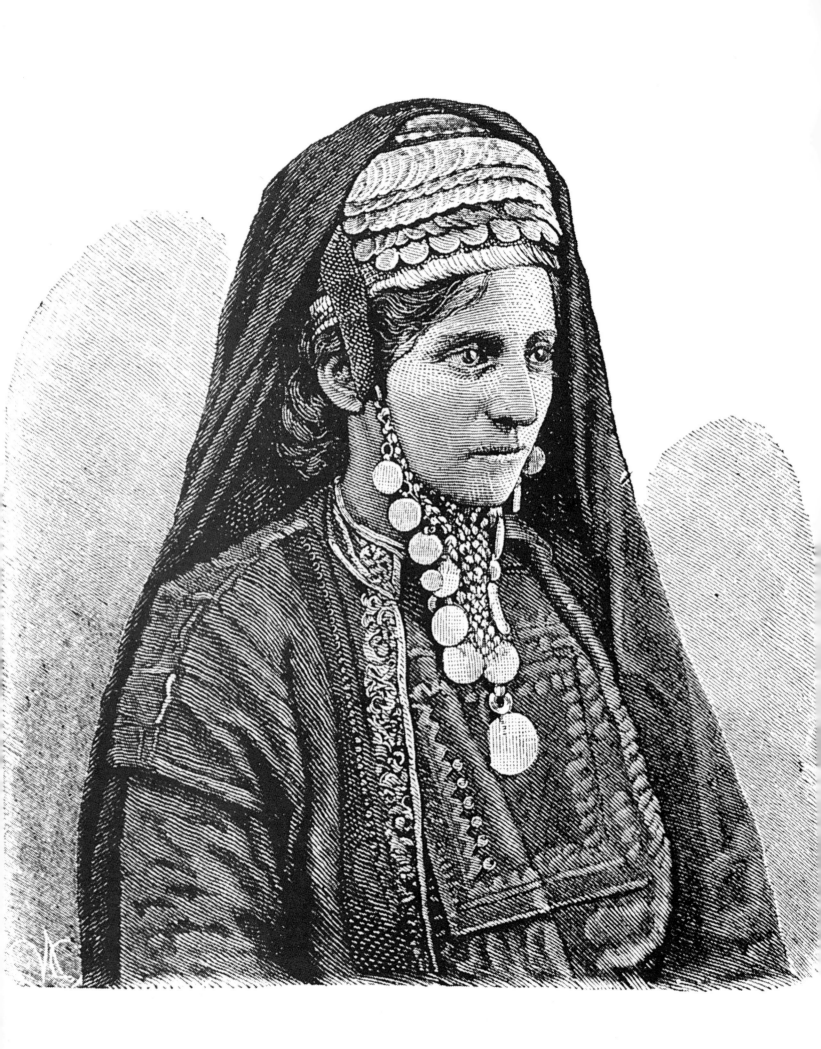

Chapter 3

Figure 39.
A Christian woman
from the Bethlehem
area, 19th century.
She is wearing a
shatweh (from
Jessup, 1873:5).

Kerchiefs, headveils and wimples

T he following chapter deals with the various lengths of cloth which can be tied, draped and knotted in some manner around the head and shoulders. Unlike the other chapters in this section it is not the way in which the garments are placed around the body which is of importance, but their sequence of arrangement. Thus the first item to be discussed is the kerchief, which is normally placed immediately on the head and hair (fig. 23). This is followed by the headscarf and the headveil which usually go over the kerchief.

It should be stressed that only a few of the many types of kerchiefs and headscarves and veils will be discussed in this chapter. In most countries of North Africa and the Near East, virtually every settlement seems to have had its own method of tying these garments. It would require an extensive study in itself to record all the forms and variations.

Kerchiefs

Women in many traditional societies can be seen wearing a small kerchief which is wrapped around the head so that the hair cannot be seen or cause a distraction. Such scarves are not restricted to one particular part of the world, age or social group, or even religious or political group.

In many Near Eastern and North African countries, small kerchiefs (often called *mandiil* or *sharb*) are worn by both Christian and Muslim women over their hair, and these have a similar function to those worn by European women, namely to protect and secure the hair. The idea of

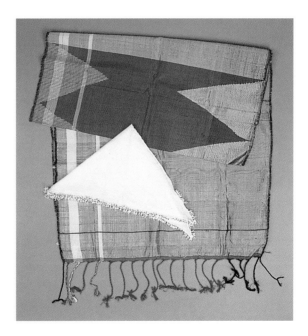

Figure 23. Group of modern kerchiefs and headveils (RMV 5825-10, 5863-5; photo. by B. Grishaaver).

the Near Eastern kerchiefs, however, is not only to secure the hair, but also to act as a foundation for headveils.

Kerchiefs are usually made out of small squares of material folded diagonally. The triangle is placed over the head and hair, while the ends are passed to the back of the head, twisted together and then brought to the front of the head where they are knotted.

There are various types of kerchiefs. In some areas of Morocco, for example, women use a rectangle of material with one corner folded inwards. It is then tied at the

Figure 24. Method for tying a Moroccan kerchief (halika and rug'a; based on Racknow 1958, pl. xxi).

Figure 25. A group of modern Egyptian kerchiefs or mandiil (RMV 5825-9,11, 5863-1; photo. by B. Grishaaver).

Figure 26. Group of modern Turkish kerchiefs (RMV 5827-6, 30,34; photo. by B. Grishaaver).

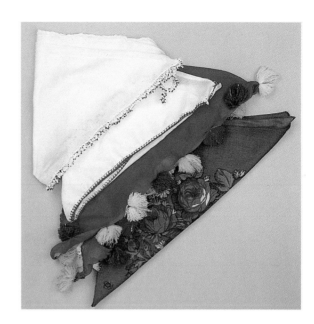

A Erstes Kopftuch, unmittelbar auf dem Haar, حليكة *hālika* auch رقعة *rug'a*, oder als سبنية عل القاس *söbnīya 'la l-qāṣṣ* bezeichnet.

Dieses Tuch A dient als Basis (sös) und Schutz für das Tuch **B** bzw. **C**.

Die Zeichnungen zeigen die Art des Zusammenlegens und der Zipfelver-Knüpfung.

Die Kopftücher I
TETUAN

Figure 27. A Turkish woman wearing a headscarf similar to one depicted in Figure 26.

back of the head. This form of kerchief is called by a number of different names, including *halika* and *rug`a* (fig. 24; Rackow 1958, taf. XXI). Another type of kerchief from Morocco is called a *mharma* and is made from a square of material which is folded in half diagonally, and then tied with a knot at the back of the head (Rackow 1958, taf. XLI). This kerchief is also sometimes tied under the chin.

In Egypt there are various types of *mandiil* (sharb; fig. 25; Rugh 1986:20-1). Sometimes they are white with small borders made out of coloured, crocheted or knotted yarn. Others have large coloured pom-poms sewn to the border. Other kerchiefs, especially those from Middle Egypt, are brightly coloured and are usually decorated with a floral motif (the colours of these kerchiefs are very similar to those used on Russian peasant shawls). Normally, the *mandiil* is folded in half diagonally, and then wrapped around the head, with the ends being brought to the front again, where they are knotted.

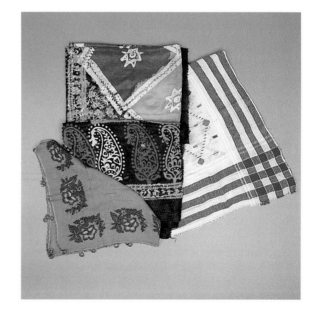

Similar small kerchiefs are worn by women in Turkey, but normally only indoors, rather than as a base for other head coverings (fig. 26). As with the other countries, there are numerous different types of these kerchiefs (*yazma*; *çember*).[20] Normally, small squares of light-weight material are bought and then decorated at home, although ready made versions are available. A *yazma tig*, for example, is decorated with crochet work, while the *yazma igne oyasi* is embroidered (fig. 27). Other forms are decorated with a form of lace (*mekik*) or beads (*boncuk*).

There are numerous different ways of wearing the *yazma*, but one of the most common ways is to fold the

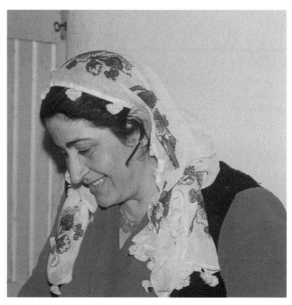

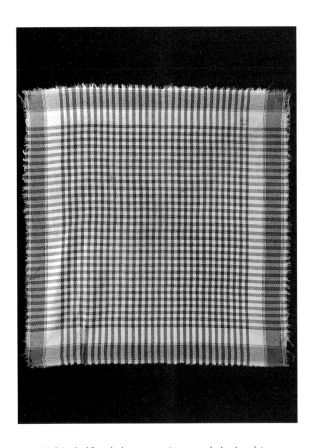

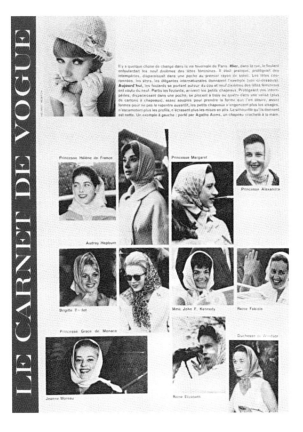

Figure 28.
A "Mother Ida"
headscarf from Sweden
(BM 24510 c. 1900,
courtesy of the Textile
Museum, Boras).

Figure 29.
Different ways of
wearing headscarfs
from a 1960's
edition of Vogue.

material in half and then wrap it around the head in a similar manner to the Egyptian *mandiil* described above.

Headscarves and Headveils

In many areas of the world women wear some form of loosely tied scarf or veil which covers all or part of the head and hair. As a generalisation, a headscarf is usually knotted or fastened in some manner around the head, chin and neck region, so that it does not come loose. A headveil on the other hand, is allowed much more movement and is usually only fastened at the top or sides of the head (see below).

There is a wide variety in the way such scarves are put onto the head. In Sweden, for instance, there is a traditional scarf called "Mother Ida's headscarf", which is named after Ida Sofia Gustavsdotter (1870-1929; fig. 28). She was a farmer's wife who sold butter (carried in her headscarf) to the lace factory in Boras in southern Sweden. The pattern of her scarf and the way she wore it (without the butter in it), became well-known and it is still used in the Boras region.

Sometimes headscarves are worn as protection against the wind, sun or rain, as for example, those used in Europe. In this case the scarf is usually a large square of material, folded diagonally and then knotted under the chin (figs. 29 and 30). A headscarf is also a well-known element of *hijab* (see Chapter 7) or Islamic clothing, but the main difference here is that most western headscarves are not worn tightly around the face with the hair hidden, while the *hijab* version is used to wrap closely the head and neck.

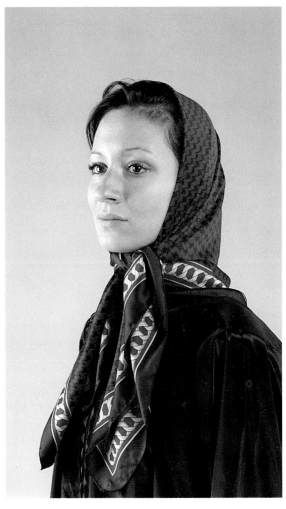

Figure 30.
European style
headscarf (private
collection; photo. by
B. Grishaaver).

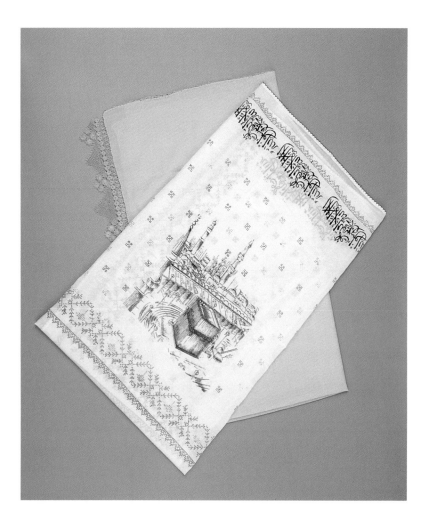

neck. The ends are then brought forward and knotted again at the top of the head. The whole ensemble is sometimes kept in place using a length of material (*harraz*) made out of a small square of cloth folded in half diagonally and then lengthwise.

Another method of tying headscarves from Morocco is called *ad-darra*. It consists of a large square of material folded in half and with the point of the triangle turned over (fig. 34; Rackow 1958, taf. LXVII). The cloth is then placed over the head, while the two long ends are tied at the back of the neck and covered with the rest of the cloth.

Headveils

A head veil is a length of material which is placed and then fastened in some manner over the kerchief or, sometimes, the headscarf. Often these garments are worn in combinations. In Egypt, for example, it is quite common to wear a small kerchief which covers the hair (*mandiil*; see above) and a larger veil which covers the hair and head (Rugh 1986:21-23). In some cases an outerwrap is placed over the top of these two garments which covers the head and upper body (*miláyeh*; see page 69).

In many areas of North Africa and the Near East, women also wear large squares of material over the head. In parts of Egypt, a *tarah*, is worn which is made from a long, rectangular length of light-weight material (usually black; figs. 35 and 36). The cloth is usually between two and four metres long. It is wrapped several times around the head in various ways and then the remaining cloth is allowed to hang down the centre of the back (Rugh 1986:22).

There are various forms of the Moroccan version of this final covering. One particular form (*al-mandiil*) is worn when travelling and on special occasions. It takes the form of a large rectangle of material which can be white, red or blue (Rackow 1958, taf. XLI). It is placed over the kerchief (*mharma*) and then draped around the head in an intricate Z-motion (fig. 37).

In Egypt the final head covering is often called a *shaal*. These headveils are often used to give a more finished look, especially on more formal occasions (fig. 38; Rugh 1986:23). They come in various forms, and may be of fringed cotton, rayon or even velvet. In Lower and Middle Egypt they are normally between one and two metres square. Because of their size and weight these garments are normally folded diagonally and then wrapped around the head and shoulders rather than tied. In Upper Egypt the *shaals* are often rectangular in shape with fringed ends. There are often bands woven into the material near these fringes. These garments are usually draped over the head and allowed to fall over the shoulders of the wearer.

Another area where headveils are commonly worn is in Palestine. Here there has been a very long tradition of wearing headveils of a wide variety of shapes and colours, and patterned in various traditional forms.[21] The veils are usually worn over an elaborate headdress of some kind

Figure 31. Two modern Turkish headscarves (RMV 5827-15,18; photo. by B. Grishaaver).

Figure 32. A Turkish woman wearing a kerchief with headscarf.

Headveils are usually draped loosely over the head and allowed to hang down over the shoulders and back. Here the intention is usually to hide the hair and disguise the shape of the head and shoulders, while at the same time allowing some movement of the cloth.

Headscarves

There are numerous ways of wearing a headscarf. They depend upon where a person comes from, the shape of headscarf (square, triangular, rectangle), and what it is made from.

In Turkey, for example, there is a wide range of scarves available which reflect different social and ethnic groups, ages, as well as function (every day, morning, evening, festival, etc; figs. 31 and 32; Akkent and Franger 1987:205ff). In addition, the way in which a scarf is tied can vary according to the time of year. In winter, for instance, a much heavier scarf is worn which is tied closely around the head and neck, while during the warm summer months a light-weight scarf is worn which is fastened at the back of the head (Akkent and Franger 1987, bl. 16, 18).

In northern Morocco there is a great diversity in the tying of headscarves. In some cases large fringed squares of cloth (*sabniya d'albhar* or *sabniya maslula*) are folded in half (fig. 33; Rackow 1958, taf. XXII). The triangle is draped over the forehead and knotted at the nape of the

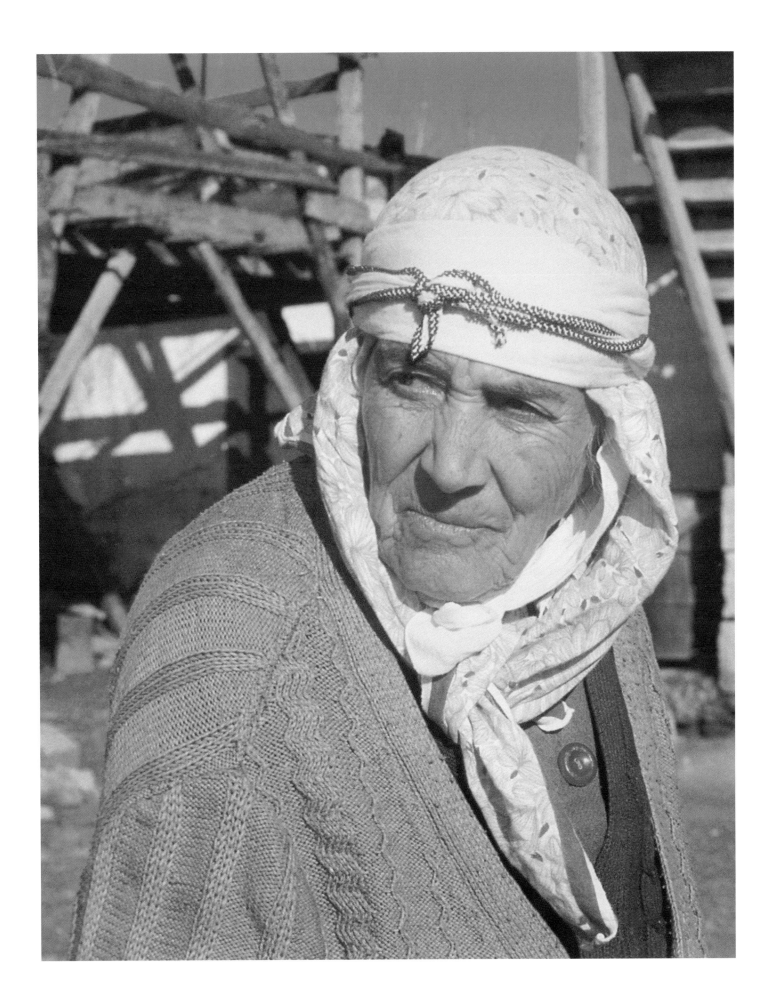

Figure 33. Method for tying a Moroccan headscarf (sabniya d'albhar; based on Racknow 1958, pl. xxii).

Figure 34. Method for tying a Moroccan headscarf (ad-darra; based on Racknow 1958, pl.lxvii).

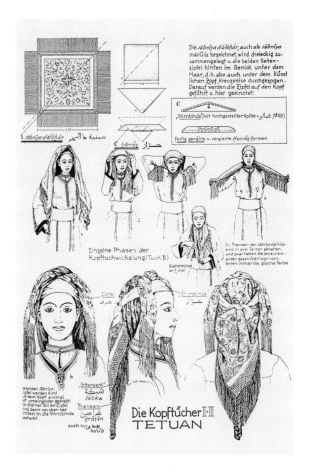

Figure 35. An Egyptian woman wearing a black headveil (tarah; photo. by the author).

(such as the *shatweh*, *smadeh*) or a small bonnet (*wuqa*), and allowed to cover the shoulders (fig. 39). Each region had its own particular form of headveil. In the Jaffa region, for instance, there were white head covers made from two lengths of material sewn together and then decorated with embroidery along the two short edges. Traditionally in Ramallah, on the West Bank, this type of veil was made of two long lengths of material. These were sewn together and then embroidered, usually with red and black yarn. The Ramallah veil was called a *khirqah*. Finally, the women of Bethlehem were known by their tall, very distinctively shaped *shatweh*, which were worn covered with a large white veil.

Some mention also needs to be made of the headveils worn by Muslim and Sikh women living in Pakistan and Northern India. Instead of wearing the sari (see page 69), women in these regions tend to wear trousers (*salwar*, *shalwar*), with a blouse (*kurta*) and a long shawl (*orhni*) or veil (*dopatta*)[22]. The *dopatta* is a large rectangle of fine cloth (silk or muslin), about two to three metres long and one metre wide. It is draped over the breasts and left shoulder and then allowed to hang over the right arm (fig. 40). The veil can be raised to drape the head or it can be drawn across the face to screen the wearer when in public.

Headbands and Headropes

In order to keep head veils in place some societies have developed various types of headbands and headropes. A

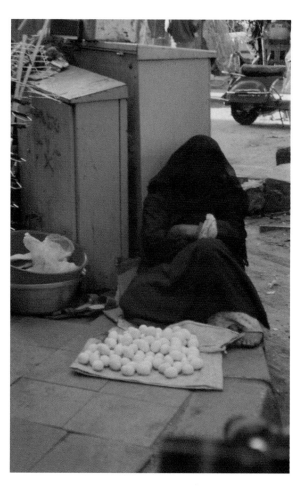

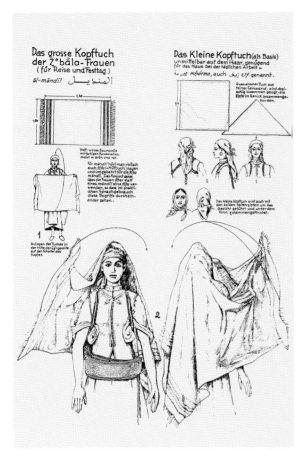

headband is literally a length of material which is tied around the head. It is often used to keep one or more other pieces of cloth in place. As may be expected there are various forms of headbands. During the beginning of the twentieth century, for instance, nomadic women of the Rwala region in northern Yemen traditionally wore a large dark headveil (*makrûna*). This is a large square of material which was folded in half diagonally. According to writer and traveller, A. Musil, it was worn in the following manner:

> "Holding the left lappet to her left cheek, she throws the kerchief over her head in such a way that the middle lappet falls on her back; the right lappet she then passes under the chin, covers with it the left lappet on the left cheek, and folds it over her head again" (Musil 1928:123)

The *makrûna* was kept in place with a kerchief or *mindiil*. This was a dark cotton kerchief folded into a band about five centimetres wide which was wound around the *makrûna*. In place of an ordinary *mindiil*, a band of some fine material was sometimes used. This band was called a *safa`a* (or *mer`ez*). Another type of band was called a *krajsa* which was made of a fabric so loosely woven that it stretched. The complete wrap made from these finer materials was called a *sitfa*.

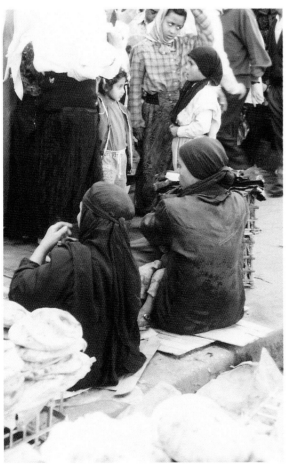

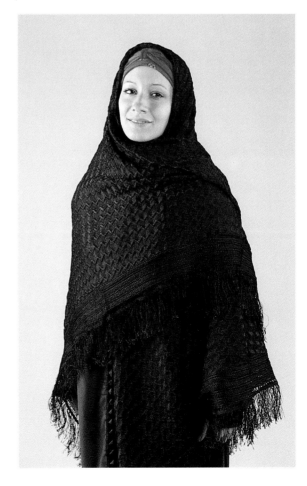

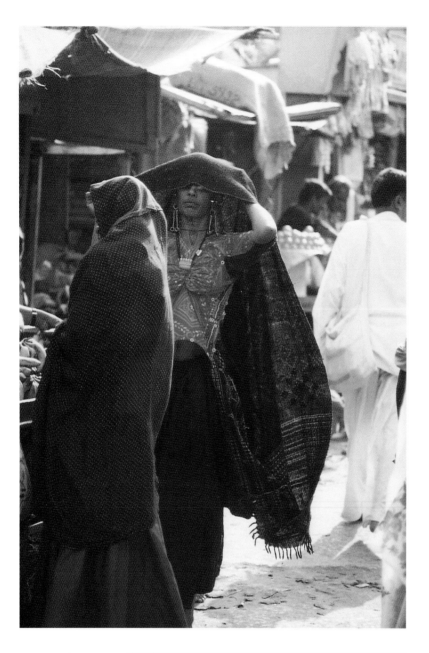

Another form of headband was worn by Bedouin women from the Galilee region. Traditionally these women have worn a black crepe headveil (*shambar* or *milfa`*) bound with a headband called an *`asbeh* (fig. 41; Weir 1989:160). The latter were made out of a square of material folded and rolled diagonally, and then wrapped round the forehead and knotted at the back of the head. More elaborate versions of this garment have fringes or tassels which hang down the back. According to the anthropologist, S. Weir, brides often wore an *`asbeh* on their wedding days, while their female guests would wear another type of headband called a *zamliyeh* decorated with green, yellow and black stripes (Weir 1989:161, 163).

A headrope is literally a rope tied around the head in some manner. It is usually made of one or more cords covered with a spun sheep's wool, goat hair or camel hair yarn or some other form of cord (fig. 42). Called an *`aqal* (*`egal*) in Arabic, it is one of the most characteristic forms of Arabic clothing. During the nineteenth century the rope worn by the Bedouin was relatively thick, but it gradually became thinner. Normally, an *`aqal* is worn by men, but occasionally it is used by women. In general (but it should be stressed, not always), a form of *`aqal* with only one cord is worn by women, while the man's *`aqal* may have two or more cords. In addition, the woman's version is black, while the male form can be black or multi-coloured and decorated with metal threads of various kinds, for example, gold (*`aqal mqassab*; Weir 1989:66-8).

The *`aqal* is traditionally associated with nomadic tribes. However, since the 1930's it has become an accepted part of male clothing worn in settlements and towns throughout the Near East.[23]

Medieval European Wimples

Some word should be said at this point about the medieval European wimple and its different forms. It is included in this study because during the medieval period there was a direct relationship between the form of headcovering used in Europe and that worn in the Near East.

As described in the previous chapter, women used to cover their heads in various ways. Similarly in Northern Europe headveils were worn. During the early medieval period (from about the tenth century onwards), the headveils were simply a piece of material held in place by a fillet or ribbon encircling the brow or by being pinned to the hair.

A major change in the headcovering worn by women took place in the twelfth century when the wimple (guimple) was introduced. A wimple consisted of a piece of linen or silk, usually white, which was fastened to the hair on the crown or on each side of the head just above the ears (fig. 43; Yarwood 1988:447-8). It was then draped to cover the chin, neck and throat.[24] The lower edge was often tucked into the gown neckline. This garment appears to have been introduced into Europe by the Crusaders following their sojourn in the Middle East. It is known from other fields that the Crusaders brought various ideas and technology back to Europe, including

Figure 40.
A woman from Gujerat Bhuj wearing traditional North Indian clothing (courtesy of K. de Vries).

Figure 42.
A man's headcovering with headrope (RMV 398-2c,d; photo. by B. Grishaaver).

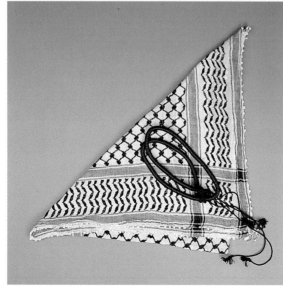

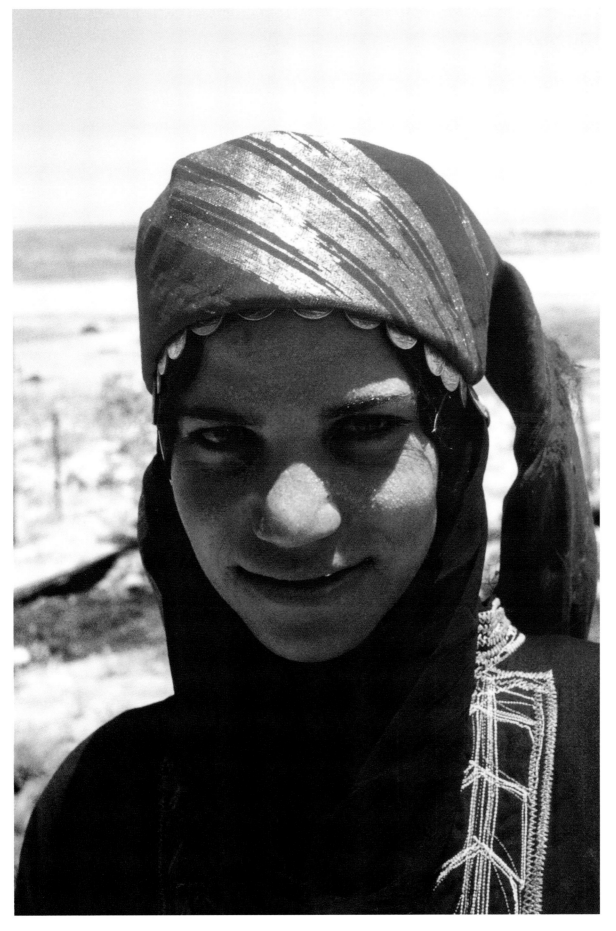

Figure 41.
*A Druze woman from
the Galilee region
wearing a headband
(asbeh; courtesy of
Shelagh Weir).*

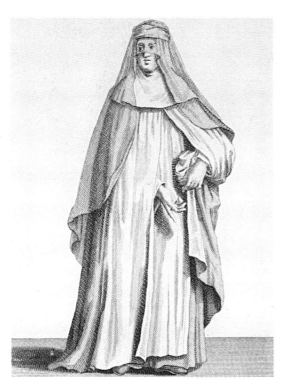
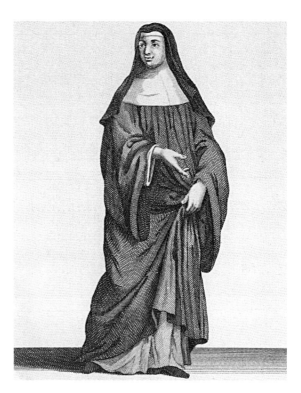

Figure 44a-b.
Nun's clothing
from Germany,
mid-18th century.
(a) cloister sister
from Jungfernberge
in ordinary clothing,
(b) cloister sister
from Font Evraud
in choir clothing
(courtesy of
D. Stuart-Fox).

various types of loom (Laver 1995:56). So it should come as no surprise that clothing was affected by these new influences. Certainly, the fact that the wimple was tightly wrapped around the neck and covering the hair indicates that it belongs within an Islamic, rather than Western tradition.

The wimple (guimple) was worn mainly from the late twelfth to the mid-fourteenth century and, less fashionably, in the fifteenth century (Yarwood 1988:447-8). It was often worn with different types of head veils including the *couvrechef*. This garment is the same as the Anglo-Saxon headrail (coverchief, headrail, kerchief), which was a veil draped around the head and hung loose or was tucked into the neckband of the gown (Yarwood 1988:122-3). The Norman term *couvrechef* was anglicized into coverchief (the present-day kerchief). It was largely discard by the upper classes in the fourteenth and fifteenth centuries in favour of the more shaped, stiffened headdress. The draped head coverings remained the everyday wear for peasant and working classes throughout the centuries, becoming later the kerchief worn in the nineteenth century in industrial towns in Europe, as well as in the country districts to this date. It has now become the headscarf.

The survival of the medieval wimple can be seen in Europe in the form of traditional nun's clothing (fig. 44a-b). "To take the veil" is an accepted way of saying that a woman has entered a convent in preparation of becoming a nun. Similarly, the removal of her veil can be taken as a sign of disapproval. One intriguing source of information about this subject is the Medieval *Register of Archbishop Eudes*, which is an account of ecclesiastical events in northern France over a period of twenty-one years. In this account there is the case of one nun, Alice of Rouen (who first appeared in the *Register* in AD 1255), who was

accused of having borne a child fathered by a priest from Beauvais. As a punishment for her behaviour her veil was taken away, so demoting her to the ranks of 'normal' women (Johnson 1991:121).

The clothing of a nun was strictly defined. The habit, for example, was necessary as a sign to the outside world and a reminder to the wearer of her special position. Similarly, the veil was used to cut-off the wearer from the outside world and to prevent vanity by hiding the hair. Sometimes the position of the veil was abused as can be seen in the Villarceaux Case, which concerned the inhabitants of a small Benedictine priory north of La Roche Gudent. The lax behaviour of the nuns towards their veils was described in the *Register* of July 9th 1249: "We decree that no more saffron shall be placed on the veils, that the hair be not arrayed in vain curls ... nor shall the hair be allowed to grow down below the ears: (Johnson 1991:117).

The short wimple worn by modern nuns is a sad remnant of the original version, yet the fact that it has survived indicates the great symbolic value of this garment.

Notes:

20 Information about Turkish headgear has been provided by A. Voeten, CNWS, Leiden University.

21 For a detailed discussion of the various types of head coverings used in Palestine, see Weir 1989, and Völger *et al.* 1987.

22 The trousers were adapted from Turkish style trousers called *chalvar*.

23 The wearing of the `aqal may even date back to the time of Tutankhamun (c. 1325 BC; Vogelsang-Eastwood, forthcoming).

24 In medieval France this throat veil was called a *barbette*. It is also known as a *gorget*.

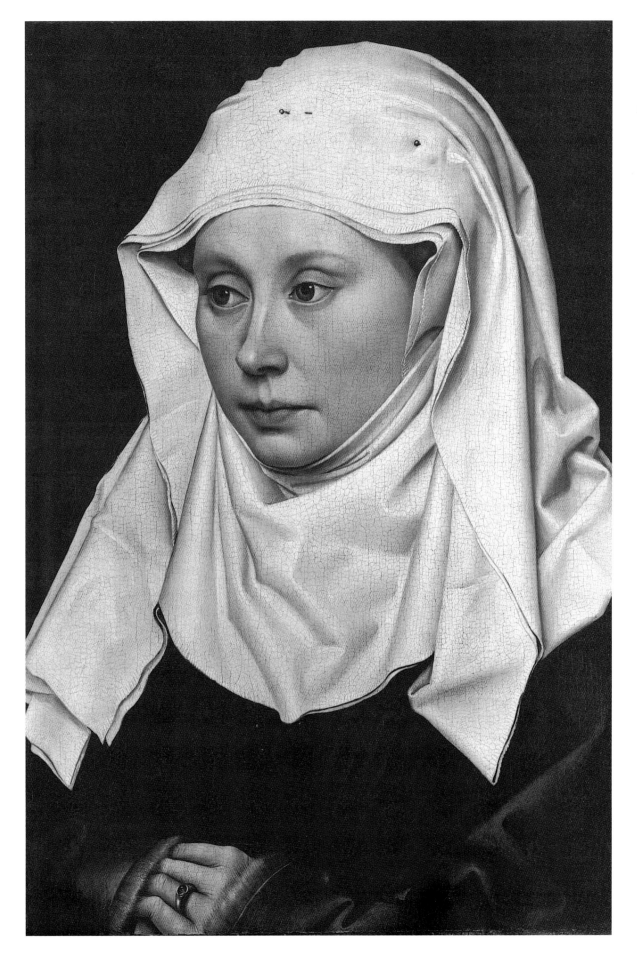

Figure 43. An unknown woman wearing a tightly fitting wimple, painting by R. Campin (1378-1444; courtesy of the National Gallery, London).

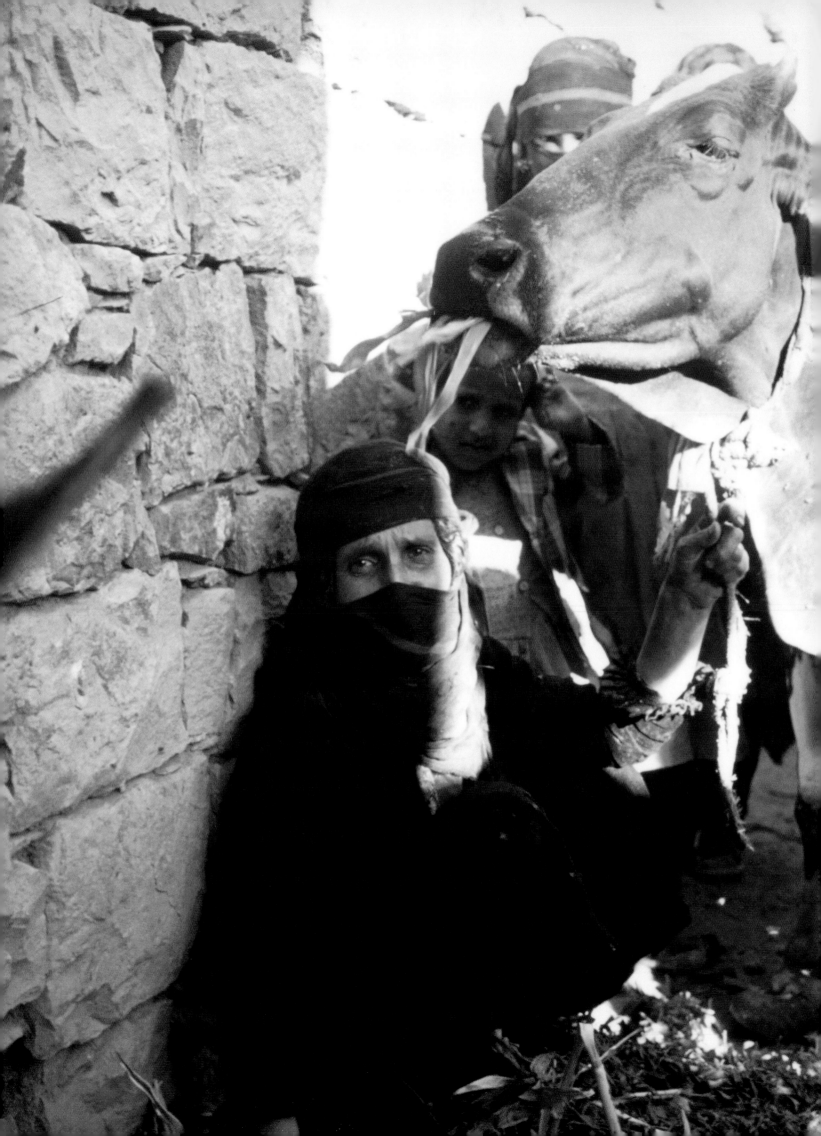

Chapter 4

Face veils

In this chapter a description will be given of the various basic types of face veils which can be found in North Africa and the Near East. For the purpose of this study, a face veil is defined as a length of material or some other substance, which is specifically designed to cover part or all of the face. It is a separate item from the headscarf which is used to cover the head and hair and sometimes the face as well.

Face veils can vary considerably in materials used, their form and their size. In Nubia, for instance, some women wear veils made out of their own hair, while Turkmen brides of the Khiva region, south of the Aral Sea wear veils made out of strings of beads. The part of the face concealed by a face veil can also vary considerably. Small, shaped lengths of cloth or leather are used to cover the nasal region by women in Oman. In contrast, in Yemen large lengths of material are used to hide all of the face.

Independent of materials used, there are many types of face veils. The differences can indicate the origins of the wearer, her family, whether she lives in an urban settlement or belongs to a nomadic group. Other factors include her social position, wealth and age. The effects of such elements on the development of veiling will be discussed in later chapters.

Below a description is given of various types of face veils. This has been organized according to how the veil is fastened to the head, for example, wrapped, draped or tied. Thus, the main types of face veils can be divided into three groups. Firstly, there are those forms which are made from lengths of material that are wrapped around the head. Secondly, face-panels or lengths of cloth which are draped over the face. Finally, there are the face veils such as the *burqa`* and *niqab*, which are tied to the head.

Wherever possible the local name for a veil is used, but it should be stressed that there would seem to be no consistency in (local) terminology. In many cases the term *burqa`* is used by both modern authors and their sources of information to mean a face veil without specifying what form of veil they mean.

All the veils discussed in this chapter date from after the tenth century AD. Indeed most examples cited belong to the twentieth century. Over the centuries some types of face veils have vanished or their names have been changed. It is, therefore, sometimes extremely difficult to understand what sort of veil is being referred to in older sources. During the medieval period in Egypt, for instance, various terms for veils were in general use, such as the *niqâb*, *khimar* and *miqna`a* (Stillman 1972:222-3). Of the medieval veils, only the *niqab* and *burqa`* seem to have survived to the present day.

Wrapped face veils

The wrapping of the face and head with one or more pieces of cloth is a common practice in many parts of the world. There seem to be two basic types of facial wrappings. The first is where only one piece of cloth is used. The whole of the head may be enveloped in the

Figure 50.
A woman from San`a, Yemen, wearing a face veil (lithma; copyright, R.E. Kon).

Figure 45.
A woman wearing
a Syrian shanbar
(c. 1880; from
Ohne, 1980).

Figure 46. Two
women from
Xinjiang, in the
Kashgar region of
China. The women
are wearing veils
over their heads and
faces (courtesy of
K. de Vries).

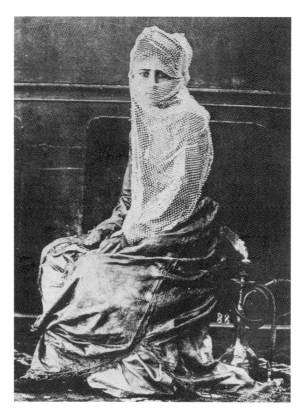

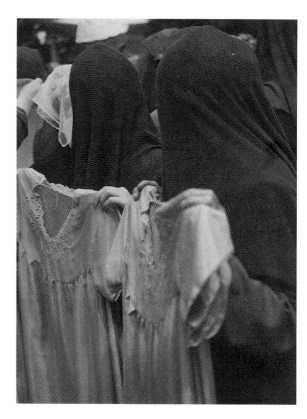

cloth (head wraps), as is the case in nineteenth century Syria and present-day north India. In other cases only the lower part of the face is covered, such as with the *lithma* worn by women in countries as far apart as North Africa and Yemen. The second basic type includes the use of two or more lengths of material which are used to cover the forehead and the lower part of the face, including the nose, mouth and chin.

Head wraps

The use of a single piece of material to envelop the head can be found in a number of countries. Urban women in nineteenth century Syria sometimes wore a length of cloth known as a *shanbar* around their heads (see Kalter 1992, figs. 546-9). Various types of material were used for these veils, but in general a light coloured and semi-transparent cloth was favoured. In some cases these veils were decorated with tiny, printed motifs, or embroidered with silk or metal threads or provided with small beads or coins.

The cloth could be passed around the head in a variety of ways. In Figure 45, for example, the cloth is wrapped around the head and then brought over the left shoulder before being fastened near the right ear.

Another method of wearing a length of material as a face veil can be seen in present-day India. Some married Muslim women living in urban areas such as Delhi, wear a long length of material draped over their heads. It is often made out of a fine, semi-transparent black material which is decorated with a variety of geometric motifs such as spots or interlocking circles. Other methods of decorating these cloths include printing, embroidery and applique.

Finally, parts of eastern China has a high muslim population. In these areas, women can be seen wearing a large, brown cloth over their heads (fig. 46).

The lithma or single face-wraps (chin wraps, chin bands)

In many regions of the Middle East and North Africa women wear a single length of material or *lithma*, which is wrapped the lower half of the face (chin wraps, chin bands). The upper half of the face is either left uncovered or hidden by another garment, notably a mantle or outerwrap of some kind.

In North Africa there are various forms of the *lithma*. In northern Morocco, for instance, women from the Tutuan region use a square of material which is folded diagonally to make a triangle. Part of the long edge is then folded under (fig. 47; Rackow 1958, taf. XXIII). The veil is used to cover the mouth and chin, with the long ends tied at the back of the head.

Another form of North African *lithma* is found in north-eastern Morocco and is made of a wide rectangle of material which is wrapped around the face and then knotted at the back of the head (fig. 48). This type of veil often has some form of decoration (embroidery or crochet) along the lower edge.

But perhaps one of the most famous forms of the *lithma* is that worn by Tuareg men (fig. 49). The Tuareg veil or *tegelmust* (*tagoulmoust, teguelmoust* in Berber and *lithma* in Arabic) is a combination of veil and turban.[25] It is made from a lightweight cotton cloth (*aleshu*) which varies in width between 25.0 and 50.0 cm and between

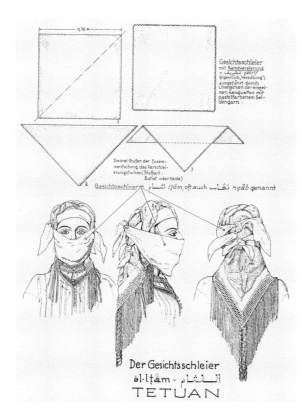

Gesichtsschleier
mit Randverzierung
... ...(eigentlich Veredlung)
ausgeführt durch
Umstechen der einzel-
nen Langwetten mit
pastellfarbenem Sei-
dengarn.

Die drei Stufen der Zusam-
menfaltung des Verschlei-
erungstuches (Stoffart)
Batist oder Seide)
Gesichtsschleier لثام lṭām, oft auch نقاب nqāb genannt

Der Gesichtsschleier
əl·lṭām - الثام
TETUAN

1.5 and 4.0 metres in length. Although it is traditionally dark indigo blue in colour, black or white versions can be found. There are various forms of veils which are known after their colour or the material used to produce them, for instance, *aleshum*, *eshash*, *takarut*, *tegeneut* and *tekerheyt*.

The band is wound around the head and face leaving only the eyes and a small patch near the back of the scalp exposed. The lower edge of the cloth is often doubled over the middle so as the cloth can be drawn tightly across the bridge of the nose, thus preventing the veil from slipping. On formal occasions the eye opening is made as narrow as possible. Sometimes a second, smaller veil of fine bleached cloth is wound over the *aleshu*.

A *lithma* is also used in Yemen as a form of "indoor veil" for unmarried girls and for married women while working at home or on informal morning visits (fig. 50; Makhlouf 1979:24, 30). It consists of a long piece of thin material or muslin which is brightly coloured. It is draped around the head in such a way as to cover the hair and forehead, while the lower part covers the mouth and chin. It can be pulled down to uncover, or pulled upwards to cover the whole face except the eyes.

When there are no men in the room, the *lithma* is worn down, but a woman must cover her face in the presence of a man who is not her husband or a close relative (Makhlouf 1979:30).

Another form of *lithma* was worn during the first half of the twentieth century by the women of some nomadic tribes in northern Arabia. Unlike their urban counterparts, nomadic women did not wear face veils which totally covered the face, but instead they wore a thin black length of material which was drawn across the lower features of the face including the mouth and chin. According to Dickson this type of face or chin wrap was worn by women of the Sulubba and the Mutair tribes (Dickson 1949:155, 160).

Figure 47. The tying of a Moroccan lithma (based on Racknow 1958, pl. xxiii).

Figure 49. A Touerag from wearing a lithma-style headcovering (courtesy of R. Munneke).

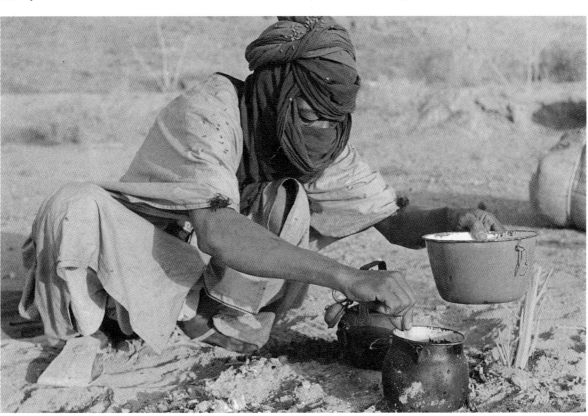

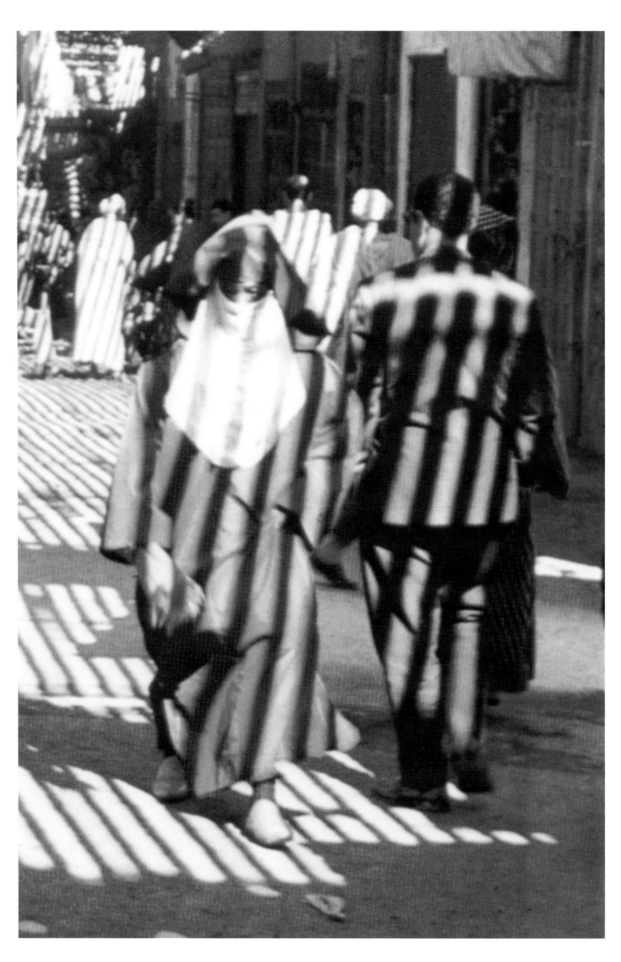

Figure 48.
A Moroccan woman
wearing a face veil
(lithma; from
Gloudemans,
1975:21).

Multiple face-wraps

The veils described above are made out of one piece of cloth which is wrapped around the head and face. In some areas of the Near East, however, women have traditionally worn two or more pieces of material for this function. The most famous of these face veils is probably the Turkish *yashmak*, which used to be worn by women living in or around the Turkish capital, Istanbul.

Depictions of Turkish women wearing *yashmaks* can be traced back to the sixteenth century, although the tradition is probably much older than this. One of the clearest examples of the use of two pieces of material can be seen in a drawing from an English traveller's handbook which dates from about 1588 (fig. 51).[26] The woman is wearing a headdress which is concealed by a *yashmak*, namely two white veils, one of which is draped and fastened to the pillbox cap, while the other covers the face from nose to chin.

An early description of virtually transparent *yashmaks* was given in a work called *Saadabad*, by the seventeenth-century Turkish writer, Sinan Chelebi:

> "Two beauties, one in lemon yellow, the other in pink, were going towards the green meadow in their glittering picnic carriages. Their yashmaks were crystal clear, their cheeks like roses, their necks like silver, their hair like hyacinths" (quoted in Croutier 1989:78).

At the beginning of the eighteenth century, an English traveller, Lady Mary Wortley Montague, visited Turkey and wrote in a letter (dated 1st April 1717):

> "'Tis very ease to see they [Turkish Ladys] have more Liberty than we have, no Woman of what rank so ever being permitted to go in the streets without 2 muslins, one that covers her face all but her Eyes and another that hides the whole dress of her head and hangs halfe way down her back" (Montague 1965, I, 7).

At the end of the nineteenth century, Lucy Garnett gave a description of a group of women from Istanbul wearing *yashmaks* in her study of Turkish women:

> The feridjes ... of the wealthy are of fine cloth or silk, the younger and more fashionable ladies affecting light tints such as pink or lilac, often with trimmings of lace on the rectangular cape, and the elderly ladies more sober tints. The yashmak is composed of two squares of white tarlatan folded corner-wise. A small cap made of some bright coloured material and decorated with pearls, or diamonds, is placed on the top of the head and serves as a foundation for the upper part of the veil, the doubled edge of which is brought down to the eyes, the ends being pinned together at the back. The other and larger square is then placed with the folded edge upwards across the mouth and lower part of the nose the ends being pinned to those of the upper square" (Garnett 1890-91:209).

During the nineteenth and beginning of the twentieth century, the *yashmak* was normally worn with the *feraje* (*feridjes*, *ferace*), which was a voluminous street robe with a collar.[27] As noted above, the veil was made from two pieces of fine white muslin, which were worn in such a way as to leave the eyes uncovered (fig. 52). The effect was such that the head appeared to be completely swathed in a single length of white gauze.

There would appear to be two basic ways of tying the *yashmak* (Tuglaci 1984:86). The first is known as the "closed *yashmak*", while the other is called the "open *yashmak*". In each case, the lower section of veil was always put on first. The *kapali yashmak* or closed yashmak was made from a length of material folded in half lengthwise. It was placed over the nose and just under the eyes. It was then allowed to hang down over the lower part of the face. The material was tied at the back of the neck. The upper piece of cloth was also folded in half and wrapped around the head and forehead, just over the eyebrows, leaving only the eyes and eyebrows visible.

The *açik yasmak*, or open yashmak, is basically identical to the closed version except that the two pieces of cloth were not folded in half. This gave the veil a semi-transparent appearance. One piece of cloth was tied around the lower part of the face, while the upper piece went around the edge of the forehead. The join at the temple where the two pieces of cloth met often remained visible and sometimes part of the woman's hair would be (deliberately) revealed.

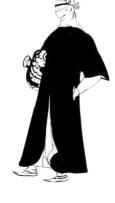

Figure 51. Turkish woman wearing an outdoor costume including an early form of the yashmak face veil (AD 1588; based on MS Bodl. Or. 430, fol. 90b).

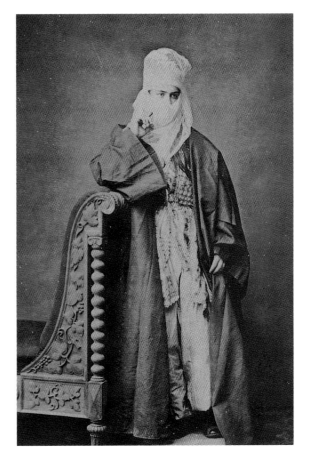

Figure 52. A Turkish woman wearing a yashmak, c. 1885 (Hotz Collection, 20:42; courtesy of the Library, the University of Leiden).

Figure 53.
A Turkish woman
wearing an early
form of the yashmak-
style face veil
(AD 1553; based on
P. Coeck van Aelst
Moeurs et fachons de
faire les Trucz).

The lower edges of both types of *yashmak* were normally tucked into the collar of the *feraje*. Sometimes the lower *yashmak* would be slightly starched and this style became known as the *sarayli yasmagi* or "palace yashmak".

Although the yashmak was virtually translucent and revealed, if not enhanced, the facial features, women were careful never to show their tip of their noses as this would be taken as a sign that the wearer was either an infidel or a prostitute (Croutier 1989:78).

During the eighteenth and nineteenth centuries fashion trends in Istanbul were copied in other parts of the then vast Ottoman Empire. Turkish women living in Salonika, for example, wore the *feraje* and *yaskmak* in both the open and closed forms. Veils were also adopted by Christian women, as can be deduced from the following description of the outdoor dress of fashionable Greek women during the early nineteenth century:

> "When abroad the Greek ladies are muffled up in a wrapping-cloak, much like the Turkish, except that they have not a square merlin hanging behind, and, instead of a hood over the face, generally wear a long veil, which, however, they frequently throw aside when not in the presence of any Turks" (Broughton 1855, I, 447-9).

In general, the wearing of the *yashmak* started to disappear following the proclamation of the Turkish republic in 1923 (see Chapter 12).

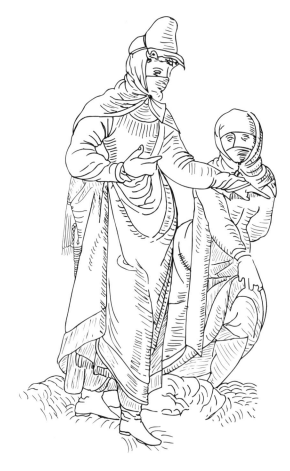

Face-panels

Instead of a deliberately shaped piece of cloth wrapped around the head (such as the *lithma* or the *yashmak*), some women wear a length of material which hangs down from the top of the head. In some case the draped veil has slits or holes cut out for the eyes, in other examples however, the material was regarded as sufficiently sheer without any need to pierce it.

Unpierced face-panels

Where fine and semi-transparent material is available it is not uncommon for face-panels to be made out of a single length of material which is not pierced. One of the earliest descriptions of this type of veil as worn by Turkish women is given in a book by the Italian Bassano da Zara called *I Costumi et i modi particolari de la vita de Turchi*, written in 1545:

> "They wear a towel round the neck and head, so that one can only see their eyes and mouth, and these they cover with a thin silk scarf a palm's width each way, through which they can see and not be seen by others. The scarf is fastened with three pins to a suitable part of the head above the forehead, so that when they go through the streets and meet other women, they raise the scarf that hangs over their faces and kiss one another" (quoted in Croutier 1989:76-7).

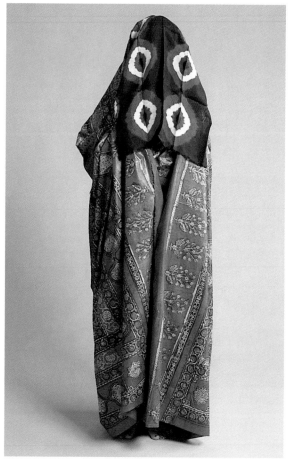

This type of veil can be seen in several near-contemporary woodcuts such as one depicting a group of Turkish women which was made by P. Coecke van Aelst, during the first half of the sixteenth century (*Sitten und Gebräuche der Türken*, 1533-50.[28] In this case, however, ties have been used, rather than pins, to keep the veil in place (fig. 53).

Nowadays, some urban women in Saudi Arabia, for instance, wear a simple veil called a *milfa* or *shella* (Topman 1981:104). It is made out of a long black rectangular piece of sheer chiffon or muslin which is placed over the head and covers the face. It is kept in position by the *abaya* which is placed on top of it (see fig. 94). Sometimes the *milfa* is decorated with embroidery, mother-of-pearl buttons, metal beads, as well as with tassels and fringes.

Traditionally, women in northern Yemen have worn a long, wide piece of material which covers their whole face.[29] The garment is normally hung from the top of the head and is kept in place by the outer wrap or a headpiece, rather than being tied with strings. Various forms of face-panels are worn in Yemen. Women living in the ancient Yemeni city of San`a, for example, wear a face-panel (*maghmuq*) made up of a piece of silk or similarly fine material (fig. 54). Normally, this cloth is sufficiently transparent for the wearer to remain capable of seeing the world around her. This cloth is normally tied dyed in such a way as to form large red and white

circles. The dyeing takes place in San`a itself. It is generally worn by married women with an outerwrap (generally called a *sitara*), which is a large piece of cotton material printed in red, blue and green (this specific type of cloth is called *ghanami*).

Until relatively recently women in San`a, Jemen, also wore a headdress or *qarqush* over the *sitara* and *maghmuq*.[30] This is a bonnet made from a square of material folded in half and heavily decorated with silver amulets, metal thread, coral and small hanging chains (fig. 55). A simpler version of the *qarqush* was worn by unmarried girls. This was discarded on their marriage night.

Another type of face-panel called a *khunna* is worn in a number of settlements and towns (including San`a) in northern Yemen. It is made up of a length of thin black muslin (fig. 56). It is worn with a long pleated skirt worn over the indoor dress (*zinnah*) and a waist-length cape which covers the head and shoulders. Both of these garments are made out of black silk-like material. The whole ensemble is called a *sharshaf*.[31]

Pierced face-panels

In order to make the world slightly more visible to the wearer some face-panels had small eye holes or grills set into them. This type of veil is also worn by young girls in Yemen (Mundy 1983, fn. 49). At home a girl would wear a *lithma*, but while outdoors she would wear over it a black face-panel (*burqa`*) with holes for the eyes. These

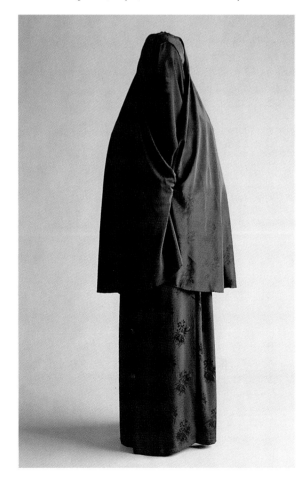

Figure 55.
A qarqush from Yemen (private collection; photo. by B. Grishaaver).

Figure 56.
A modern outfit (sheshaf) from the Sa`na region of Yemen (RMV 5865; photo. by B. Grishaaver).

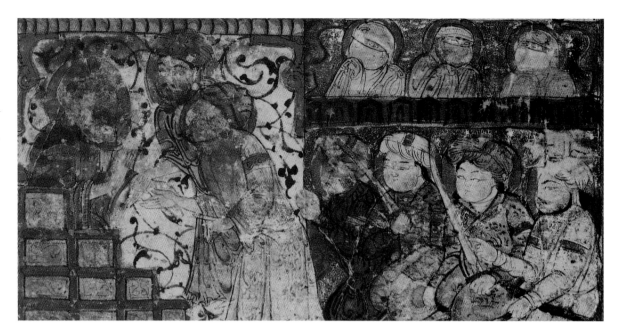

are decorated with shells, coral, buttons and other hanging ornaments. Over this was thrown a *futah* or shawl which covered the head and back.

At the turn of the century women also wore a face-panel similar to the girl's *burqa`* described above. It was worn with a *ras maghmuq*, an elaborate headpiece embroidered with gold and silver. The woman's face-panel was hung from the *ras maghmuq*. This garment has now virtually disappeared and has been replaced by the *maghmuq*, described previously.

Finally, a face-panel was worn by women in the city of Kashgar in Chinese Turkestan during the nineteenth century. A description of this veil being worn by the Kashgari women is given in the memoirs of Lady Catherine Macartney, wife of the British representative to Kashgar at the beginning of the twentieth century:

> "A thick veil made of cotton material beautifully worked all over in a pattern of drawn thread work, is worn down over the face, or thrown back over the cap or hat. Some women were very particular to keep their veils down, but I always suspected that it was the plain ones who were so modest, while the pretty ones did not want to hide their charms" (Macartney 1985:70-1).

The veil was worn with a thick white coat which was worn over the head with the sleeves hanging down the back (see page 77).

Nowadays married women and brides (see Chapter 10) in some areas of Turkestan still wear long lengths of materials over their heads and faces. In the case of married women these veils take the form of a piece of patterned material. Sometimes they are part of the mantle covering the head, on other occasions they are a separate piece of cloth. In addition, some veils have a grid for seeing through, but this is not always the case.

Tied Face Veils

Tied face-veils are another form of face veil being worn by women in the North Africa and the Near East. This type of veil can be divided into three main groups based on their construction and the way in which they are worn, namely, the *burqa`*, *niqab* and *batalu*.

Burqa`

There are two forms of *burqa`* (also spelt *burqu`*, *burko*). The first is made from a single length of material which is used to cover the nose and lower half of the face. It is normally tied with a cord which passes over the ears and is fastened at the back of the head. The second form of *burqa`* is made from two pieces of material, one of which forms a headband (*`isaba*), while the other covers the face, apart from the eyes. Normally there is a link of some kind between the headband and veil at the two sides and in the middle (over the bridge of the nose). The *burqa`* is kept in place with two ties that are fastened at the back of the head, or with one continuous loop of material.

Both types of *burqa`* are now worn by a wide variety of mainly nomadic people throughout northern Arabia, Syria, Jordan, Israel and Egypt.

A simple burqa`

One of the simplest forms of *burqa`* is made out of one piece of material and a cord to tie it around the head. Normally this type of *burqa`* is used to cover the nose and lower half of the face.

One of the earliest depictions of women wearing this type of veil can be found in a manuscript of the *Annals of al-Tabari* which dates to the late thirteenth century (fig. 57; Freer Gallery of Art, Washington, MS.30.21). In this particular example, three women are shown wearing *burqa`s* which are covered by all-enveloping chadors. The veils cover their noses, mouths and chins.

In a poem by Nizami of Ganjeh (AD 1115-1202) called *Iskandarnameh* (written AD 1200), the poet describes a fictitious journey of Iskandar (Alexander the Great) through Khifchak in western Turkistan. According to Nizami, Iskander was astonished to see that the women of Khifchak were unveiled and remonstrated with the local elders. In order to shame the women of Khifchak he set up a statue of a veiled woman, and as a result of his actions veiling was introduced to Turkistan:

In this splendour-place, a bride of new regulation
made of hard [black] stone, he set up on the road.
On it, a sheet [a veil] of white marble,
Like the leaf of the lily on the head of the musk-willow.
Every woman who used to look at its modesty
Used, through its shame [its being ashamed], to
become face-concealed;
Used, through shame [of herself], to lower the veil on
her face;
The cheek concealed and the face hidden.
The Kifchak woman bound her face from that day.
(Nizami 1881, v. 54-58)

A later Persian illustration to the above poem depicts two women wearing white chadors (outerwraps) but no face veil (fig. 58).[32] After looking at the veiled statue, who was wearing a black *chador* with black *burqa`*, one of the shamed women pulls her *chador* over her face.

Nowadays, this type of face veil can be found in many regions of North Africa and the Near East. In present-day Tunisia, many women wear a large outerwrap called a *haik* (see Chapter 5), with a small face veil (fig. 59). The veil is usually made out of a light weight piece of material and is fastened to the head with two ties. The lower half of the veil is often slightly oval in shape and decorated with lace.

The Iranian picheh

The basic 'modesty' garment traditionally worn in Persia is the *chador*, a semi-circular piece of material worn over the head and allowed to drape to the floor. According to the costume historian, J. Scarce, by the thirteenth century AD, the chador was worn with a *burqa`*, but by the fifteenth century, a second form of veiling had been developed, namely, a black horsehair face veil or mask called a *picheh* (Scarce 1975:6). This form of veil is fastened to the head with two ties and can thus also be classified as a *burqa`*.

The use of the *picheh* was noted in Tabriz by Ruy Gonzales de Clavijo, the Castillian ambassador to Timur between AD 1403-1406: "These women go about, covered all over with a white sheet, with a net made of black horse hair before their eyes" (Clavijo 1859, V, 89). In AD 1471 Caterino Zeno, the Venetian ambassador to Uzun Hasan Khan wrote: "they cover their faces with nets woven of horsehair, so thick that they can easily see others, but cannot be seen by them" (Zeno 1873:13).

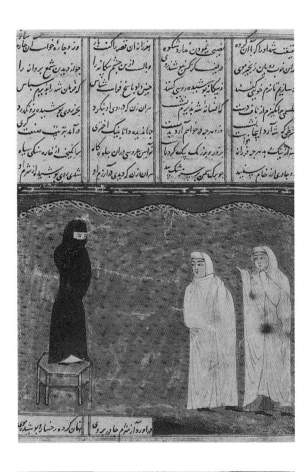

Figure 58. A Persian story about a statue of a veiled woman set up by Alexander the Great (O. Vet. 82; courtesy of University Library of Uppsala, Sweden).

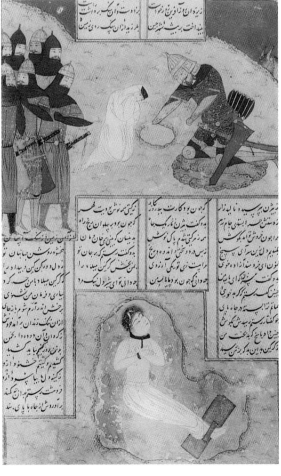

Figure 60. Bizhan rescuing Rustam from a pit (MS Ouseley Add. 176, fol. 186r; courtesy of the Bodleian Library, Oxford).

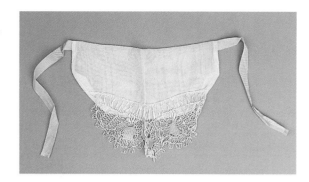

Figure 59. A Tunisian veil (private collection; photo. by B. Grishaaver).

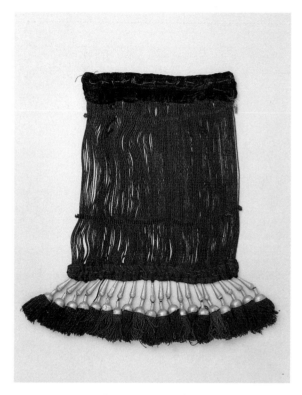

Figure 63. A face veil (shamena) made from cords and weighted with silver ornaments (RMV 5000-165; photo. by B. Grishaaver).

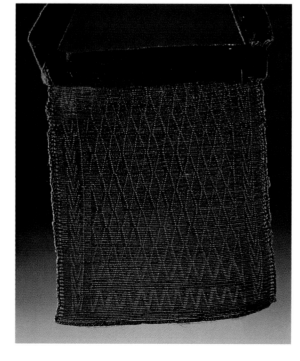

Figure 61. A 19th century example of a horsehair veil from Iran (pecheh 41291; courtesy of the Volksmuseum, Rotterdam).

The horsehair mask can also be seen in a medieval miniature of Bizhan rescuing Rustam from the well (fig. 60).[33] In this example, Bizhan is wearing a white, all-enveloping chador with a small black *picheh*. The veil is represented as having been turned back, away from Bizhan's face. Whether this depiction of her veil should be seen as an artistic convention to treat an awkward piece of clothing or because the artist was trying to give a sense of the urgency in the situation is not clear.

The use of this type of veil continued well into the nineteenth and early twentieth centuries. It is not clear exactly when it ceased to be worn, but it is likely that this occurred following an edict from 1936 by the then Shah which banned the use of veils (see Chapter 10).

The Turkish peche

During the nineteenth century a *burqa*`-type veil called a *peche* or *petçe* was worn by Turkish women living outside of Istanbul. This type of veil was made out of a stiff black mesh (fig. 62a-b; Tuglaci 1985:86).

The form of the veil, as well as method of construction is very similar to the Iranian *picheh*. In addition, the similarity of the two words, peche and picheh, indicates that they are of the same origin. Given the long history of the Iranian version, it would seem likely that the Turkish *peche* was an adaptation of the Persian form.

The Turkestan shämenä

Another type of *burqa*` worn in Turkestan and northern Afghanistan, namely, is the beaded veil (*shämenjä*).[34] This form of veil is made up of an elaborate silver and coral head band which covers the forehead. Various forms of beads are hung from the band in order to form the veil (fig. 63). The strings can vary in length from ten to fifteen centimetres to one which completely covers the face and neck. In the case of the longer versions they are usually lines of weaving across the width of the beads in order to keep the stands of beads in place. The beads may be black in colour or a mixture of large and small black and coloured beads. This sort of veil is usually worn by newly married women.

Two-piece burqa`

As noted above, a *burqa*` can often be made up of two pieces of material, one used as a head band, while the other covers the face.

One of the earliest surviving examples of a two-piece *burqa*` comes from the Egyptian site of Quseir al-Qadim (Eastwood 1983). It was excavated in a Mamluk rubbish level which was dated by the excavators to about AD 1250-1350. The veil is made from two pieces of white linen (fig. 64). The forehead band was hemmed along all four edges, while the lower piece was only stitched along the tip and for about nine centimetres down each of the long sides. A small corded tuck was stitched down the centre of the forehead piece and over the nose

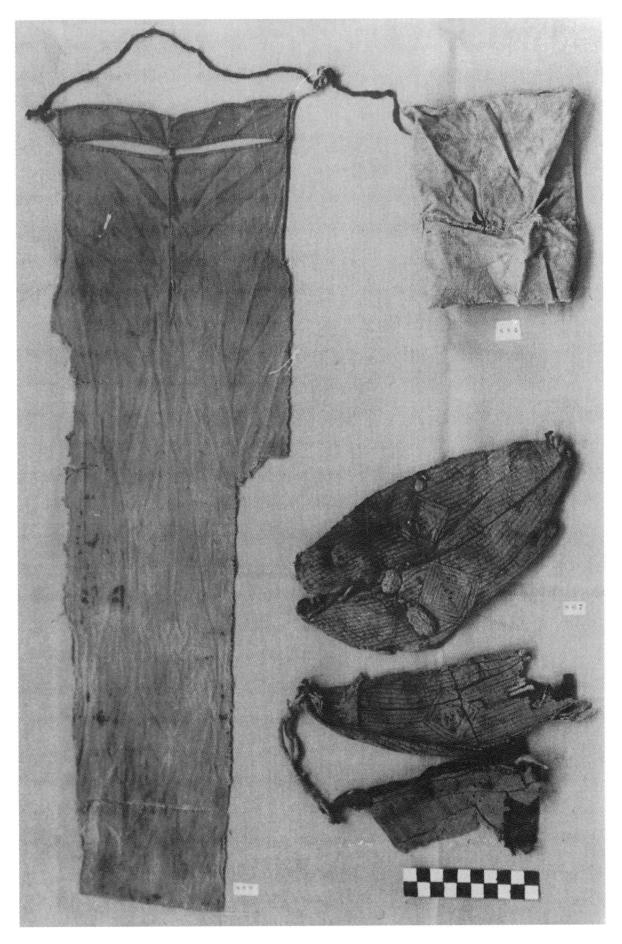

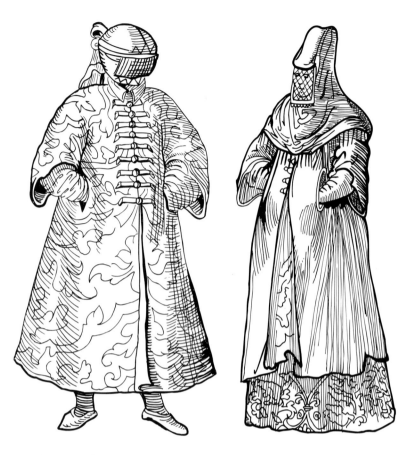

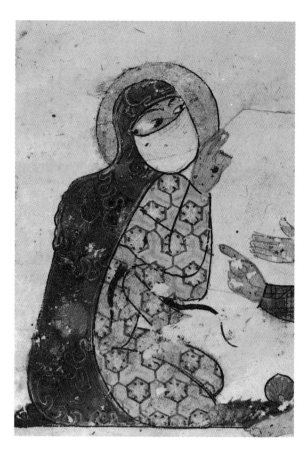

region. This had the effect of producing a ridge along the bridge of the nose, so fitting the veil to the face. At the join between the two sections there was a cord wrapped with a linen thread. The veil was secured by a single, plaited linen cord which was slipped over the head.

Representations of women wearing this type of veil can be found in a number of contemporary illustrations, for example, in a thirteenth century manuscript of Matari's *Maqamat*, which depicts Abu Zaid and his wife before the Cadi of Taliz (British Library, OR 9718; fig. 65). The woman is wearing a long checked *izar* (see Chapter XXX) or outerwrap with a coloured veil which fits closely over her face. A similar veil was depicted in the thirteenth century work called the *Dacwat al-Atibba* by Ibn Bultan. In this case a woman is shown wearing a white *izar*, with a short gown (*thaub*), black boots (*khuff*) and a close fitting white *burqa`* (fig. 66).

During the early nineteenth century, Cairene women wore a two-piece *burqa`* made from a thin crepe-like material, in either cotton or wool (fig. 67). A description of this veil is given by the Arabist E.W. Lane, who was living in Egypt at that time:

"Next is put on the "burko", or face-veil, which is a long strip of white muslin, concealing the whole face except the eyes, and reaching nearly to the feet. It is suspended at the top by a narrow band, which passes up the forehead, and which is sewed, as are also the two upper corners of the veil, to a band that is tied round the head" (Lane 1895:53)

A second form of "burko" noted by Lane was worn by lower class women (fig. 68):

"a burko' of a kind of coarse black crape ... the upper part of the burko is often ornamented with false pearls, small gold coins, and other little flat ornaments of the same metal (called "bark"); sometimes with a coral bead, and a gold coin beneath; also with small coins of base silver; and more commonly with a pair of chain tassels, of brass or silver (called "'oyoon"), attached to the corners" (Lane 1895:55)

Lane also noted that the *burqa`* and shoes were most common in Cairo and were worn by women throughout Lower Egypt. However, in Upper Egypt, the *burqa`* was seldom seen, and "shoes are scarcely less common" (Lane 1895:57).

By the end of the nineteenth century the metal ornaments between the forehead tape and the main section of the veil had become a decorated copper or brass tube which contained an amulet in the form of a coin or inscribed object (fig. 69). Similar metal tubes are still attached to the face veils worn by nomadic women in the Sinai to this day.

Modern nomadic women in many regions of Saudi Arabia also wear various forms of two-piece *burqa`* (Stillman 1981:104). The simplest versions are made out of a single piece of black cotton or rayon which is folded in half to make a double layer of material over the face (figs. 70 and 71). A headband (sometimes made out of

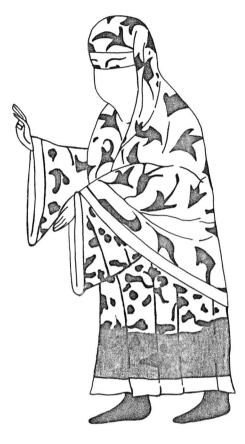

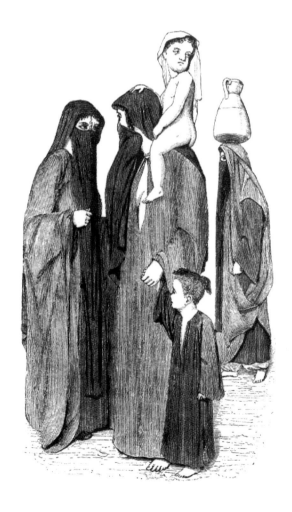

Figure 66.
*Medieval figure of
an Egyptian woman
wearing a face veil
under a long
outerwrap (from the
Da`wat al-atibba',
by Ibn Bultan).*

Figure 67.
*A Cairene woman
wearing a long face
veil (burqa`; after
Lane 1895:53).*

Figure 68.
*A lower class
Cairene woman
wearing a face veil
(burqa`; after Lane
1895:56).*

satin ribbon) is sewn in three places along the upper edge in order to form eye slits.

The Egyptian and Saudi *burqa*`s described above are characterised by their use of a minimum amount of decoration. In Palestine, however, the two-piece *burqa*` worn by married, nomadic women has a very different appearance. It is regarded as a facial decoration rather than a disguise (Weir 1989:188-91). This form of *burqa*` is made up of a band which is normally embroidered or made from a patterned material (fig. 72). The band is fastened around the forehead, while the lower section of the *burqa*` is often ornamented using a mixture of coral, beads, embroidery and coins (both real and fake). In some cases, the *burqa*` is literally encrusted with coins which are sewn onto two embroidered cloth bases. In such cases two rows of coins are suspended from each side of the central nose section and then looped up at the sides (see fig. 1).

Niqab

Another type of face veil worn in many Arabian countries is the *niqab*. It is a single length of material which has eye holes cut out of it. This type of veil is often referred to by the term *burqa*`, although technically this is incorrect.

One of the earliest known examples of a *niqab* comes from the Egyptian site of Quseir al-Qadim, which also produced the earliest known example of a two-piece *burqa*` (see above; fig. 74). The *niqab* veil was found in the rubbish layers dating between AD 1250-1350. It was made out of a single piece of cotton. Unlike the *burqa*` from the same site, however, the material was decorated

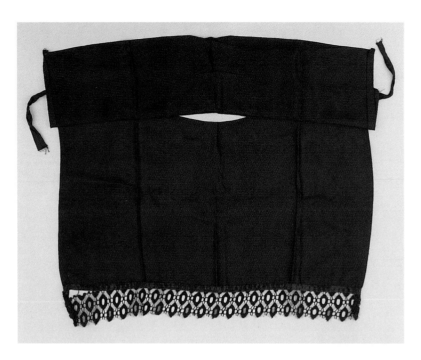

with a blue and white checked design. The eye holes were made from a long slit which was neatened with stitching. The bridge over the nose was made from a bound linen cord. Like the *burqa`* from Quseir al-Qadim, a tuck was sewn down part of the lower section in order to fit it more closely to the face.

The remains of a *niqab*-style veil were also found at the Nubian site of Qasr Ibrim. It dates slightly later than the Quseir example (Eastwood 1983:35-6). The Ibrim veil was made from a single piece of crimson silk which was cut across its width to produce the eye-slit (fig. 74). All of the edges of the veil were strengthened and neatened by a narrow dark brown wool braid. In the centre of the veil there was a knot from which a small iron ring with a leather plait was probably attached. Hanging from the plait were five blue beads which would have hung down over the nose.

Modern nomadic women in central and eastern regions of Saudi Arabia also wear various forms of *niqab* (locally called *burqa`s*; Stillman 1981:104). These veils

Figure 70. Face veil (burqa`) from Saudi Arabia (private collection; photo. by B. Grishaaver).

Figure 69. Two, late 19th century face veils (burqa`), from Cairo (RMV 1029-4,5; photo. by B. Grishaaver).

Figure 71. Figure wearing a complete outdoor outfit from Saudi Arabia (private collection; photo. by B. Grishaaver).

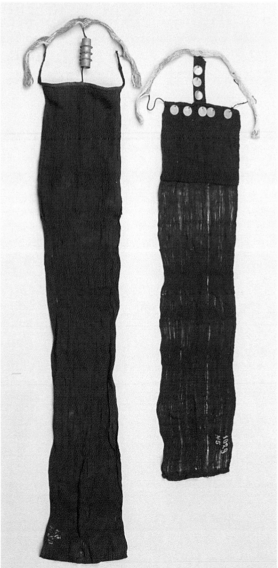

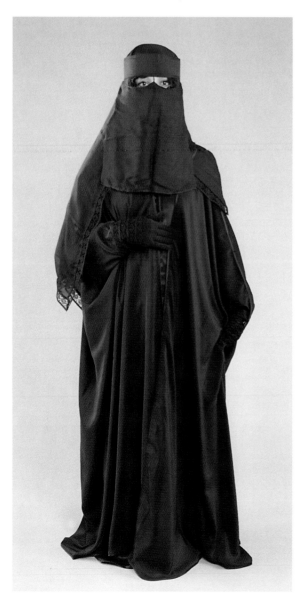

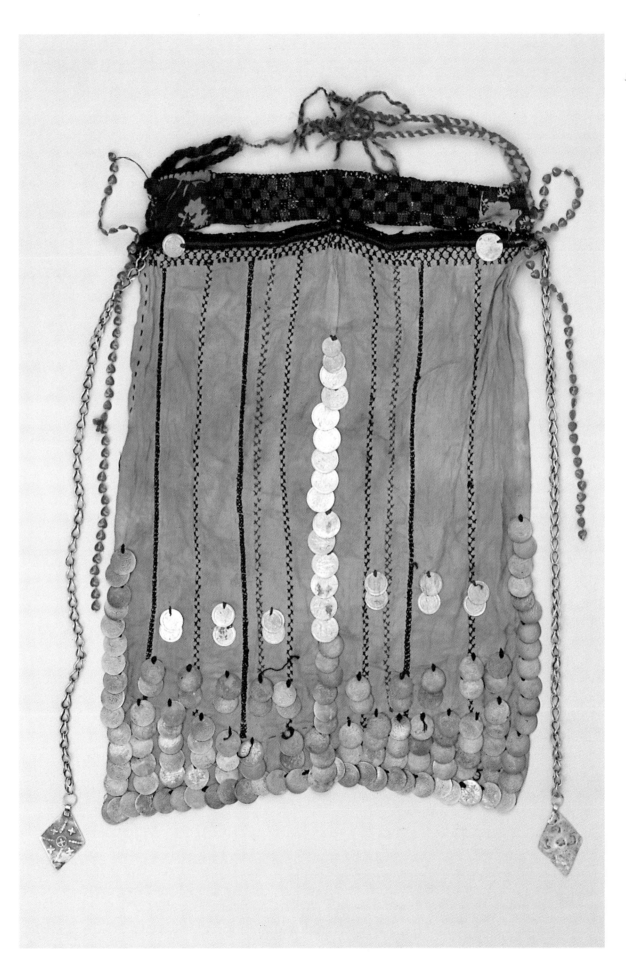

Figure 72.
*A nomadic woman's
face veil from North
Sinai (private
collection; photo. by
B. Grishaaver).*

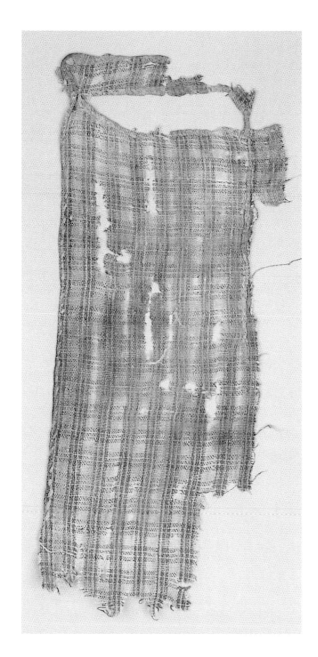

Figure 73. *A face veil (niqab) from the Egyptian site of Quseir al-Qadim (c. 1300 AD; courtesy of the Oriental Institute, Chicago University).*

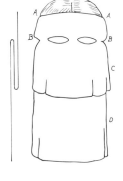

Figure 76. *An Arabian face veil worn by some nomadic women (niqab; after Dickinson 1949:154-5).*

Figure 74. *A face veil niqab) from the Egyptian site of Qasr Ibrim (c. 15th c. AD; courtesy of the Egypt Exploration Society, London).*

are normally made out of a single piece of cloth which is folded in half in order to produce a double thickness of material. The length of such veils may vary from thirty centimetres to nearly one metre long. The slits for the eyes are cut out and may vary quite considerably in size.

The simple versions of this veil are usually made out of black cloth, although more elaborate versions may be made from blue or red material. Other versions are made of stiff heavy leather stained with ground henna. This sometimes comes off on the skin of the wearer giving her face a reddish hue.

The more elaborate versions are decorated with a variety of different substances including appliqued braids which outline the sides and eye openings. Sometimes coins are attached down the centre of the veil along the nose line. In addition, mother-of-pearl buttons, metallic threads, fringes made of metal beads and other forms of tassels may be used as decoration (fig. 75a-c).

A form of *niqab* from Arabia appears to have been noted by the English traveller H.R.P. Dickson, who travelled to this part of the world during the early twentieth century (Dickson 1949:154-5). He describes a veil, which he calls a *burqa`*, worn by nomadic women from various eastern and central Arabian tribes.[35] The veil was made out of a length of coarse, black silk (*jezz*) which had slits cut into it for the eyes. Thus it is of a *niqab* rather than *burqa`* construction (fig. 76). This form of veil was kept in place with three cords, one of which was tied around the forehead, the second was tied at the temples, while the third thread was tied around the neck. Part of the material was folded upwards making a denser veil around the lower half of the face and neck.

Batalu

Yet another form of face veil, related to the *niqab* type of veil is the *batalu*. this veil is known from lands on both sides of the Persian Gulf. Basically, the *batalu* is made from a single piece of material. It has a tube down the middle front, which shapes the garment so that it fits the contours of the face (fig. 77).[36] Some form of stiffening is usually placed down the middle of the veil to create a 'nose' (see below). The veil (many people describe this item as a mask, the so-called 'black masks') is kept in place either by a long length of cord which passes over the top of the head, or by two shorter lengths which are hooked over the ears. Normally, a *batalu* is made out of a thick black mercerised cotton or a shiny silk.

This type of garment was noted by Dickson as being worn by women on the island of Failaka and those of the 'Ajam tribe of eastern Arabia (Dickson 1949:155). It is currently worn by women in what is now Oman and the eastern United Arabic Emirates (UAE). There it is generally known as a *burqa`*, although technically it is made out of one piece of material with a stiffened nose section.

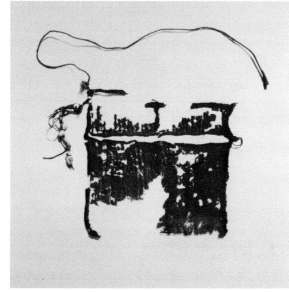

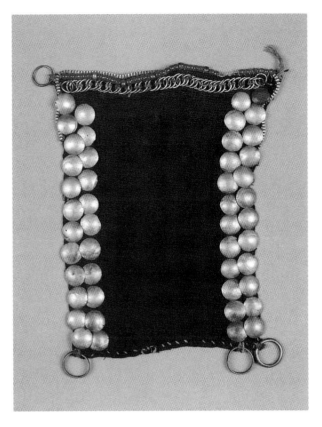 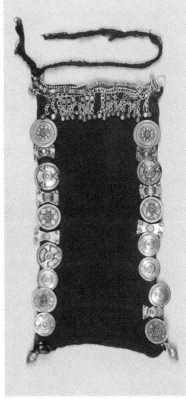 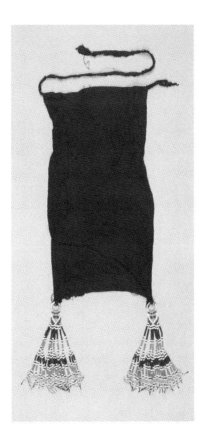

Two different versions of this type of veil are worn in the region.[37] There is a form worn by urbanised women living in and near the city of Sohar and a form worn by nomadic women. The urban version is made from a single, roughly rectangular shape of cloth. The lower angles are transformed into curves, while approximately one half of the contents are cut away to form two eye holes. The inner contours of the lower part are heart shaped, the upper part straight, while the sides slant inwards. The height of the nose corresponds to the width of the headband. The whole length of the *batalu* corresponds to the width of the woman's face, plus about three centimetres. According to Wilken, the nose section is made out of a stiff stay (about three centimetres wide, made of wood or bone) which runs the whole breadth of the veil (about 20.0 cm).

The veil is kept in place by four strings. Two are attached at a level slightly above the ears, while the other two are attached below the eyes. The strings are tied together at the back of the head, in a running-noose knot on top of the inner head scarf (*leeso*; Wikan 1982:89).

The colour of the 'black masks' is produced from indigo which leaves a bluish stain on the faces of the wearer. A gold coloured *batalu* or one decorated with gold rings was used on special occasions.

Similar veils are worn by urban women in the eastern parts of the United Arabic Emirates. Patricia Holton, who regularly visited this region in the 1980's, described this type of veil being worn by women from the Dubai region as a "stiff, black burnished gold canvas veil" and later as "black harlequin masks" (Holton 1991:13).

The nomadic version of the above type of veil is much simpler. It is made out of a single piece of cloth which covers the whole face, with the exception of slits cut into the material for the eyes (fig. 78). Down the middle of the veil there is usually a 'nose' which is again padded in order to produce a rigid effect. Holton described a woman wearing such a veil:

"It covered her face from the top of her forehead to the bottom of her chin. It was made of a dark blue, rough, woven material and left only two small oval slits for the eyes" (Holton 1991:111).

Both forms of the *batalu* are also worn in remote areas of southern Iran (Wikan 1982:107-8). There is a strong trade link between Iran and this region of the Arabian peninsular which can be traced back for many hundred of years. In addition, following the attempts by the Shah of Persia in the 1930's to westernize the country (see Chapter 10), many Persians fled to what is now Qatar, Oman and the Emirates. It should come as no surprise, therefore, to find these influences are reflected in the garments people from this region wear.

Veils with Grids

This type of veil is very similar to the face-panels described earlier in this chapter. However, instead of being draped over the face and kept in place by friction, they are deliberately tied to the head in a manner similar to the *burqa`*, *niqab* and *batalu*.

Figure 75a-c. Group of face veils (niqabs) from northern Yemen (modern; 2489.64b, 4991.117, 451.2; courtesy of the Tropenmuseum, Amsterdam).

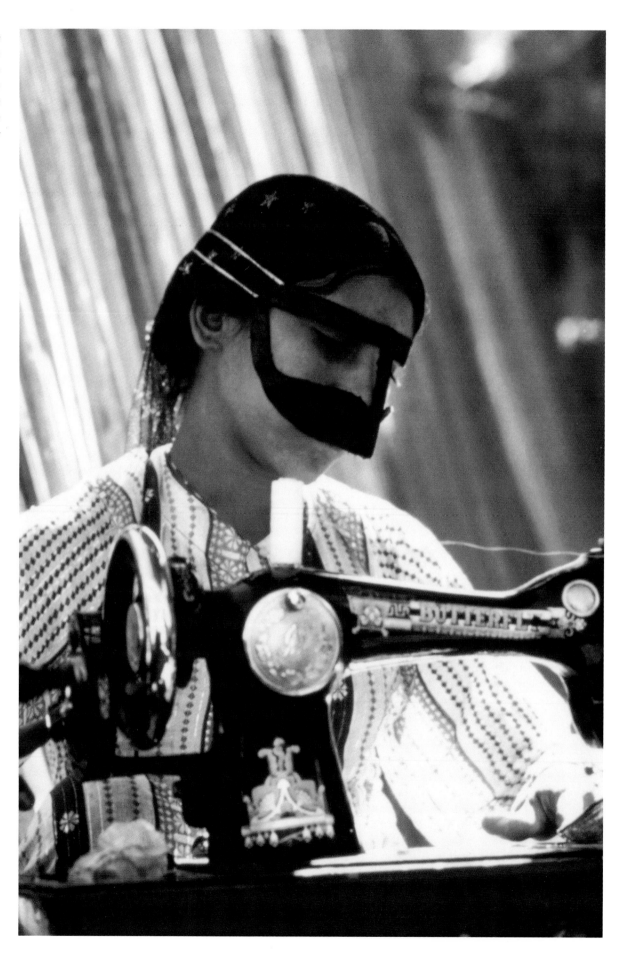

Figure 77. *A face veil (batalu) worn by urban women from Oman (photo by L. Abercrombie courtesy of the National Geographic Image Collection).*

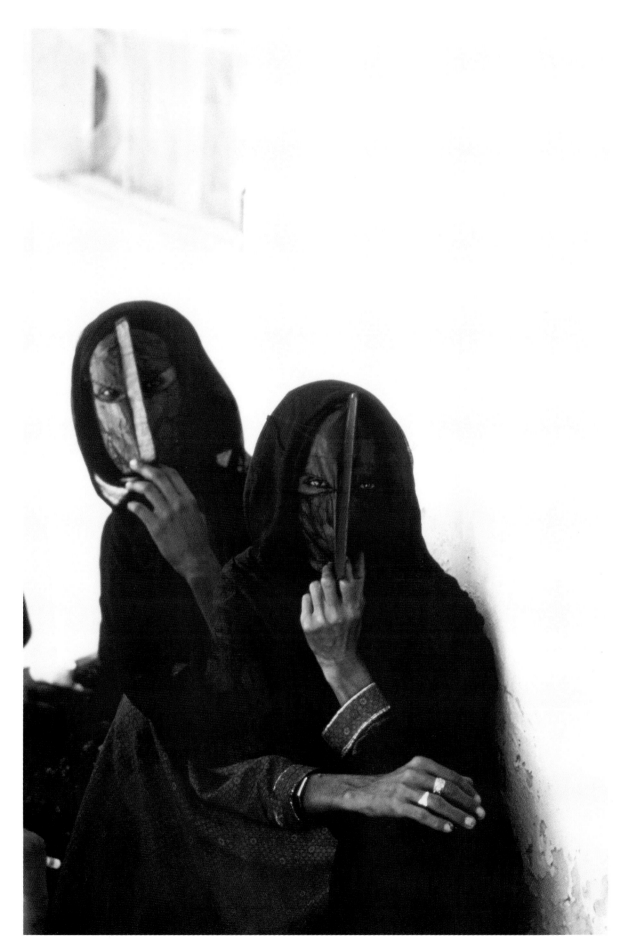

Figure 78. *A face veil (batalu) worn by nomadic women from Oman (photo by L. Abercrombie courtesy of the National Geographic Image Collection).*

Figure 79. A late 19th century face veil (ru-band) from Persia (RMV 5389-33; photo. by B. Grishaaver).

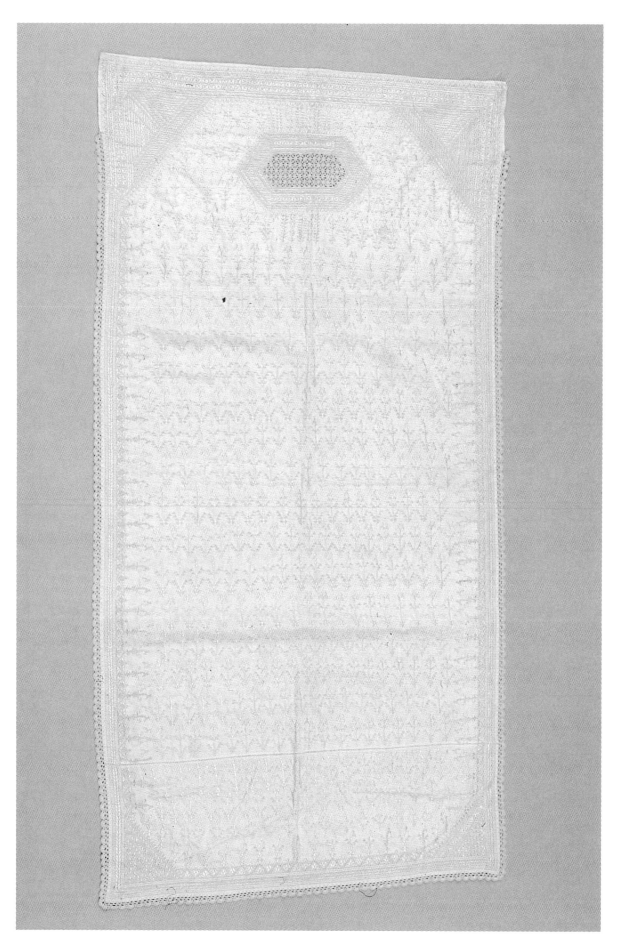

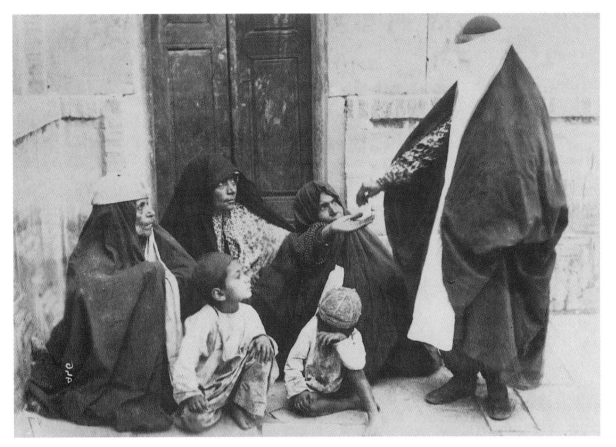

Figure 80.
A Persian woman
wearing a dark
outerwrap (chador)
and face veil
(ru-band; Hotz
Collection 16:98;
c. 1885; courtesy
of the Library, the
University of Leiden).

The wearing of the *pecheh* with the *chador* (see the next chapter) by Iranian women has already been noted. In addition to this form of veil, by the seventeenth century a new form of veiling seems to have been introduced called a *ru-band* (Scarce 1975:7). The veil takes the form of a rectangular piece of white fabric with either a slit or grid for the eyes (fig. 79). The veil was worn over the *chador* and could be flipped back over the head when the woman wished to reveal herself.

Sir John Chardin, writing in the late seventeenth century, described the outdoor dress of a Persian lady:

"The third [veil = the *chador*], is the White Veil, which covers all the Body; And the fourth is a sort of Handkerchief [*ru-band*], which goes over the Face, and is fasten'd to the Temples. This Handkerchief or Vail, has a sort of Net-work, like old Point, or Lace, for them to see through" (Chardin 1927:215-6)

The use of the *ru-band* continued well into the nineteenth century (fig. 80). The *ru-band* with its mesh is being described in the following account by Dr. Willis, who was writing about his life in Persia between 1866 and 1881:

"The outdoor costume of the Persian woman is quite another thing; enveloped in a huge blue sheet, with a yard of linen as a veil, perforated for two inches square with minute holes, the feet thrust into two huge bags of coloured stuff, a wife is perfectly unrecognisable, even by her husband, when out of doors" (Willis 1891:325).

Nowadays most women in Iran wear a black version of the chador which covers all of the body, including the hands, while leaving the face uncovered.

Notes:

25 Briggs 1960:151; Cupers 1994:132-3.
26 Bodleian Library, Oxford, MS Bodl. Or 430.fol.90r.
27 Tuglaci 1984:83; Scarce 1987:779, 85.
28 Wien Graphische Sammlung Albertina 1957/350-1-10.
29 The information about Yemeni veils is based on information provided by Prof. R. Kruk, Leiden University; Makhlouf 1979:30-1; Mundy 1983:535-6; von Bruck 1987:396.
30 According to Prof. Kruk, the *sitara* can also be worn over the *qarqush*.
31 It is possible that the *sharshaf* was introduced into northern Yemen by the Turks. According to Mundy it only became common in Yemen after 1962 (Mundy 1983:539).
32 AD 1439; Royal University Library, Upsala, O.Vet.82.fol327b.
33 Bodlean Library, Oxford MS Ouseley Add 176 fol 186r. Scarce 1987:144, pl. 99.
34 Jowzjan 1977:146, fig. 4; Kalter 1984, pl. III.114.
35 Such as the Utair, Harb, 'Utaiba, Sbei, Rashaida, Bani Khalid, Beni Hajiir and 'Awazim, as well as the Murra and Manasir; Dickson 1949:154-5.
36 Wikan 1982:88-91; Holton 1991, figs. p. 256, 254; fig. 35.
37 The following description is based on Wikan 1982:88-91; Dickson 1949:154-5; Holton 1991, figs. p. 246, 254.

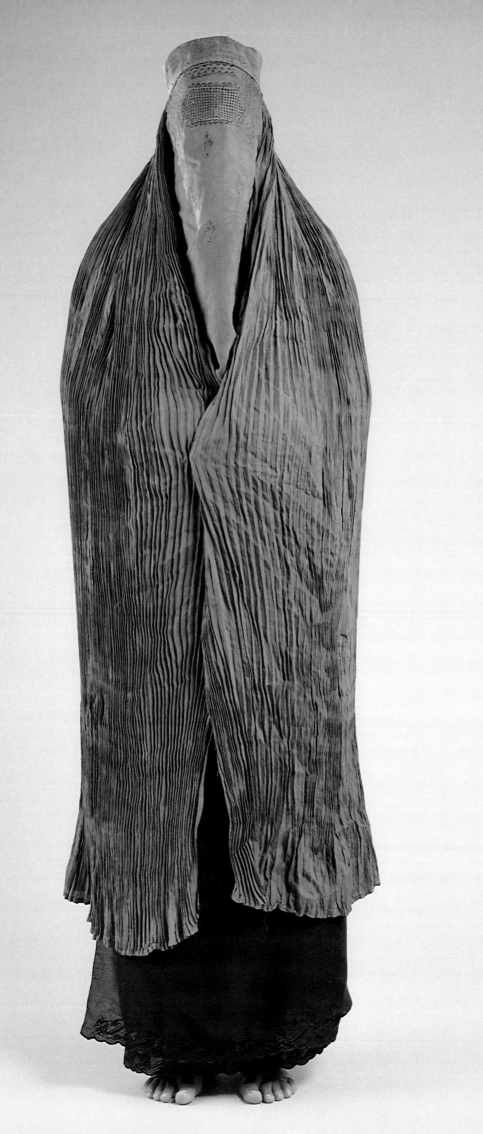

Chapter 5

Outerwraps and garment veils

This chapter deals with some of the types of outerwraps worn by North African and Near Eastern women when out-of-doors. An outerwrap should not be confused with a mantle, such as the Spanish *mantilla*. Although both garments are made from large lengths of cloth, a mantle is usually draped loosely over the head and allowed to hang down over the wearer.[38] Normally there is no intention of hiding specific parts of the body. An outerwrap on the other hand, is usually close fitting around the head, neck and upper body and has the express intention of concealing and disguising these regions. Outerwraps are worn by draping or wrapping the material around the person. Sometimes pins and brooches are used to fasten the material together, but this is not widespread.

In addition to outerwraps, attention will also be focused on the so-called garment veils, which are items of apparel, usually a coat of some kind, which are deliberately placed over the head and hang down over the body.

Outerwraps

There are various ways of wearing an outerwrap. They may be draped over the body, wrapped around it, or fastened with ties, pins or tucks. In the following section, various types of outerwraps will be described, including the *haik* from Morocco, the *sari* from India and the *melaya* from Egypt.

The Moroccan izar/Algerian huik

Women from the Maghreb (Morocco, Algeria, Tunisia), wear an outerwrap called the *izar* in Morocco and the *haik* in Algeria.[39] The *izar/huik* is not strictly speaking an outer garment, as it is not worn over a dress or trousers. However, it is worn in such a way that the body, and more especially the head, can be totally covered when outside the house.

There are various methods for wrapping the *izar/huik* around the body. The following description is based on the instruction given by E. Rackow, *Beiträge zur Kenntnis der materiellen Kultur Norwest-Marokkos* (1958).[40] It is based on the *izars* worn by urban women living in the Hlot region of Morocco. Their *izar* is made from two pieces of material about 4.50 metres long, which are sewn together (fig. 81). Part of the material is folded over. Then about 40 cm is placed over the right shoulder and the rest is carried around the back (to about the left elbow), about 50 cm of the material is then turned over, brought back towards the chest and fastened on the left shoulder. The folded material is subsequently brought across the chest and fastened with a pin on the right shoulder. The folded material creates a sort of bib across the chest (Rackow 1958, taf. LX-LXII).

The bulk of the material is then passed over the head. A pinch of cloth is taken from about 50 cm down the outer edge and fastened to the left shoulder, either using the existing pin or a new one. The excess material is

Figure 92. A modern Afghan chadri (private collection; photo. by B. Grishaaver).

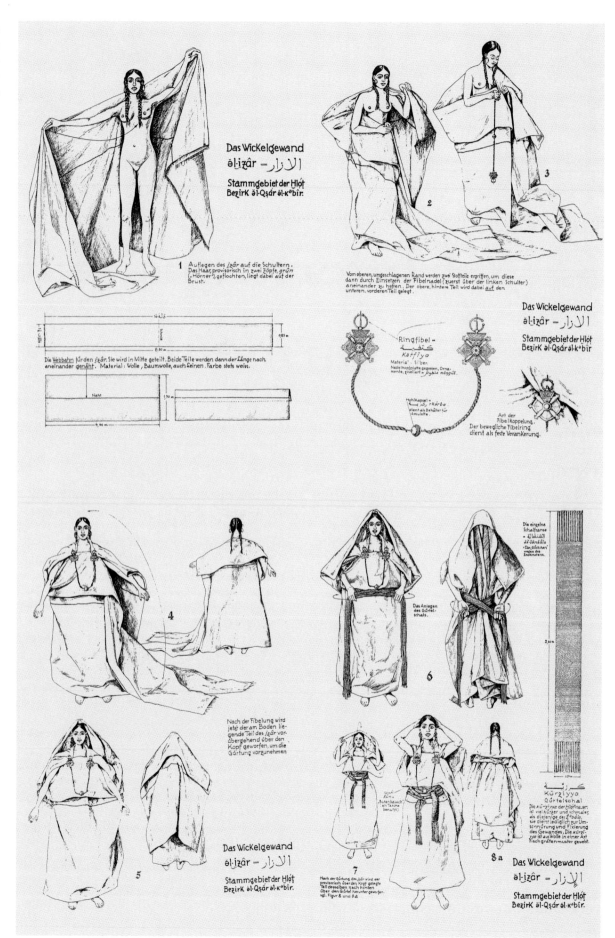

brought forward and used to hide the arms, hands and front of the body.

In Morocco a belt (as-sansala) is tied several times around the waist to fasten the garment (Rackow 1958, taf. LXII). Such a belt is not normally worn with this garment in Algeria.

The modern Tunisian huik

The *huik (haik)* which is currently for sale in various Tunesian cities is different from the Algerian *huik*. It is made from a large semi-circular piece of light-weight material and usually has a pale colour (white, cream, yellow). The *huik* is placed over the woman's head and allowed to cover the body down to the calf or ankles (fig. 82). It is normally worn with a small *burqa`* type mask (see page 52).

The Indian sari

One of the most elegant wrap-around garments currently worn, is the Indian *sari*. Strictly speaking it is not an outer garment, since it is not worn over a dress, gown or trousers, nor at first sight does it appear to be an Islamically inspired garment. However, the use of the *sari* derives from the Mogul period in Indian history, and has certain characteristics in common with outerwraps from Southwest Asia.2

In early Indian literature there are no direct references to women's clothing. Instead there are allusions to the *vasah antaram* (undergarment) and the *paridhanam* (upper garment; Joshi 1992:218). Both of these garments were worn while a woman was in public. In addition, upper class women probably also wore the *drapi* or mantle on special occasions.

Following the eleventh century, with an increasing number of invaders and others migrating to India, a number of new garments were introduced, notably the *kancuki* (bodice); the *choli*, a tight-fitting half-sleeved dress; the *dukul* or *dupatta*, which is a scarf used to cover the head and shoulders and a similar garment called a *orhni* which was used to cover the breasts, back, shoulders and head. It was during this period that women were advised to dress more modestly.[41]

During the sixteenth century most Hindu women in northern India wore a half-sleeved bodice (*choli*), an ankle length skirt (*ghagra*), and a headscarf (also called an *orhni*). After about 1790 the *orhni* had become a much larger garment that covered much of the body, eventually including the head. Passing over the breasts, part of the garment was tucked in at the waist, while the rest of the material ended in graceful folds from the navel down to the ankle.

At the beginning of the nineteenth century, the *ohrni* had developed into what we now call a *sari*. It is currently being worn throughout the whole of northern India, from Rajasthan in the west to Bengal in the east and from the Punjab hills to Bombay in the south (fig. 83).

The basic, modern sari can vary in length from 5.0 m to 8.2 m, depending upon the fashion and the style of wearing. All styles of wearing a *sari*, however, begin in the same manner, namely one end of the material is placed in front and tucked in to a petticoat of some kind, then the *sari* is drawn around the waist and tucked into the petticoat. At this point draping and folding plays an important role as the material is pleated, tucked in and wrapped around the body.

The end of the Gujarati-style *sari* is normally allowed to hang loose and is thrown over the right shoulder so that the decorated border is displayed at the front. Married women wearing the Bengali-style of *sari*, on the other hand, wear the end over their heads, while in the Uttar Pradesh form the *sari* goes over the head with the decorative end finishing at the front.

With all of these styles, however, should the need arise the face can be concealed by passing the end section of the *sari* over the head. Sometimes it is held across the face with the hand, or held in place with the teeth.

The Egyptian Miláyeh

There is a long Egyptian tradition of wearing outerwraps. Their use seems to have been introduced by the Greeks. Basically the outerwrap worn in Egypt consists of a long length of material (sometimes made from two widths of cloth sewn together), which was placed over the head and draped over the body.

During the medieval period the outerwrap was called an *izar*.[42] In Mamluk representations which date to the thirteenth century women are shown wearing a long length of material which is draped over the head and which reaches to the ankles, in a similar manner to the *chador* worn in Iran (see figs. 88 and 155). This garment continued to be worn by high and middle class women well into the nineteenth century. According to E.W. Lane, who was writing about Egyptian life during the 1830's, three types of outerwraps (*miláyeh's*) were commonly used by Egyptian women, namely the *habarah*, *eezár (izar)* and *tarah*.

During the early nineteenth century, wealthy married ladies wore the *habarah*, which, according to Lane, was made out of:

> "two breadths of glossy black silk, each ell-wide and three yards long. These are sewed together, at or near the selvages (according to the height of the person), the seam running horizontally, with respect to the manner in which it is worn. A piece of narrow black ribbon is sewed inside the upper part, about six inches from the edge, to tie round the head. Unmarried ladies wear a habarah of white silk, or a shawl. Some females of the middle classes, who cannot afford to purchase a habarah, wear instead of it an "eezár", which is a piece of white calico, of the same form and size as the former, and is worn in the same manner" (Lane 1895, 53-54).

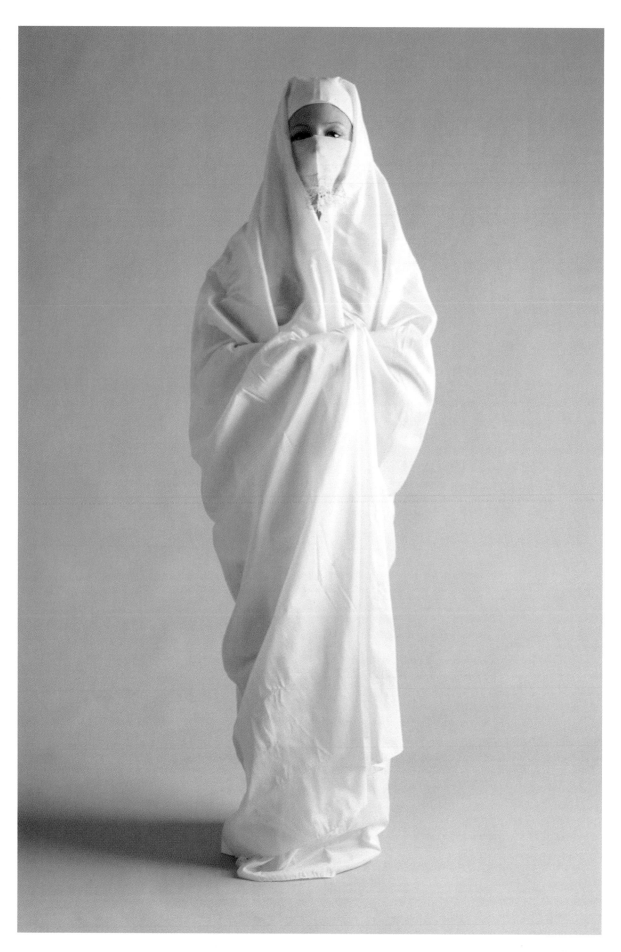

Figure 82.
A Tunisian huik
and veil (modern,
private collection;
photo. by
B. Grishaaver).

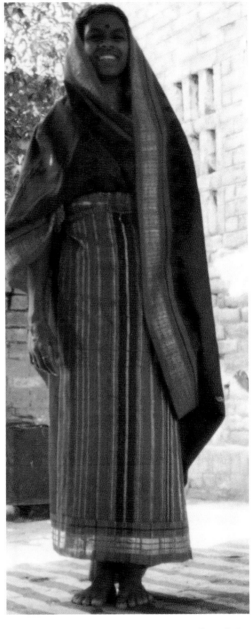

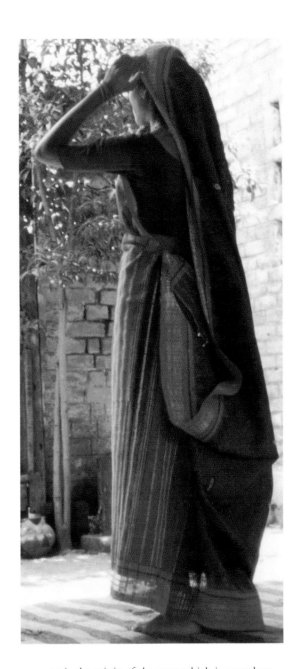

Figure 83.
A modern sari from
India (private
collection; photo. by
B. Grishaaver).

Lane also noted that another variation of the *habarah*, which he called a *miláyeh*, was made out of blue and white check cloth (fig. 84). Again medieval and nineteenth century representations of women wearing such checked garments can be found. This garment has survived in regions of Upper Egypt, especially around Assyut, in the form of the *shugga* (Rugh 1986:36). A wide flowing, floor-length cloak which completely envelops the wearer and "gives the impression of a floating balloon in full motion" (Rugh 1986:36).

During the eighteenth and nineteenth centuries, the *tarah*[45], another type of *miláyeh* was worn by *baladi* or peasant women. It consisted of a large piece of material (usually dark), which was wrapped around the body in various ways (fig. 85). Sometimes it was wrapped several times over the head and then the shoulders. On other occasions it was placed over one shoulder, wrapped around the body and then placed over the head. This

garment is the origin of the wrap which is nowadays called a *miláyeh laff* (Rugh 1986:108-9).

Miláyeh laff literally means "wrapped cloth", and it is draped *sari*-like over a house dress (fig. 86). It is used to cover the hair and body. The ends of the *miláyeh* are tucked under the arms.

Some people regard the *miláyeh laff* as a provocative and it is certainly used in Egyptian films to show *baladi* or peasant girls talking with young men. 'Accidentally', part of the *miláyeh* may slip to show her brightly coloured garments underneath:

"a series of alluring gestures ... walk(ing) coquettishly in a manner that makes her hips seem to roll to the rhythm of her clicking slippers, tinkling bracelets, and the little bursting noise of chewing gum bubbles ... Both glamour and modesty are combined in the bint al-balad's wearing apparel, the melaya liff, which

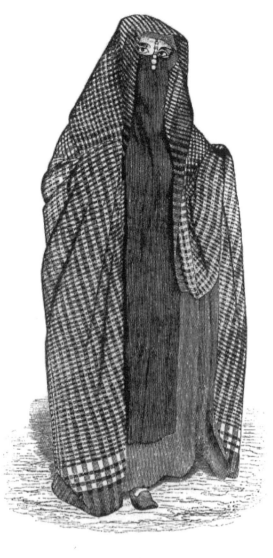

reveals the graceful bodily curves (particularly of the midriff), yet covers what should not be revealed or what is shameful" (el-Massiri 1978:526, 529).

As the use of *galabiyehs*, western clothing and *hijab* or Islamic clothing, becomes more popular in Egypt, the use of the *melaya* and *miláyeh laff* is gradually dying out. Fewer and fewer women are be seen in the streets of cities, including Cairo, wearing this traditional garment.

A garment related to the *miláyeh laff* is still found in Nubia and Sudan, where women wear a garment called a *taub* (fig. 87). This is made up of a long, light-weight length of cloth. Most of the material is wrapped around the body and then the loose end is draped over the head as a form of covering which is placed across the face when necessary.

Body covers

In some cases the outerwrap developed into another form of garment, namely the body screen. This type of garment covers the whole body, from head to ankles, with an all-enveloping piece of material. This development can be seen in eastern Iran and western Afghanistan in the form of the *chadri* or *burqa`*.

The Iranian Chador and the Afghan Chadri

In this form of garment, a large semi-circular piece of cloth is hung and draped over the body, instead of being fastened or wrapped around the person (fig. 88). In Iran, this method of covering the body developed at a very early date into the *chador*. There are various types of *chador*, depending upon whether they are worn in or out of doors.

The use of the *chador* with a face veil *(ru-band)* was described by the nineteenth century English traveller, Dr. Willis:

> "The outdoor costume of the Persian woman is quite another thing; enveloped in a huge blue sheet, with a yard of linen as a veil, perforated for two inches square with minute holes, the feet thrust into two huge bags of coloured stuff, a wife is perfectly unrecognisable, even by her husband, when out of doors" (Willis 1891:325).

Nowadays most women in Iran wear a black version of the *chador* which covers all of the body, except for the face. Some women also wear a black, triangular hood called a *maghneh* under the *chador* in order to make sure that their hair and neck region are totally covered (fig. 89).

The indoor or "prayer" chador

By the mid-Safavid period (ca. AD 1600) women had started to wear a light-weight indoor *chador*. Few representations of this *chador* exist. Nevertheless it survived into the twentieth century as an indoor or prayer *chador* (fig. 90). The religious function of the garment may in fact be the reason why it is not frequently represented. In

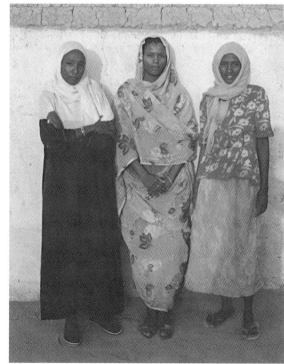

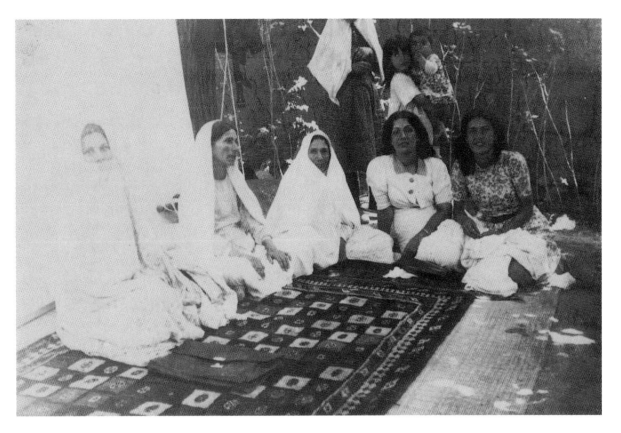

Figure 90.
A group of Iranian
women of the
Shakeri-Hendi
family, one of whom
is wearing an
indoor chador
(courtesy of L.A.F.
Barjesteh van
Waalwijk van
Doorn).

1923, C. Colliver Rice wrote about her experiences in Persia and her observations of how women lived:

> "... the custom is that a cotton prayer chadar is worn over this dress indoors, and for the street an outdoor chadar. These prayer chadars, so called because [they are] worn during the prayer ... [they have] an all-over pattern of flowers or small sprigs" (Rice 1923:160).

The wearing of the prayer *chador* or 'prayer-veil', rather than the all-enveloping *chadri* (see below), is also prevalent in parts of Afghanistan such as Herat (Doubleday 1988:64). Small coins are sometimes placed in the middle of the *chador* so that the lengths of material on either side are balanced helping it to stay in place. As noted by the English visitor, Veronica Doubleday, just before the Russian invasion of Afghanistan, the *chador* was regarded as a more fashionable, and cheaper, alternative to the *chadri* (Doubleday 1988:64): "I had thought I was buying something drab and shapeless, but they [some Afghan friends] made me see that the prayer veil was a highly coveted item of fashion" (Doubleday 1988:64).

The Afghan Chadri

The close proximity of Iran to Afghanistan and what is now Pakistan, has had an influence on regional dress, especially those of women, in these two countries. At some point in the late eighteenth, early nineteenth century the Iranian *chador* and *ru-band* were adopted into Afghan clothing tradition, from where it spread to what was then north-west India (fig. 91).

Lieutenant James Rattray, who was serving with the Second Grenadiers of the Bengal Army at the time, gave a vivid description of the garments worn by women living in the Afghan capital Kabul in the first half of the nineteenth century:

> "... When out of doors, or taking horse exercise, these ladies don an immense white sheet, reaching from the top of the skull-cap to the feet; a long square veil [ru-band] attached by a clasp of gold or jewels to the back of the head, conceals the face, across which is an opening of net-work, to admit light and air. This dress is called a 'Boorkha'. It conceals the whole figure, all outline of which is so entirely lost, that a stranger, on first viewing, a part of these shrouded

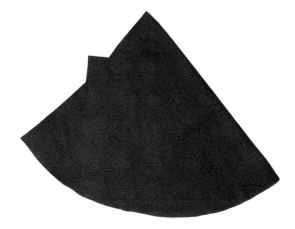

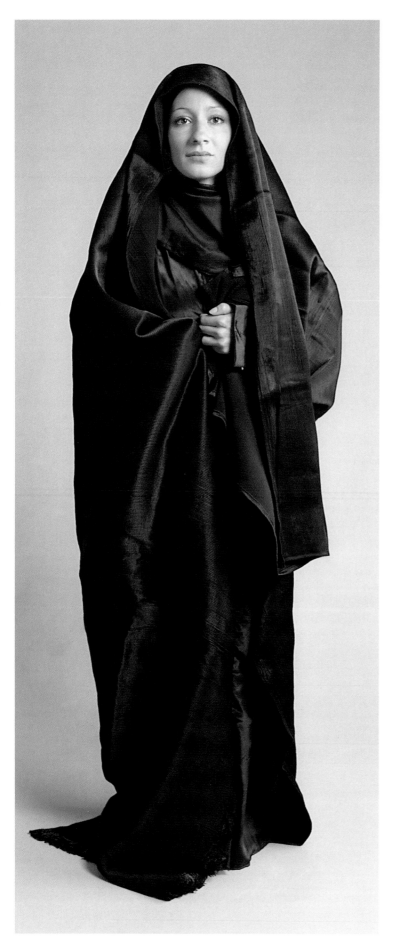
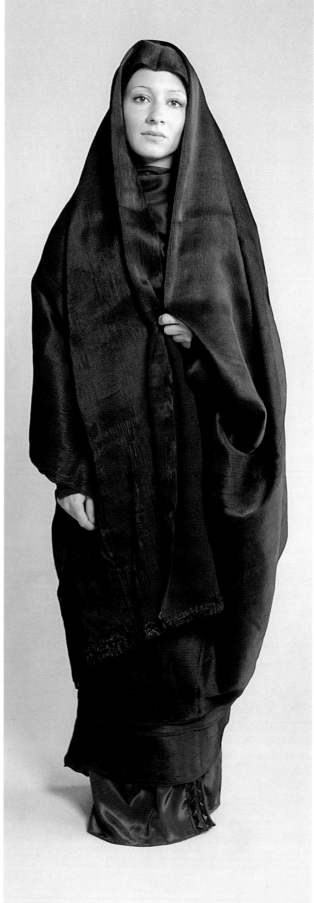

beings flitting about him in the streets, might well be at a loss to guess to what class of creatures they belong" (Rattray 1848:29).

By the end of the nineteenth century a new garment, the *chadri*, had developed which incorporated the *chador* and *ru-band* into a tent-like garment falling from the cap (fig. 92).[44] Because it completely covers the head, face and body, this type of garment may be characterised as a body screen. The basic aim of this garment is to disguise completely the appearance and shape of a woman's body, from head to lower part of the body. Such garments are now mainly worn in Afghanistan and north-western Pakistan.

At the beginning of the twentieth century Muslim women north-western India wore a slightly different form of *chadri* (Cooper (Cooper 1915, pl. facing p. 170). Instead of an area of openwork for the eyes, two holes cut out and lined with netting (fig. 93). The use of the *chadri* continues to be worn by Muslim women to the present-day in the cities of Afghanistan and in nearby Pakistan.

Garment veils

The last group of 'outerwraps' to be described in this chapter are the so-called 'garment veils'. They are normally multi-purpose garments which can be used as, for example, coats or as headveils, according to the wishes of the wearer. Examples of coats being used in this manner come from some regions of Palestine (for example, around Nablus), where it is not uncommon for the sleeved coat or *qumbaz* to be draped over the head and shoulders (Weir 1989:78). Garment veils also occur in Saudi Arabia where sleeveless coats called *abaya's* are draped over the head of nomadic women. A more elaborate, sleeved coat called a *chyrpy* or *charpy* is worn by women in Turkestan.

The Arabian Abaya

When in public many women in northern Arabia and elsewhere wear a *thawb* or dress covered with an *abaya* (*aba*) or coat-like garment, but without sleeves (Stillman 1981:96). The *abaya* can be worn with the neck opening placed over the top of the forehead, while the rest of the garment hangs down (fig. 94).

The origins of the *abaya* are unknown, but there are reports of women wearing them dating from the beginning of the nineteenth century. It would seem likely, however, that the *abaya* was being worn long before this date.

During the summer a light-weight *abaya* is worn, while in winter it is made from a much heavier cloth. In both cases, however, the *abaya* is traditionally made out of either sackcloth (vegetable fibre; *khaysah*) or some form of animal fibre such as sheep's wool (*suff al-aghnam*), goat and camel hair (*wabar*). Nowadays the *abaya* is usually black, but in the past travellers have reported other colours such as white and light blue.

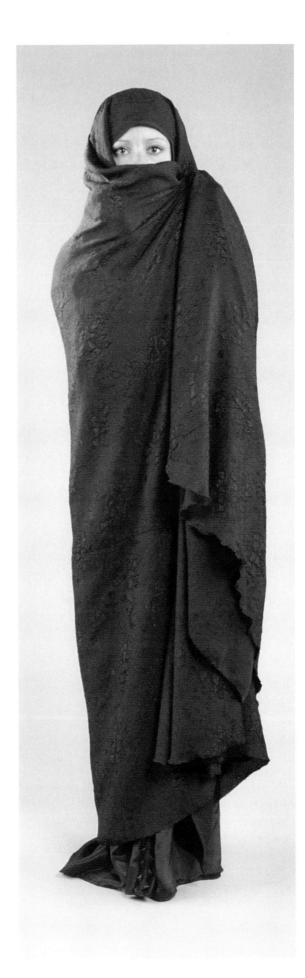

Figure 85. An Egyptian outerwrap or melaya (modern, RMV 5826-4; photo. by B. Grishaaver).

Figure 86. An Egyptian outerwrap or melaya laff (modern, RMV 5829-1; photo. by B. Grishaaver).

Figure 88. A modern Iranian chador (RMV 5832-1; photo. by B. Grishaaver).

75

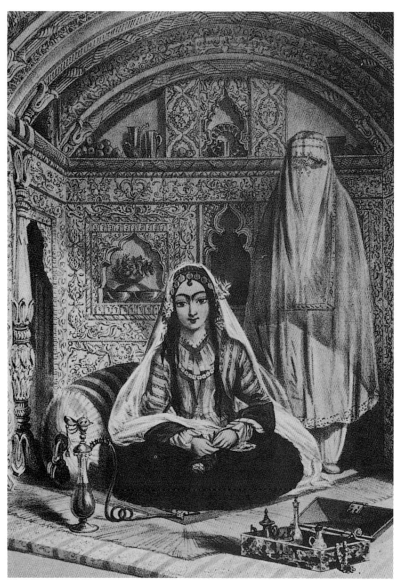

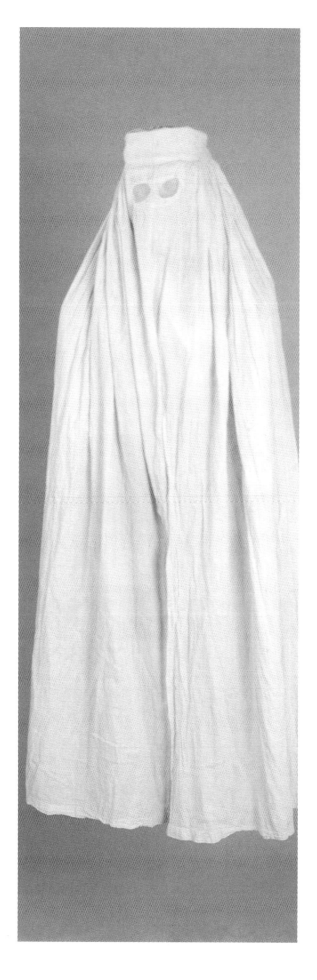

Figure 91. A 19th c. print of an Afghan woman wearing a chadri (from Rattray 1848).

Figure 93. An Pakistan/North Indian version of the chadri (RMV 465-1; photo. by B. Grishaaver).

The size of an *abaya* can vary quite considerably, but generally they are about one and a half metres wide and two metres long (Stillman 1981:102). They are made from two pieces of material, which are either sewn along the shoulder seam or sewn together horizontally at the hipline, or sometimes both. There are no side seams. Because of its almost square shape, the shoulders of the *abaya* hang down over the arms, giving the effect of sleeves. The shoulder seam and the border at the neck and front are usually decorated with braid or cord, but in the same colour as the main body of the garment. A wider braid is used around the neck and front openings, while decoratively knotted buttons are sewn on either side.

The Turkmense Chyrpy

In some areas of West Turkmen both urban and nomadic married women of the Teke tribe, wear a large, 'sleeved' coat *(chyrpy, charypy, khalat, kurthe or paranja)* which is made out of colourful cloth (fig. 95a-b). Traditionally, such a coat was made out of a warp-ikat material, although nowadays examples in pale white-striped green, brown or dark blue cloth can be found (Kalter 1984:81, 91). The colour of the coat is also used to give an indication of the status of a woman; younger women tend to wear dark colours, while an older woman would wear one with a light or white ground.

The 'sleeves' of the *chyrpy* are in fact false and are made of two long, tapering pieces of material which are sewn together and allowed to hang down the back of the garment. The coat is worn in such a way that it completely envelopes the wearer.

Comparable coats were worn by the women of east Turkestan. A description of such a coat worn by women from Kashgar was given in the memoirs of Lady Catherine Macartney:

"For going out, a long coat reaching to the heels is put on, made of velvet, silk, or chintz, as the case may be. The coats are very similar to those worn by the men, only they are longer and have bands of brocade on the chest to denote, by the number, the standing of the wearer, whether she is single, newly married, or a matron with a family. But no belt is ever worn, being considered indecent for a woman. The caps are much like the men's generally, though for full outdoor dress some of the older women wear huge pork-pie shaped hats, with broad bands of fur turned up all round. Over everything, head and all, a big white muslin coat is thrown, and held together in front with the sleeves, through which the arms are never put, hanging down behind. A thick veil made of cotton material beautifully worked all over in pattern of drawn thread work, is worn down over the face, or thrown back over the cap or hat" (Macartney 1985:70-1)

The Japanese kazuki/katsugi

Finally, in order to show the widespread use of such garment veils, it seems worth while to say something about the *kazuki* worn by Japanese women (Morioka and Rathbun 1993:138). By the time of the Lady Sei Shonagon in the tenth century AD a travelling costume had been developed which consisted of the white *kosodo* or early form of kimono, and another *kosodo*, called a *kazuki*, which was worn over the head.

The *kazuki* or 'veil kimono' was draped over the head with the sleeves hanging over the shoulders. The neck opening of the *kazugi* was placed over the forehead. If needed, the front of the garment could be pulled over the face of the wearer to prevent recognition or to offer shelter. The *kazuki* became known as the *katsugi* during the late Muromachi period (AD 1392-1568).

By the end of the seventeenth century, the *kazuki* had assumed its characteristic form whereby the neck-opening

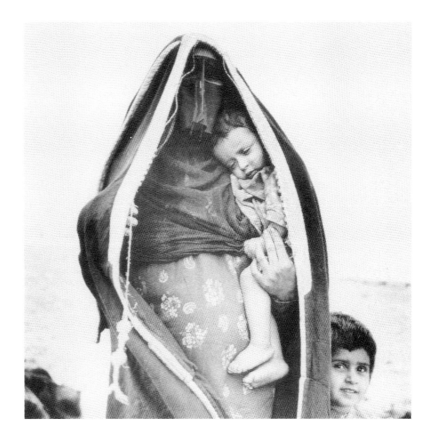

was lowered at the front by about twenty centimetres (fig. 96). This 'extra' space was needed to make room for the newly fashionable, large coiffures of Japanese women. To protect further their hair arrangement, women sometimes wore a cotton band *(wataboshi)* over their hair (Morioka and Rathbun 1993:138-139). It was kept in place with a long, wooden hairpin.

During the Edo period (AD 1600-1867), there were several classifications of *kazuki* (Morioka and Rathbun 1993:138). The *gosho kazuki* (Imperial Palace *kazuki*), for example, was generally made of dark blue silk gauze, which was usually decorated with a striped pattern in the mid-section. This form of the *kazuki* was worn by women of aristocratic families living in Kyoto.

Lower ranking women seem to have had more freedom in their choice of colour and decoration for the *kazuki* (Morioka and Rathbun 1993:138). The *machi kazuki* (town *kazuki*), for instance, was also made from silk, but came in a variety of colours and designs. At the same time, an *asa* or bast fibre (such as ramie) *kazuki* was being worn by lower class women. This form developed into the *daimon kazuki* (large cresented *kazuki*). This kazuki became the characteristic form during the eighteenth and nineteenth centuries. It is recognisable by the presence of a large, usually circular motif on the back of the robe. When the robe was worn, the motif enclosed the head (fig. 97). These large motifs were often based on the chrysanthemum which was traditionally associated with longevity.

Figure 94. An Arab woman wearing an abaya over her head (from Ferdinand, 1993, fig. 8,30).

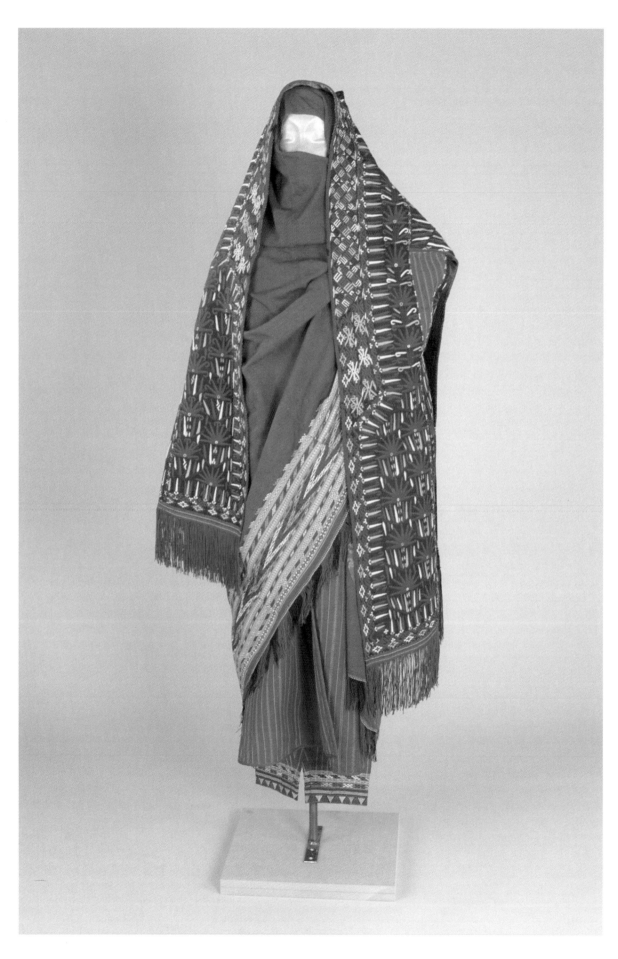

Figure 95a-b.
Figure wearing a
complete outdoor
outfit for a mature,
Turkemen woman,
including a garment
veil or chyrpy
(RMV 3830; photo.
by B. Grishaaver).

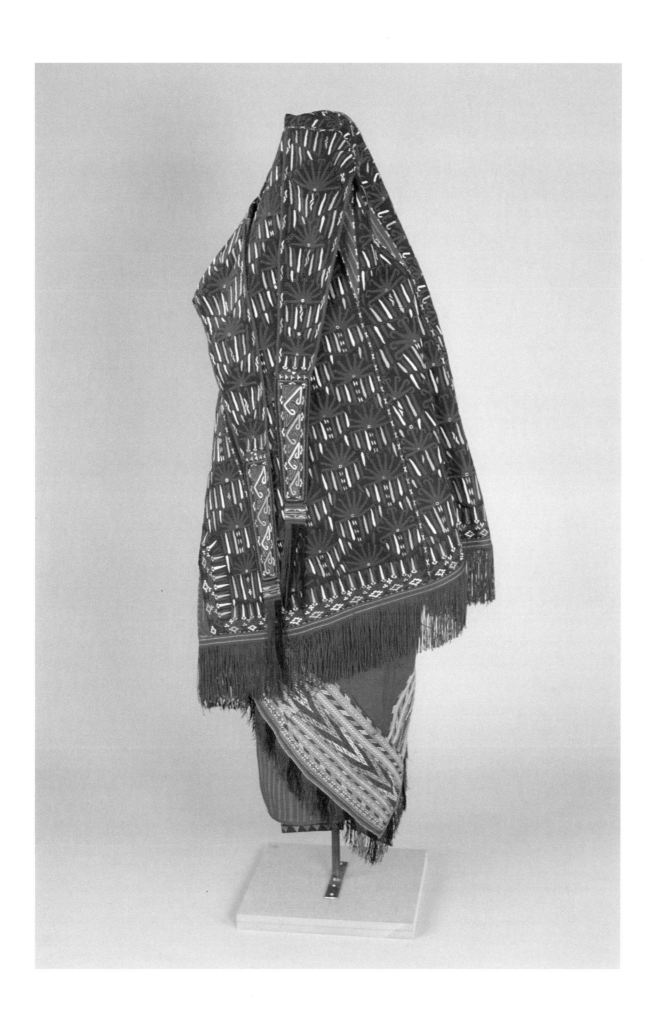

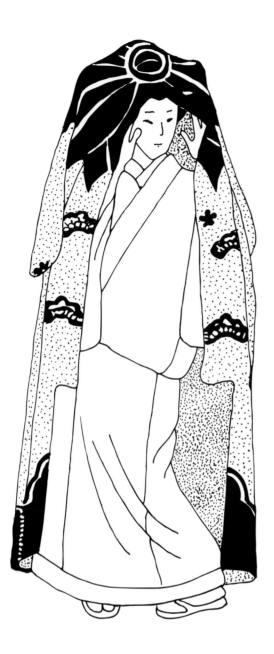
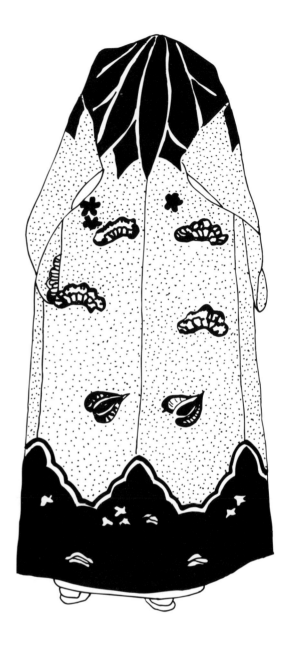

The wearing of the *kazuki* was banned in the city of Edo in the mid-seventeenth century, following an incident in AD 1652 when an unemployed samurai disguised himself under a *kazuki* and tried to assassinate a high-ranking adviser to the shogun. In Kyoto and other areas, however, its use seems to have continued until much later.

By the beginning of the twentieth century the wearing of the *kazuki* had been abandoned in most of Japan, although it has survived in some rural areas and is occasionally worn during ceremonial events such as weddings and funerals (Morioka and Rathbun 1993:138).

Notes:

38 The word mantle derives from the late Latin *mantus* and medieval Latin *mantum*, meaning a cloak.

39 The appearance and draping technique of the Moroccan *huik* will be discussed in the following chapter.

40 See also the instructions in Marçais 1930:108, pl. XXV.

41 Based on Dar 1969:27ff; Chandra 1973:135-179 and Joshi 1992.

42 The garment should not be confused with the *izar* worn by women in the Maghreb.

43 Not to be confused with the modern *tarah* which is now a much shorter length of material which covers the head and upper part of the body!

44 This garment is called a *chadri* (Scarce 1981; Dupree 1973:247), *sadar* (Ahmed 1980:104), or *burqa* (Doubleday 1988:63-64; Jeffery 1979:4).

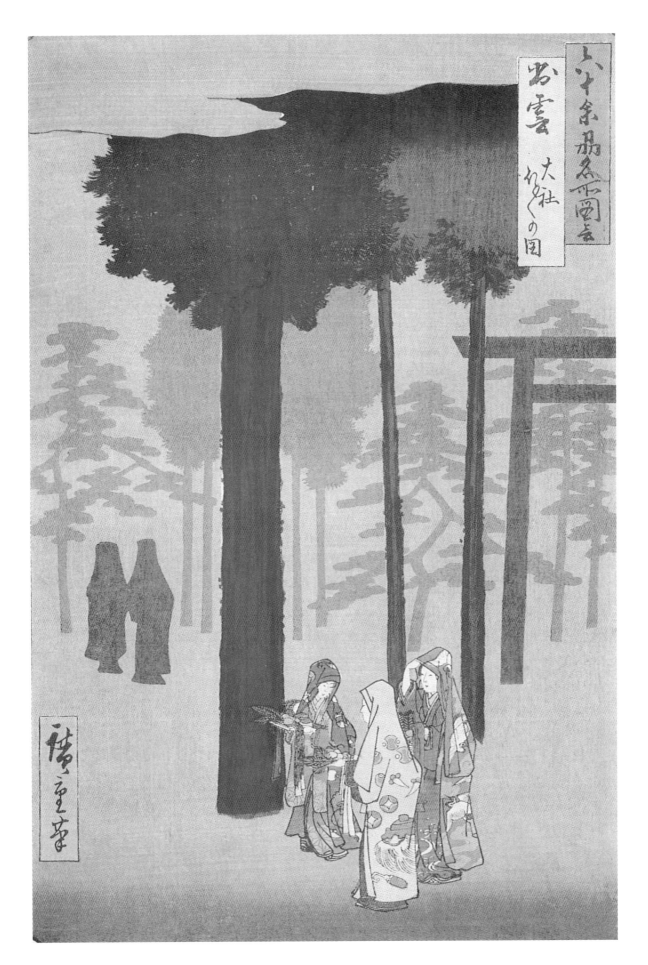

Figure 96. A group of Japanese women wearing garment veils (*kazuki*; RMV 2494-43; photo. B. Grishaaver).

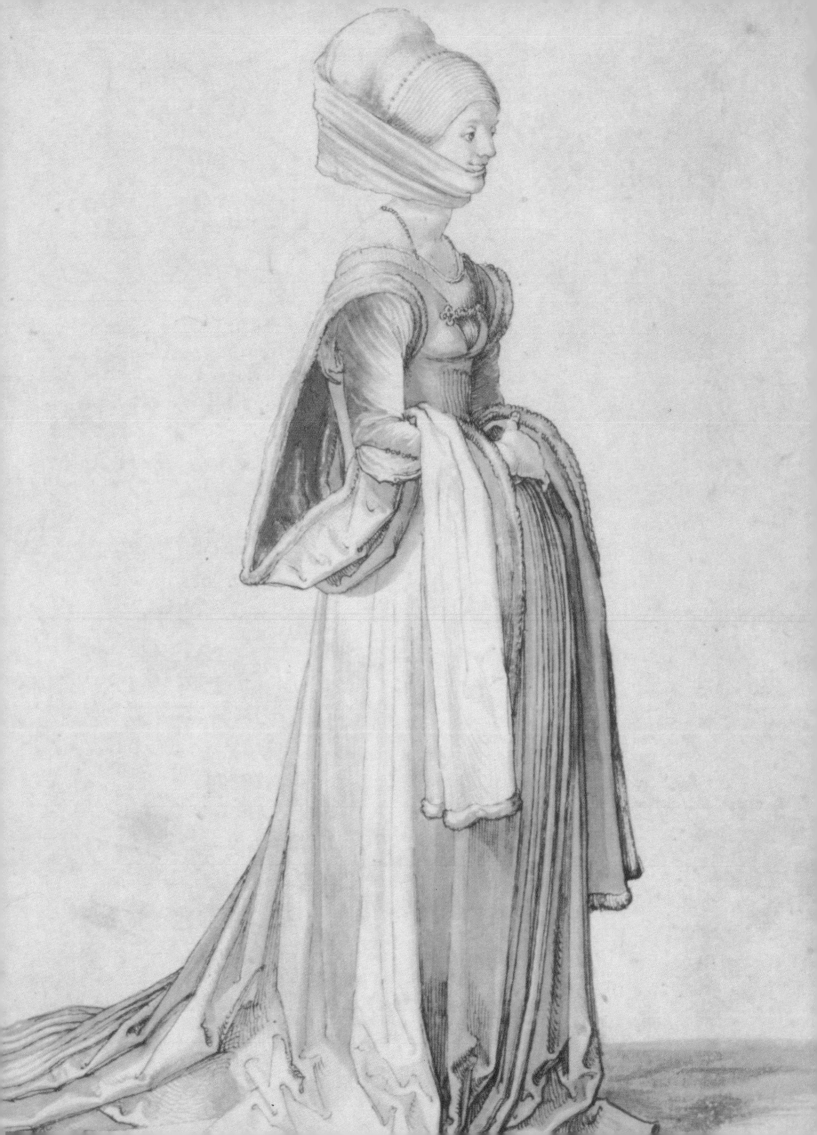

Chapter 6

The movement of veils and veiling

Throughout history garment styles have been moving around the world, become fashionable in one particular region and either adapted to local conditions or dropped. One of the most famous recent examples is the use of jeans, which were originally developed in France, were subsequently adopted by North Americans, and which during the last thirty years have virtually conquered the world.

In this chapter two examples of a garment will be described which originated in North Africa and eventually moved via the Iberian Peninsula to Northern Europe and elsewhere. The two garments in question are the so-called chin band and the mantilla. Both garments originated in North Africa as the *lithma* and *huik* respectively. The appearance and function of both of these garments have been described elsewhere (see pages 46 and 67).

The *lithma* is a length of material wrapped around the lower part of the head. At present it is worn throughout North Africa. The *huik* is a large, rectangular length of material which is wrapped around the head and body. It is worn by women in the same area.[45]

The Iberian peninsula has been dominated by many different peoples. With the collapse of the Western Roman empire, for instance, in the early fifth century AD, Spain was invaded by the Vandals. Later, the Goths founded the Visigoth kingdom with Toledo as its capital. Following the disintegration of the Visigoth kingdom, the Islamic Moors from North Africa gained control of much of the peninsula (Map 2). The Moorish influence

was to last for about eight hundred years. However, in northern Spain, Christian kingdoms persisted and during the eleventh century AD the Christian kingdoms of Leon, Castille and Aragon came into being and throughout the following centuries they enlarged their territories. Eventually, only the tiny kingdom of Granada in southern Spain, remained under Moorish rule and this was to fall by the end of the fifteenth century.

Throughout the Medieval period there were close contacts between the Moorish and Christian dominated areas of the Iberian peninsula (May 1957). These contacts included the exchange of textiles. One of the most telling sources of information are the Moorish or Andalusian textiles which were found in the twelfth and thirteenth century AD royal tombs at the Monastery of St. Maria la Real de Huelgas, Burgos, in northern Spain (Carretero 1988). The tombs include those of Leonor de Inglaterra y Maria de Almenar (AD 1156-1214); Maria de Almenar (died c. AD 1200); Leonor of Castille, Queen of Aragon (died AD 1244), and Berenguela, Queen of Leon and Castilla (AD 1180-1246), and Alfonso de la Cerda (AD 1271-1333). All of these tombs included Andalusian textiles, many with Arabic inscriptions woven into them. Thus, the Moorish period should be seen as a period of considerable influence from Moorish and Islamic textiles and costume upon Christian Iberian forms.

As noted in a previous chapter, the *lithma* is traditionally associated with women living in North Africa. One of the earliest examples of a Moorish

Figure 101.
A sketch by Albrecht Dürer of a woman from Nuremberg dressed for a dance. She is wearing a chin wrap (c. 1500; Wien, Albertina Winkler 224).

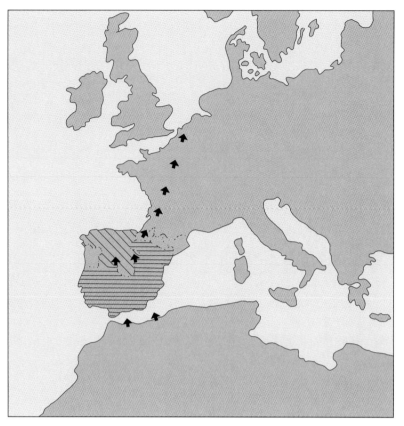

Map 2.
Map showing the geographical spread of the huik (North Africa, Spain and The Netherlands).

representation of the *lithma* can be seen in a miniature of Alfonso the Tenth, *El tratado de ajedrez*, which dates to about AD 1283. Here two Moorish ladies are depicted playing chess (Anderson 1942:72, fig. 27). Both women are wearing turbans made from narrow bands, while their lower faces are covered with the *lithma* form of veil (fig. 98).

By the twelfth century, the *lithma* began to appear in Christian Spain in the form of the chin band or *barboquejo* (Anderson 1942:51, 66, figs. 19-20). One of the earliest depictions of women wearing a broad chin wrap with pleated edge can be seen on a late eleventh or early twelfth century cloister panel in the Monastery of Santa Domingo de Silos, at Burgos (Anderson 1942, fig. 4). In each of these early examples, it would appear that the chin wrap and headcovering were made out of a length of material many metres long, which was carefully wound around the head (Anderson 1942:54).

A small number of medieval examples of chin bands have actually been found in various northern Spanish tombs. Most of them are between 11.0 and 15.0 cm wide and made out of fine material. One of the earliest surviving examples of these chin bands was found in the tomb of the Christian queen, Leonor de Inglaterra y Maria de Almenar (AD 1156-1214). Queen Leonor was buried in the above mentioned Monastery of St. Maria la

Real de Huelgas, Burgos, in northern Spain. The queen's chin band was made out of a narrow length of very fine linen which had a pleated silk border sewn onto it.

In later representations, Iberian women are shown wearing a high headdress called a toque, which was trimmed with pleats or ruches. The chin band that went with it became more elaborate and covered the mouth and in some cases the nose as well. The use of such a mouth band can be seen in the tomb effigy of Dona Leonor Ruiz de Castro (died c. AD 1275), which shows the lady with covered chin and mouth. A more elaborate version covering the nose as well can be seen in the miniature of Alfonso X (the Wise; reign: AD 1252-1284), *El tratado de ajedrez*, in which a woman is wearing a low horned hat and has her throat, chin and nose covered (fig. 99).

By the fifteenth century the use of the chin wrap had spread with the movement of Spanish fashions to Northern Europe. Women wearing chin, mouth and nose bands are depicted in a painting entitled: "A hunt in honour of Charles V at the Castle of Torgau" (c. AD 1544) by Lucas Cranach (AD 1472-1553; Prado Museum, cat. no. 2175). In the lower right-hand corner of the painting there is a small group of ladies, some of whom are hunting (fig. 100). Several of the women, but not all, are wearing bands which cover their mouths and part of their throats.

During the fifteenth and sixteenth centuries, the women of Nuremburg in Germany were noted for the wearing of such face coverings, although by now the band had become much wider. Nevertheless, the band still covered the throat, chin and mouth. Some of the ways in which these garments were worn were captured in sketches made by Albrecht Dürer (AD 1471-1528). In one example the woman has the band across her chin, while in another she has it across her chin and mouth (fig. 101).

By the late sixteenth century the wearing of the chin band, as well as the mouth and nose bands, appears to have died out, at least for secular clothing, in both Spain and Northern Europe.

The Spanish mantilla and the huik

The development of the Spanish mantle or mantilla has an even longer and more complex history than the chin band. The early history of the garment is complex and involves ancient Iberian, Medieval Islamic, as well as Germanic and South American influences.

The Spanish mantilla and its relatives

One of the longest surviving examples of a mantle can be found in Spain where it is now called a mantilla. *Manta, manto* are the Spanish words for a blanket and large shawl respectively, which have been used for centuries as enveloping outer garments. The *mantilla* is the diminutive applied more generally to the black or white lace, silk or cashmere head shawls or veils used as

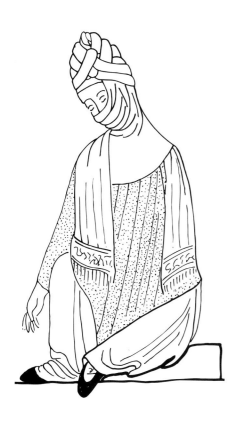 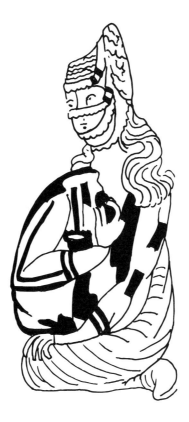 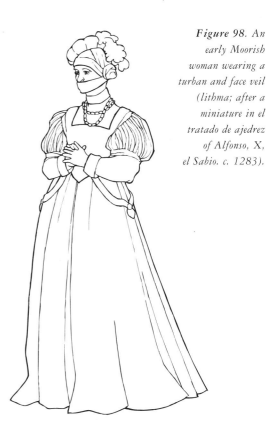

Figure 98. An early Moorish woman wearing a turban and face veil (lithma; after a miniature in el tratado de ajedrez of Alfonso, X, el Sabio. c. 1283).

accessories to fashionable Spanish dresses. The *mantilla* continues to be worn to the present day, although it is now regarded as an item of traditional rather than everyday clothing. Women going to church usually wear a black lace veil over their heads, while on formal occasions, such as weddings, female guests may also wear a token *mantilla*. Such *mantillas* were recently worn at the wedding of the daughter of the king of Spain, where the queen and other ladies of the royal household wore long black mantillas and combs with modern clothing.

The wearing of a mantle of some kind can be traced back in the Iberian Peninsula to at least the sixth century BC (fig. 102). Simpler mantles can be seen on a relief from a woman's tomb at La Albufereta (prov. Alicante; Archaeological Museum, Alicante), whereby the woman is wearing a long mantle draped over her head, which reaches down to the ground (Arribas, nd, fig. 43). The mantle continued to be worn by women throughout the Roman and Visigoth periods in Spain.

Following the disintegration of the Visigoth Empire, the Moors from North Africa gained control of much of the peninsula. Not surprisingly, it was during the Moorish period that the wearing of the woman's mantle began to take on a North African/Muslim appearance. It became larger and more closely fitting, while the head and face were deliberately covered, especially by Muslim women. There is a relief on Granada Cathedral, for example, which depicts a number of Muslim women about to be baptised. They wear an all-enveloping outerwrap which appears to a form of *haik* as worn in North Africa (see page 67; fig. 103).[46]

Sometimes, small flat hats or boards with small projectiles were worn over the top of the mantles. It would appear that the cloth was attached to the boards. These women were illustrated by Weiditz during his tour of Northern and Southern Europe in the early sixteenth century (c. AD 1529).[47] The ladies come from the Granada region. Similarly dressed women are also shown in Spanish paintings from the period, notably in an anonymous engraving from 1558 which shows the (Christian) citizens of Valladolid at an Auto de Fe (fig. 104).[48]

The North African Haik

As noted above, the Spanish mantle took a more southern Spanish/Islamic appearance in the period of Moorish domination. The mantle now had many similarities to the North African *haik*. This was, and still is, the traditional outer garment worn by many men and women in Morocco, Algeria and Tunisia. The *haik* (sometimes called a *melhafa*), is made out of a sheet of material about 4.70 m long and about 1.80 m wide. It is normally worn with a small face veil called an *ijar* or with a *lithma*-style veil (see page 46).

This garment has various Berber and Arabic names, but the Arabic *ha'ik* (*hayk, tahaykt*) is the one most commonly used nowadays. One of the earliest references to the makers of *haiks* is from the medieval work *Rawd al-Kirtas*.[49] There it was noted that the manufacturers of *haiks* were established near the fritter-fryers in the city of Fez.

Descriptions of the *haik* can be found in early seventeenth century European literature. In AD 1605 de Brèves wrote about the Algerian *haik*:

Figure 99. A woman wearing a horned headdress with chin and face wrap (after a miniature in el tratado de ajedrez of Alfonso, X, el Sabio. c. 1283).

Figure 100. Detail from a painting by Lucus Cranach Helviejo (c. 1472-1559), entitled "A Hunt in Honour of Charles V" (Prado Museum 2175). Some of the women depicted in the painting are wearing face and chin bands (drawing by K. Wilson, Rotterdam).

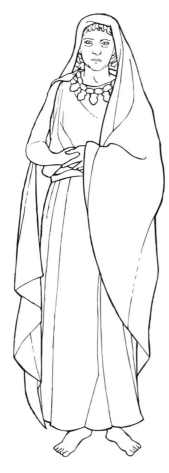

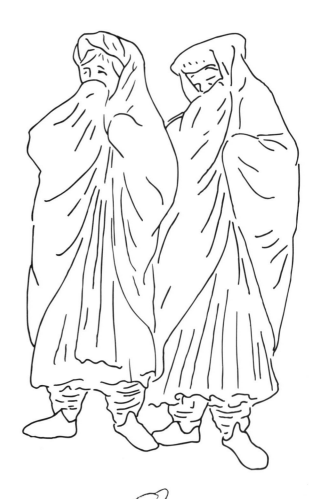

Figure 102. An Iberian figure of a woman wearing a long mantle (c. 6th c. BC; drawing by K. Wilson, Rotterdam).

Figure 103. A group of medieval Moorish woman about to be baptised, Granada Cathedral (after Marçais 1930, fig. 58).

Figure 104. A Christian Spanish woman attending an auto de fe. She is wearing a huik (c. 1558; after Bibliotheca Lipperheide, no. 2008, Berlin; drawing by K. Wilson, Rotterdam).

"Femmes allant par la ville se couvrent et enveloppent le corps d'une grande pièce de serge ou d'étamine et se cachent le visage avec deux linges: l'un (qui est plus proprement un bandeau faisant partie de la coiffure) voile le front jusque sur les paupières d'en haut et l'autre la partie inférieure de la face, tellement qu'elles ne montrent que les yeux" (de Brèves 1630:362).

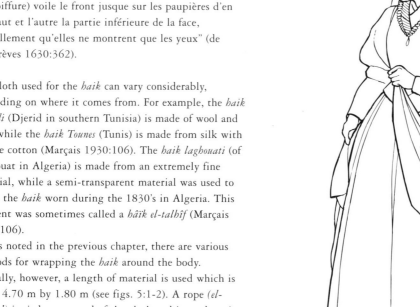

The cloth used for the *haik* can vary considerably, depending on where it comes from. For example, the *haik Djeridi* (Djerid in southern Tunisia) is made of wool and silk, while the *haik Tounes* (Tunis) is made from silk with a little cotton (Marçais 1930:106). The *haik laghouati* (of Laghouat in Algeria) is made from an extremely fine material, while a semi-transparent material was used to create the *haik* worn during the 1830's in Algeria. This garment was sometimes called a *hâïk el-talhîf* (Marçais 1930:106).

As noted in the previous chapter, there are various methods for wrapping the *haik* around the body. Basically, however, a length of material is used which is about 4.70 m by 1.80 m (see figs. 5:1-2). A rope *(el-mazdul)* is tied to one end of the cloth and is used to tie the rest of the material about at three specific points. The bulk of the material is then passed over the head. A pinch of cloth is taken from about 50.0 cm down the outer edge and knotted to the left shoulder. The excess material is

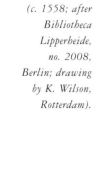

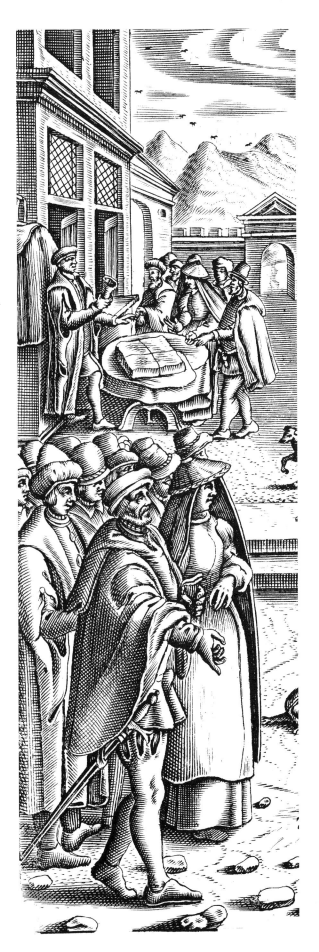

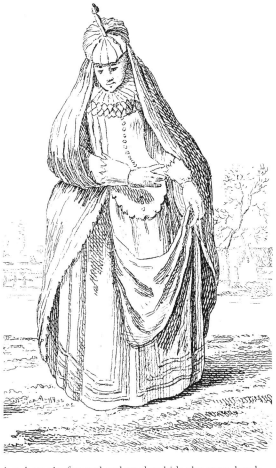

Figure 106.
*A Dutch woman
wearing a 'basket'
heuke (c. 1645;
private collection).*

Figure 105.
*A Dutch woman
wearing a pointed
heuke (c. 1750,
private collection).*

then brought forward and used to hide the arms, hands
and front of the body. This method of wrapping the huik
gives it its characteristic belted appearance which
reappears in the European versions.

The European haik/heuke

As noted above, the Moors took the *haik* into Spain where
it was seen and illustrated in its adapted form by
Christoph Weiditz in Granada in AD 1529. Several
versions developed from the purely Islamic/Moorish form
and the Christian form, but they all have certain elements
in common. For example, the covering of the head with a
large cloth which is counterbalanced by a small cap or
board of some kind. In the case of the Spanish ladies the
cap became highly ornamented. Often the *haik* was worn
fastened around the waist with a belt which was hidden
by the folds of material.

During the sixteenth century it became fashionable in
Europe to wear Spanish style clothing. Even Queen
Elizabeth I wore Spanish fashions, although at the time
Spain and England were mortal enemies. It was at this
date that a long version of the Spanish mantle became
especially popular with women in The Netherlands and
parts of northern Germany. Here it was known as the
hoyke, heuke or *huik*. It would appear that unconsciously
people were using the Arabic term.

The basic garment was made from a long length of
material which was draped over the head. Sometimes it

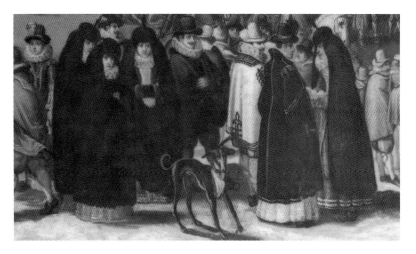

Figure 107.
*Painting by Denis
van Alsloot called
"Skating during
Carnival". The
women in the
foreground are
wearing heukes
(courtesy of the
Prado Museum,
1346).*

hung straight to the ground. On other occasions it was fastened around the waist or just under the breasts.

There were several different types of *heuke*, but the main types are the peaked *heuke*; the *heuke* with a flat hat (sometimes with a small, decorative projection), and the *hooded* heuke. The peaked *heuke* had a wood or whalebone board which projected over the face like a duck's bill while the fabric of the cloak was held in close to the face at the sides. The bill or peak acted as a counterbalance to the weight of the material of the garment. At first the bill was flat, but gradually it became higher and concave on top and convex beneath.

During the late sixteenth century a rounded hat with a spike on the top was often worn over the *heuke* and held it in place on the head so that it could be draped in folds around the figure without a peak (fig. 105). The *heuke* continued to be worn in the early decades of the

seventeenth century, when the material was often pleated causing the fabric to fall in a multitude of folds. At this time, the garments were sometimes kept in place with a basket-like hat instead of a board or bill (fig. 106).

Depictions of these garments can be seen in a number of paintings from the period. For example, the garment is shown in a painting entitled "Skating during Carnival" (c. 1620) by Denis van Alsloot (c. AD 1570-1628; Prado Museum, acc. 1346). The foreground of the painting is dominated by groups of women wearing *heukes* with flat caps and points (fig. 107).[50]

As noted above, at some point during the sixteenth century, a hooded form of the *haik* was developed which used wire or whalebone was used to stiffen the upper part of the *heuke* so that it could project in front of the head like a canopy. This form of *heuke* later became famous in the Noord Holland region of The Netherlands (fig. 108).

The Peruvian mantle

Following the Spanish conquest of the New World, the wearing of a mantle was also introduced into South America. One of the most famous examples of the women wearing this garment is that of the so-called "Veiled Women of Lima" *(the tapadas)*.[51]

It is not clear when this style of clothing was introduced into Peru, but it seems that it was being worn as early as AD 1561 when the then Viceroy Nieva, tried to have the *tapada* banned from the streets of Lima (Holmgren nd:12). By the eighteenth century the garments worn by the *tapadas* had become an important, if not essential, item of a Spanish lady's wardrobe.

Figure 108.
*Reconstruction of a
mid-nineteenth
century funeral
procession from
North Holland. The
women are wearing
mourning heukes
(copyright
J.H. Boersen,
Hippolytushoef).*

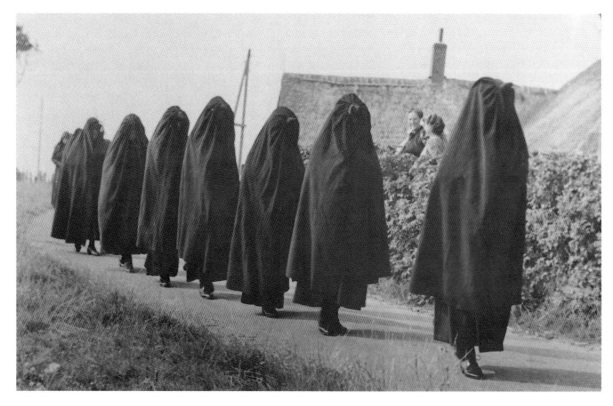

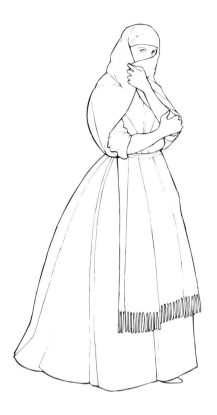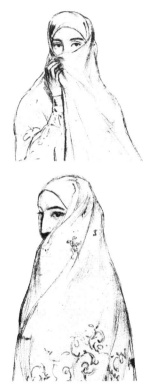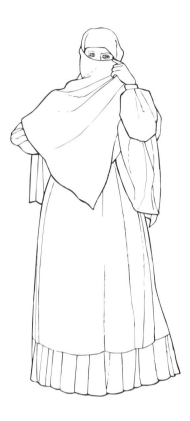

Curiously it was only worn in Lima, and veiled women were not seen in nearby towns such as the port of Callao.

The costume of the *tapada* was made up of three pieces, a skirt *(saya)*; a cloak *(rebozo* or *manto)* and a shawl (fig. 109a; Fuentes 1866:98-9). Originally the skirt was worn tightly fitted to the body from the waist to the ankles. Later it became much larger and had numerous thick pleats *(despledgada)*.

The cloak or *manto* was made out of a large piece of black or dark coloured material such as silk or fine cotton. Unlike other examples of mantles, however, part of it was either fastened to the skirt or in some cases tied around the waist. The cloth was then drawn up to cover the head, shoulders and arms. In this way material was used in the fashion of a hood rather than a mantle, and as such it is a closely related to the *huik* and the Flemish *heuke* described above. The shawl was worn under the cloak in such a way that the waist was visible. The whole ensemble was simply called a *saya y manto* and was worn over a dress.[52]

There would appear to have been several unwritten laws concerning the wearing of this outfit. For example, there was the tradition that no one uncovered the wearer's face (Leon 1982:52). If the *tapada* wanted to conceal her identify even further, then a poor and ragged skirt *(de tiritas)* was worn. Finally, it was the custom that when night fell the *tapadas* disappeared and 'normal' clothing, with the face uncovered, was assumed.

Because of the concealing nature of the garments, they allowed women to go out into the streets and meet men and have a rendezvous which otherwise would have been impossible. As a result, both the Catholic church as well as the government tried to prohibit the wearing of this ensemble, but without success. During the beginning of the nineteenth century the *Lima manto* had started to disappear, probably due to the importation of new fashions from Europe, but in its place the *manto chilena* (Chilian *mantilla*) was adopted (fig. 109b; Fuentes 1866:101). This is a larger piece of dark coloured material, usually silk or cotton, which was draped over the head, part of it being allowed to cover the face (from right to left). In this respect it can be regarded as a veil form of mantle. This form of veiling seems to have died out at the beginning of the twentieth century.

Notes:

45 For a fuller description of these garments, see pages 67 and 69.

46 Weiditz 1927 ed., tafels LXXXIV-VI; Marçais 1930:180, fig. 58, pl. XXV.

47 Weiditz 1927 ed., tafel. CXXXVI; CXL, XCIII-IV, L.

48 Bibliotheca Lipperheide, no. 2008, Berlin.

49 Ali b. Abdallah b. Abi Zar al-Fasi (trans. Beaumier 1860:58).

50 See also a painting by Hendrik Avercamp, called a "Winter Landscape with Iceskaters" (Rijksmuseum, Amsterdam, SK-A-1718), whereby a woman wearing a *heuke* is depicted in the bottom right-hand corner of the painting.

51 See Fuentes 1866:98-100; Quesada 1968:108, 112; Kadinlar 1987:149-50.

52 According to Leon, there were various different ways of wearing it according to the political and economic climate (Leon 1981:52).

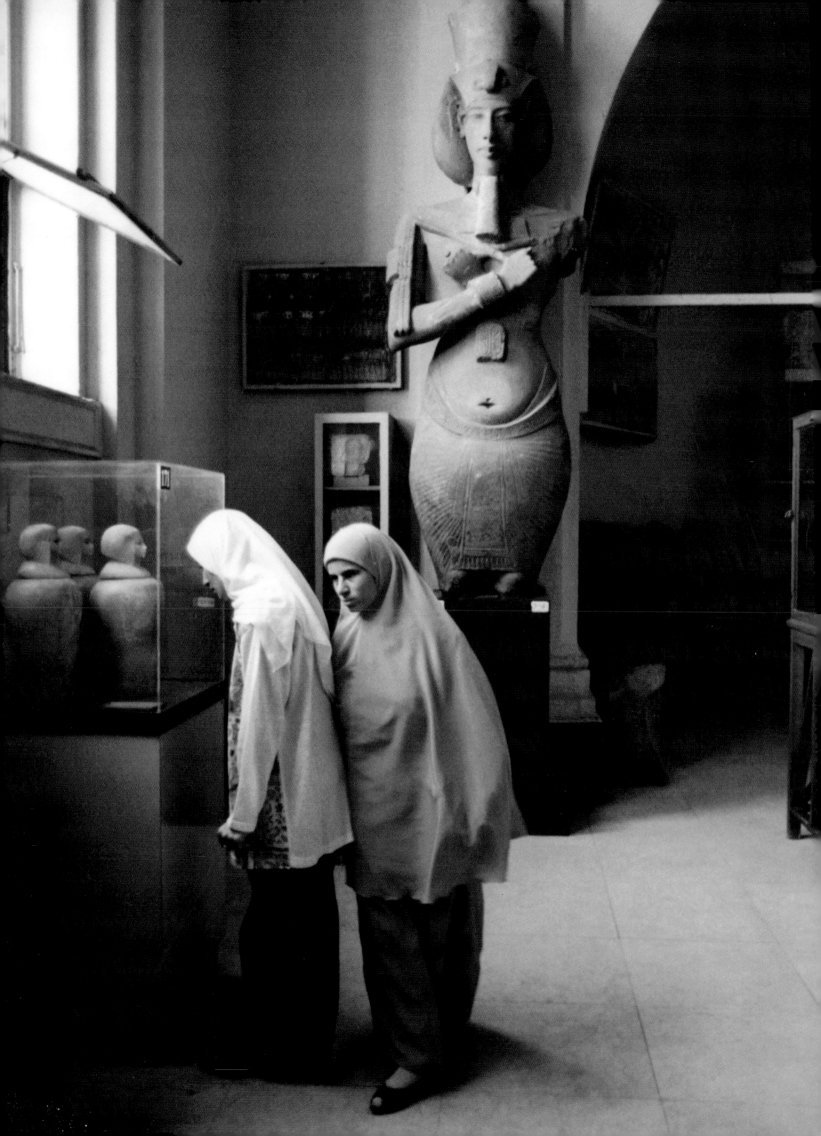

Chapter 7

Hijab, "Islamic" clothing

Religious beliefs can have a strong influence upon the appearance and even cut of clothing. Within Christian cultures, for example, there is a difference between traditional Protestant and Catholic styles of dressing. Even within the Protestant tradition there are significant variations between members of 'low' and 'high' churches. The former tend to be more 'puritanical' and plain in dress, while the clothing of the latter is regarded as being more liberal and sometimes even, frivolous. Similarly, the concept of traditional dress and what is 'allowed' has been interpreted quite differently within the Islamic world. The traditional clothing of Muslim men and women from Indonesia, for instance, is very different from the garments worn in Sudan. In recent years the spread of fundamentalism in the Muslim context has led to the development of a clothing type which is not seen as traditional to a particular region, but which conforms to Islamic principles. This type of clothing is called *hijab*. There are several versions of *hijab* for both men and women, but in each case the emphasis is on concealing the shape of the body and on simplicity in style and colour. In the case of women the reasons behind the wearing of *hijab* can be quite complex.

Hijab

The word *hijab* can be taken to mean a partition separating two objects, a screen or a curtain. It was used in the Koran as an instruction to believers in the time of the Prophet, Muhammad, on how they should deal with the prophet's wives:

> "If you ask his wives for anything, speak to them from behind a curtain. This is purer for our hearts and their hearts" (Sura 33:53).

The Koran's instructions for women outside the prophet's household were not as restrictive:

> "Tell the believing women to lower their gaze and be modest, and to display of their adornment only that which is apparent, and to draw their veils over their bosoms" (Sura 24:31)

Based on these two verses it would appear that women from the Prophet's household were expected to refrain from making public appearances and to keep behind a curtain when indoors. Other women were expected to behave modestly and to draw their "veils over their bosoms". The veil in question was thus a mantle not a face-veil.

Depending upon the interpretation, the above statements can be taken to indicate that modesty should be observed by conforming to conservative norms of dress, thus refusing to wear see-through blouses or short mini skirts. Or it can be taken further by interpreting "that which is apparent" to mean only a woman's face and

Figure 111. Two young Egyptian women wearing hijab.

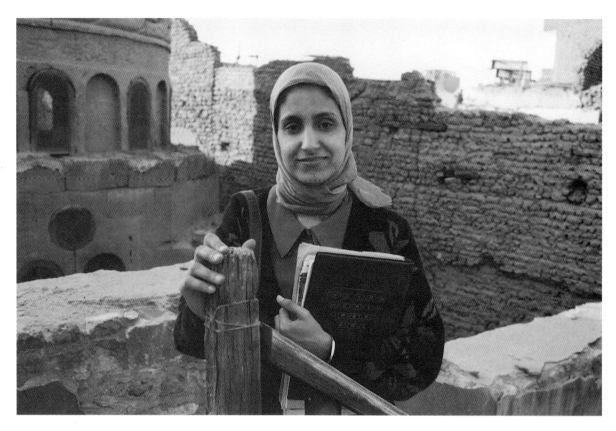

hands. The rest of her "adornment", (including the so-called erotic zones of ankles, wrists, neck), are expected to be hidden from all men except a carefully selected few.

The "few" are defined in the Koran as: husbands, fathers, brothers, fathers-in-laws, nephews, sons and stepsons (Koran, Suras 24:31; 33:55). It is also possible to be unveiled in front of prepubescent boys and "male attendants who lack vigour", namely, in the time of Muhammad, eunuchs or old slaves.

In some cases, women go one step further in search of *hijab*, and when in public they cover the body completely, including hands and faces.

Hijab clothing

There are various types and levels of *hijab* clothing. The first steps can be seen when a woman starts to wear a scarf or veil over her head (fig. 110). In Egypt, for example, there are various levels to veiling. A woman who wears a scarf or veiling is called a *muhaggaba*. Initially the scarfs tend to be short and decorative, but gradually, as the wearer begins to understand and accept the ethical code, the clothing becomes longer, larger, more shapeless and plain (fig. 111). The idea is that eventually the wearer will become completely swathed in a black cloak, gloves, shoes and face veil.

There are some subtle differences in these garments. Married women who are veiled, for example, may cover their mouth and nose, showing only their eyes. On the other hand unmarried women can leave their whole face showing. Gloves seem to be regarded as optional for both single and married women (Early 1993:120).

Colours used for *hijab* clothing tend to be either black or light and muted browns, blues, greys and greens in southwest Asia, while in Africa colours tend to be much brighter. The more subdued colours tend to be regarded as restful colours, which do not draw attention to the wearer. In addition, they are seen as being consistent with a wife and mother's role of bringing peace and contentment to a household.

It should not be forgotten, however, that there is also a degree of fashion in the wearing of *hijab*. There are a growing number of Near Eastern fashion houses, especially in Cairo and Beirut, which provide the latest *hijab* fashions in long skirts and coats with attention being paid to details such as pockets, necklines and colours. In Cairo, for instance, there is the Salam Shopping Centre for Veiled Women, which sells Islamically correct clothing. These garments include "training *hijab*" with colour coordinated long skirts and scarves, long jackets (including some with shoulder pads and studded with rhinestones). There is also Islamically correct evening wear for sale. On the second floor, tucked away in the back, there is a section which sells more sober garments, as well as sets of veils.[35]

The Egyptian television presenter, Kariman Hamza, briefly ran a televised fashion show in which Islamic styles for women were shown (Goodwin 1994:342). The garments were made in rich fabrics and colours and were frequently decorated with beads, flowers and embroidery. After the show had been discontinued, Hamza turned the format into a successful Islamic women's fashion magazine.

With respect to the concept of fashion, it should also be remembered that the wearing of *hijab* can be much cheaper than trying to follow vagaries of fashion, whether Eastern or Western. The cost of a *hijab* set in Cairo (kerchief, cover and veil) in 1995 was 33.5 Egyptian pounds (about 17 guilders; fig. 112). In addition, a number of mosques and other religious establishments used to give grants towards the purchasing of *hijab* garments, or had them available at a reduced price (Rugh 1986:154). This is in contrast to the price of a pair of jeans which can be over eighty or more Egyptian pounds. For many girls who come from country areas to study in Cairo, it is simply financially and morally easier to wear *hijab*. The other side to the coin is that, since *hijab* has become fashionable, some women have many outfits, which are all Islamically correct, but which would seem to be more inclinded towards the concept of fashion than religion.

The acceptance and rejection of hijab

Throughout the world and over the centuries there have been numerous laws regulating the wearing of specific types of clothing. To date there would seem to be no general ruling that says that all Muslim women have to wear some form of *hijab*. Yet such clothes provide one of the major sources of dispute and discontent by Muslims and non-Muslims alike.

With respect to *hijab*, the headscarf worn by many Muslim women is now seen in the West as one of the most visible and obvious symbols of (militant) Islam. As will be discussed below there are various reasons given for the wearing of *hijab*, some of them religious, while others are social and economic in origin.

Some women embrace *hijab* from deeply felt religious reasons. Often the wearing of full *hijab* is carried out with a sense of pride. In return the wearer expects and is given honour and respect. Indeed, honour and respect are the two most frequently given reasons why women wish and should wear *hijab* (Amrouche 1994:138).

In a recent article in *The Independent* (April 28th 1994) by Asla Aydintasbas on the growing trends towards the wearing of *hijab* in the East End of London, she noted that ten years ago pressure on young Muslim women to accept a stricter Islamic dress code came from parents. This situation has now changed and it is peer pressure which is more dominant. Asma (aged 16) recalled in the article, how she was harassed by groups of Muslim boys for not wearing a scarf:

> "They tell us that we show no respect for our parents by wearing these Western clothes and that we should all cover our heads in order to be true Muslims. While some boys are more coercive, telling girls that they would only be 'truly beautiful' under the scarf, others have gone further, accusing them [unveiled girls] of being 'slags'".

It was also noted in the article that a new Muslim identity was developing amongst the young female members of Britain's Islamic community. In the East End of London, teenagers of Turkish, Bengali and Middle Eastern backgrounds were coming together as Muslims whose religious approach differed from the traditional practices of their parents. They regard themselves as followers of Islam rather than, for example, Turkish Muslims. For some of the girls the wearing of *hijab* has become a symbol of their new awareness of being followers of Islam.

It is not only girls of Muslim families who find the wearing of *hijab* attractive. According to the article by Aybintabas, she interviewed one girl from an English Christian background who had converted to Islam. Samia, as she is now known as, had come to terms with wearing a full form of *hijab* including scarf, a long coat, gloves and a veil across her face, leaving only her eyes uncovered. When asked if she missed the freedom of Western clothes she replied in the negative:

> "It's not a question of what I want to wear. When you accept Islam, in a sense you have to give something up for it. There isn't a choice. Allah says women have to cover up."

Thus, for some women the wearing of *hijab* indicates both their religious and their cultural identity. At another level, for some Muslim women living outside of their own country, the wearing of *hijab* becomes a statement of both their 'eastern' identity and, more importantly, an expression of their religion. It provides a barrier against a foreign, 'Western' way of life, as well as telling other Muslims that here is a sister who is to be respected and treated correctly.

It should also be noted that it is not only women who accept Islamic clothing to emphasise their religious beliefs. It is stated in the Koran that men should also behave and dress modestly:

> "Say to the believers, that they cast down their eyes and guard their private parts; that is purer for them" (Sura 24:30).

As an extension to this idea, in some countries men have taken to wearing Arabic costume as a sign of their Islamic faith. One example can be taken from Malaysia, where some young men have adopted the practise of wearing Arabic style dress: "In public gardens and in other places in this new town can be seen young village Malays dressed as Arabs, with turbans and gowns. The Arab dress - so far from Pakistan, so far from Arabia - is their political badge" (Naipaul 1982:229).

For many Muslim women who choose to work outside the home the wearing of *hijab* means they can do so

Figure 112.
A figure wearing a
modern hijab outfit
from Egyptian
(RMV 5826-3a-c,5;
photo. by
B. Grishaaver).

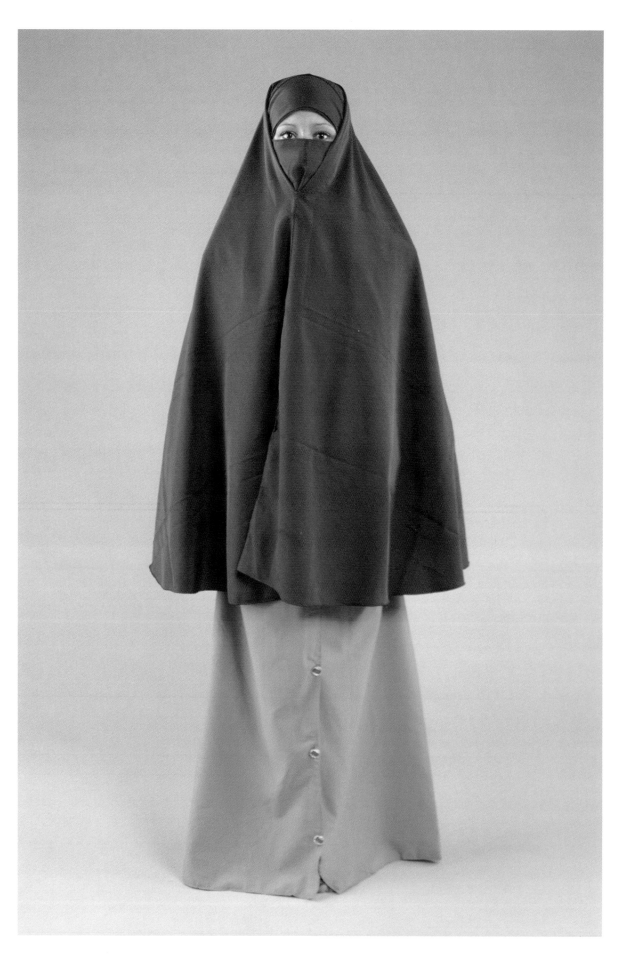

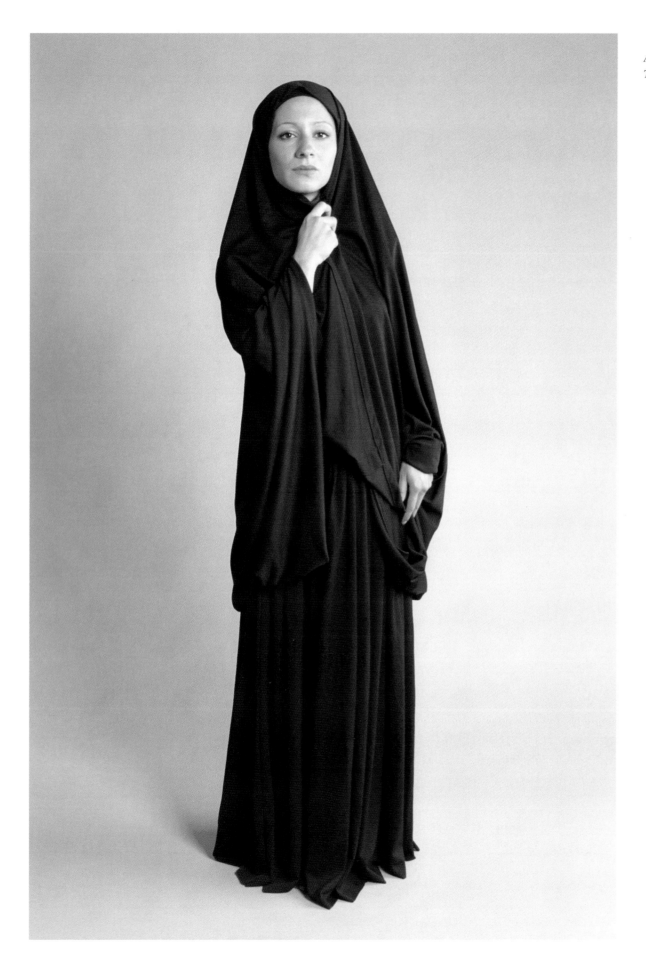

Figure 113.
*A figure wearing a
Turkish hijab-style
garment (carsaf:
RMV 5817-25:
photo. by
B. Grishaaver).*

without embarrassment or shame, while at the same time adding to the family's financial and social situation. By wearing *hijab* they are stating that they conform to Islam and present no threat to the social role of men. In return, veiled working women receive minimal censorship from inside and outside the family home.

It was noted by the Iranian writer Nesta Ramazani that the wearing of *hijab* has become the means of more social activism:

"By wearing the badge of purity, women can move about freely. By wearing the badge of modesty, they may fight for women's rights. By wearing the badge of moral rectitude, women compel the state to back up its claim to the equality of men and women within Islam" (Ramazani 1993:424).

Veiling has also been used as a reaction to a particular political situation. In 1980, for instance, the Turkish government banned the wearing of Islamic dress in universities (fig. 113). More specifically, women were forbidden to wear a headscarf (Moghabam 1993:161). As a result of this prohibition many women started to wear turbans as a form of protest. The "Turban Movement" has now become a major part of the Islamic movement within Turkey, and one of its rallying calls is for the return to Islamic clothing.

There is a more extremist view that includes the idea that anything to do with the West, namely cars, music centres, televisions, money, are representatives of the "Great American Satan" or the "plague from the West" (the Iranian concept of *gharbzadegi*; Moghadam 1993:141). The claim has been made that by depriving women of chastity, modesty, and honour through ideas of independence and sex appeal, western influences have weakened Islamic societies, especially those of Algeria and Iran. Thus, it was seen by some that the:

"Main antidote to the virus of *gharbzadegi* is *hijab*. Furthermore veiling must be compulsory in order to protect the cultural identity and integrity of the group and of its female members" (Moghadam 1993:141-2).

Thus the veiling of women can be seen as representing a partition between a woman and her immediate surroundings, as well as the evil (Western) world and, in the last instance, the woman's acceptance of her traditional role as mother and housewife, who stays within the confines of the home (Djura 1994:138-9). For some women, the act of wearing *hijab* has specific negative connotations, notably that this act represents an acceptance of a woman's legal inferiority to men as laid down within Islamic law. These imbalances can be seen in inheritance laws, laws regarding witnesses, as well as a woman's rights regarding marriage and divorce.

On a social and economic level there is also a view expressed by some people, usually of the upper echelons of society, that it is only lower and middle class women who wear *hijab*. The wearing of such clothing is seen as an expression of their unsophisticated nature and their inability to withstand family pressures and in particular that of their male relatives.

Protests against the wearing of hijab have taken a number of different forms. While there may be a public acceptance of hijab, there is simultaneously the concept of the 'mini-revolt'. In such cases, some women wear hijab in public, but privately protest by wearing miniskirts or deeply cut blouses under their veils (Djura 1994:138). There have also been a number of articles in Egyptian newspapers about the subject of veiling and it has been noted that there is now strong criticisms of hijab from the side of older Egyptian women. In particular, they feel that the newly veiled younger ones have betrayed them and the gains they made over the past seventy years (MacLeod 1991:138).[54]

In some countries the wearing of *hijab* has been accepted with a minimal of conflict and numerous women have embraced the wearing of this type of clothing system. According to some writers the wearing of *hijab* became one of the signals of the Islamic revival which began in 1967 following the Six-Day War with Israel. Muslim philosophers pointed to the secularism of Nasser's government and urged Egyptians to return to the Islamic laws they had abandoned. Since then there has been an upsurge in the wearing of this type of clothing, especially by lower middle class women. But although there has been considerable peer pressure, there has been a minimum of violence.

In other areas of the world, however, there is a deeply felt resentment against its instalment. In lands where militant fundamentalism is strong, many women feel they have been forced into the decision of either staying at home or wear *hijab*. Veiling has long been used by governments for various political ends, as will be discussed in Chapter 12. But it is worthwhile quickly highlighting some other examples of this form of (mis)use of *hijab*, namely the return to *hijab* in Palestine and the use of the 'black veil' in Algeria.

The lack of political success is one of the reasons given for the return to *hijab* in the Palestinian region. Ziad Abu Amer, a political science professor at Bir Zeit University, noted: "people resort to cultural references, like the veil, especially when they perceive their whole national existence is threatened".[55] During the 1980's a Palestinian Islamic group called *Mujama* suggested the return to a stricter, Islamic moral and social code (Moghadam 1993:163). One of their main targets was women's appearance; at first they encouraged and then threatened women into covering their hair. Graffiti, as well as physical and verbal violence were used. Apparently by December 1988 it became impossible for women to walk around Gaza without wearing some form of headcovering.

In North Africa, especially in Algeria, there is still greater and more open pressure on women to wear *hijab* and not to appear in public without wearing suitable garments. According to one leaflet: "The *hijab* is a divine obligation for the Muslim woman: It is a simple and modest way to dress, which she has freely chosen" (Moghadam 1993:153). At the same time there was a movement to stop women using public transport, because men and women were not separated on buses and trains. In many cases this pressure has taken on a violent aspect. It is reported by the Algerian writer, Djura, for example, that one member of the *Front Islamique du Salut* (FIS) burnt his younger sister alive because she did not wish to give up her work as a nurse and take on a traditional Islamic role for a woman namely mother and home maker (Djura 1994:117).

Many Algerians have objected to the introduction of *hijab* or the 'black veil', because they regard it as the imposition of an Eastern (Arabic) way of dressing upon their own traditional forms of costume. As noted in Chapter 5, the traditional city clothing of Algeria was made up of a *haik*, a long length of material which was often of a soft, light silk which was embroidered. Some women felt they were being forced to wear "the large, black mantle" which reached down to their feet (Djura 1994:127). Further it was felt by some that:

"The fundamentalists involved themselves in endless discussion about the ideal length, colour and form of the veils in place of being busy with basic problems facing people ... Now was all the very feminine clothing changed for the long, black veils" (Djura 1994:127).

The extreme nature which the veiling question has taken in Algeria can be seen in the fact that a number of women have recently been killed because they were not veiled. One such example is the case of a 16-year old student called Katia Bengana. In February 1994 she was shot dead by Mefta because she was not wearing *hijab* clothing. In revenge, the Organisation for Free Algerian Youth put out a statement that for every woman who was killed because she was not wearing a veil, twenty veiled women and twenty "beard wearing fundamentalists" would be executed (Amnesty International 1995:45). Shortly afterwards two veiled women were shot dead at a bus halt.

In conclusion, *hijab* clothing can be seen as a religious statement, but it should also be seen as the result of traditional practices, financial considerations, peer pressure, politics, and the desire by women to work with its related social prestige. In some instances women freely accept *hijab*, but there are also examples where this is not the case and these usually involve threats, violence or even death.

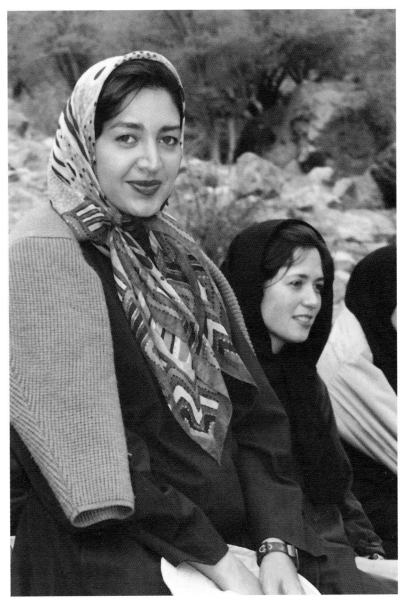

Figure 114. Two Iranian women (Sahar Khosravani and Lisa Barjesteh) wearing headscarves (courtesy of L.A.F. Barjesteh van Waalwijk van Doorn).

Notes:
53 The sets include a head kerchief (*mandiil*), a head cover (*muqnah*) and face veil (*burqa`* type).
54 The veil was abandoned by many urban women in Egypt in 1919 following the return of the feminists Huda Sha'arawi and Saiza Nabarawi from a women's conference in Rome. On arriving at Cairo railway station they tore off their veils in order to participate in anti-British demonstrations. See Philippi 1978.
55 Sabra Chartrand, "The veiled look: its enforcement with a vengeance; *New York Times*, August 22, 1991.

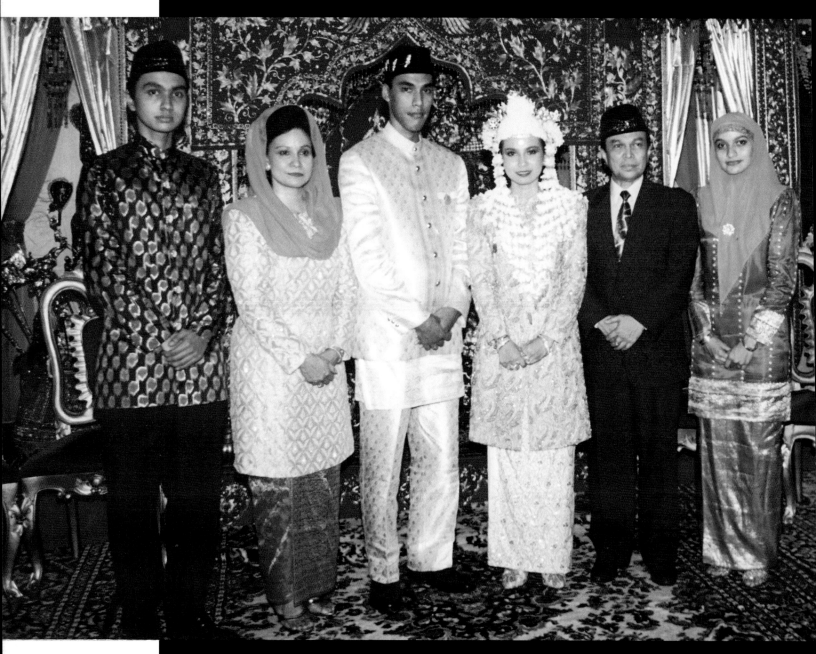

*A bride and bride's family from the Aceh
region of Java (courtesy of S. Wurian, Leiden).*

Some of the reasons given for veiling

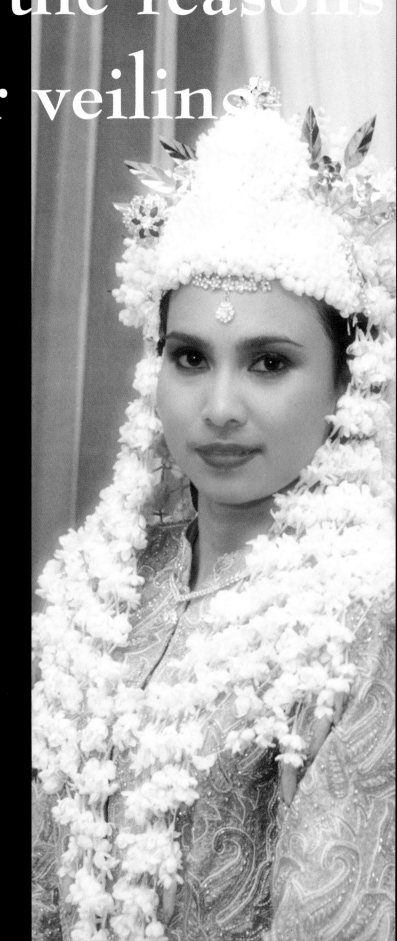

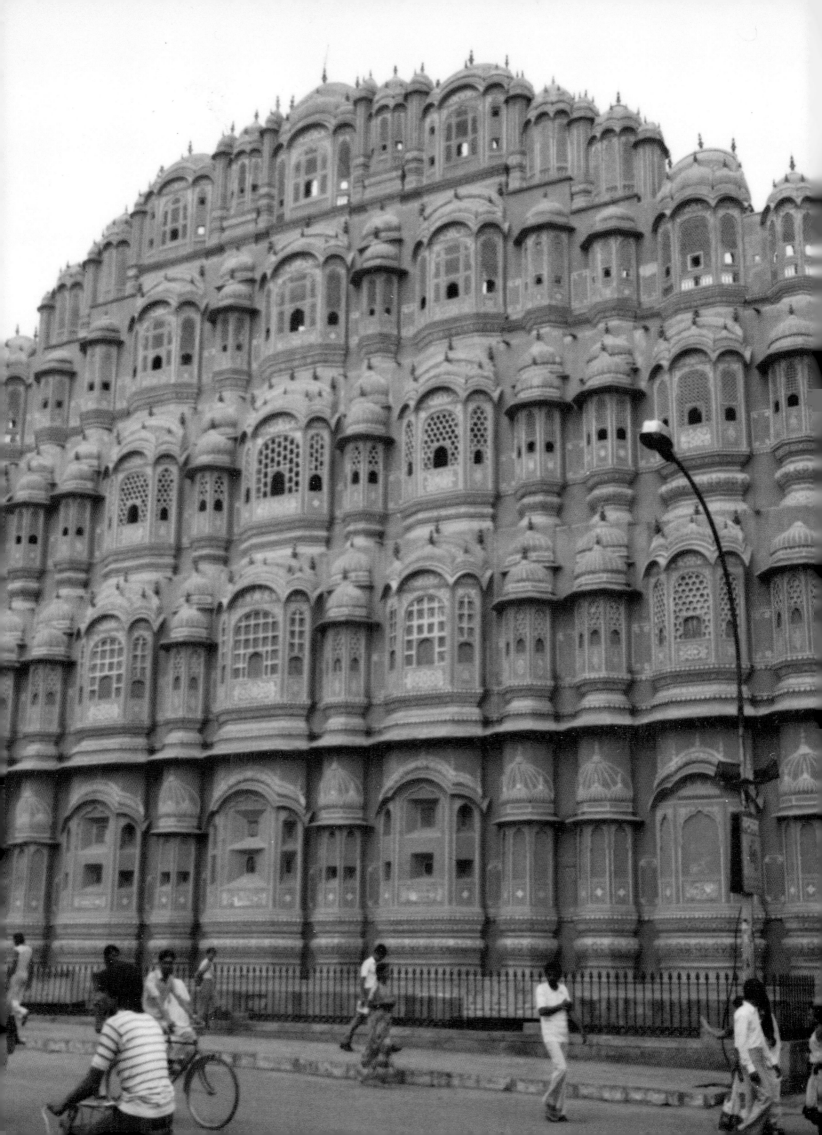

Chapter 8

Veiling, honour and seclusion

Throughout the world various methods have been developed to separate the roles, positions and living spaces of men and women (fig. 115). In some cases this is done out of economic necessity, in other examples, however, the structure of society may be based on a particular system which only endures because of the accepted dominance of one group over another. One such type of society is particularly associated with veiling, namely, the patriarchal society.

Patriarchal societies

Before discussing the influence of patriarchal societies upon the use of veiling it is first necessary to define a patriarchal society. This is not as easy as it may seem, as there are numerous definitions which appear to depend upon the social, political and sexual nature of the definer.[56]

In general, a patriarchal society can be seen as one whereby the public authority to make decisions is held by the oldest, 'acceptable' males. Within a family unit this usually means that the grandfather or father takes responsibility for making all the major decisions which affect the life of the family group. Further to this, a patrilinear family is one whereby the authority, property, wealth, goods, of a family descend through the male line of a family, usually with the oldest male taking the lead. In some cases this means the father, or father's brother, in other societies, it is the mother's brother. Finally, patrilocality means that the centre of the family lies with father's or father's brother's family unit. For example, a bride would become a member of the husband's family, rather than the other way around.

It is no coincidence that the veiling of women is especially prevalent in strong patriarchal societies where a woman is generally seen as someone who is dependent upon the male members of her family.

Ironically, because of a woman's ability to bear children they are sometimes seen as a threat to the patriarchal society. This situation appears to have arisen because there is the need to identify the father of a child and that the father acknowledges the existence and legitimacy of the child. At the same time, too many girls can threaten the structure of a family because as brides they move away from the family thus weakening it. As noted by Lila Abu-Lughod: "The family is as strong as the number of male members who make it up" (Abu-Lughod 1988:122). As a result of a woman moving to another group there is also the possibility of divided loyalties. Often, a bride who is not a direct member of the family (such as a first cousin, preferably from the father's side) remains an outsider, someone from another group or tribe.

One way of removing the threat of women and their potential fertility is to hide it behind an actual and symbolic cover, the veil. Lila Abu-Lughod noted in *Veiled Sentiments*, that:

Figure 115. *The harem area of the "Rose Palace", Jaipur (courtesy of J.I. van Waning).*

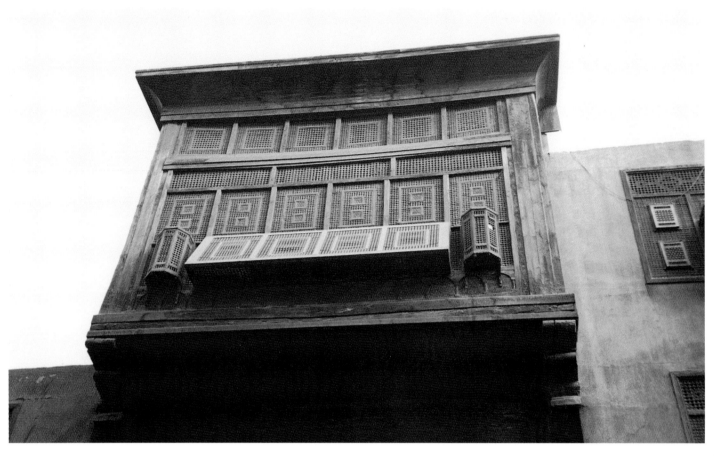

Figure 116. A so-called harem window from the old quarter of Cairo (courtesy of N. Monastra).

"Sexuality is the most potent threat to the patrilineal, patricentered system and to the authority of those who uphold it ... to show respect for the social order and the people who represent it, women must deny their sexuality. They do so by denying sexual interests - avoiding and acting uninterested in men, dressing modestly so as not to draw attention to their sexual charms, and veiling. By distancing themselves from secularity and its antisocial associations, they escape moral stigma and gain the only kind of honor open to them: modesty, the honour of voluntary deference" (Abu-Lughod 1988:165).

Thus, the concept of gender seclusion is a fundamental aspect of veiling, both for men and women. As a generalisation, women are veiled in order to express their modesty and to hide their sexuality. Men are expected to respect and support women who behave in this manner.

Modesty and honour
The concepts of 'modesty' and 'honour' are important elements in the reasons given for the veiling of women. Exactly what constitutes modesty and honour varies according to the differences in society and rank, for example, urban versus rural, settled versus nomadic. However, again as a generalisation, an honourable male (within a strong patriarchal society), may be seen as someone who is independent of character, assertive and fearless, and totally in control of his emotions. On the

other hand, women are expected to show deference, modesty, self-control and even shyness, especially when in public. A woman has to have a social sense of self-control, and not only show that she knows her position within any social group, but that she can act in a reasonable, well-behaved manner. Thus, a respectable woman knows how to act properly in social life, knows when to speak and when to listen and is at all times deferential, especially to her male relatives. In some communities, small-scale businesses are allowed such as fruit and vegetable growing, rabbit or chicken raising, sewing, weaving, but enterprises which involve considerable travel or contact with strangers (men) are not normally encouraged.

As a result of these and similar influences, it has become accepted that women have to be controlled in order to minimise their chances of contacts with outside men. As a part of this control, the myth developed that women are a source of evil and sexual temptations which need to be kept strictly within set limits. The traditional story of Adam and Eve is a prime example of the temptress myth, whereby Eve persuades Adam to eat the apple from the Tree of Knowledge. As a result, they were expelled from the Garden of Eden and women came fully under the control of men:

"To the woman he [God] said, I will greatly multiply your pain in childbearing; in pain you shall bring forth children, yet your desire shall be for your husband, and he shall rule over you" (Genesis 3, 16).

In the Koran the category of control of a woman by a man is further extended by the list of males whom she may come in contact with after puberty. This list is based on Sura 24:30

> "... their husbands, or their fathers, or their husbands' fathers, or their sons, or their husbands' ones, or their bothers, or their brothers' sons, or their sisters' sons ... or such men or children who have not yet attained knowledge of a women's private parts".

In a more extreme commentary on the above passage, the Pakistani religious writer, S. Abul A'La Maududi, notes that women were only allowed to be seen by a limited circle: "so as to reduce to minimum the chances of emotional excitement or sexual anarchy on account of the female charms and decoration" (Maududi 1979:187). Further to this view, Maududi is of the opinion that all women should be kept firmly within the bounds of their family home and not allowed out, except to go to Mecca.

In certain Islamic groups strict limits have been set concerning where a woman may or may not go. These limitations are based upon a Koranic verse where it is written that the wives of the Prophet should: "Remain in your houses" (Sura 33:33).

According to one of the *Hadiths* or Traditions, it was noted that Hazrat `Umar, one of the women of the Prophet's household, was seen coming out of her house by the Prophet. He commented that it was only permitted to go out of the house in cases of genuine need. Inevitably, the interpretation of what constitutes genuine need varies. Another *Hadith* notes that it is better for a woman not to go to a mosque, but to offer her prayers in her closet or better still her hiding place. As a result of these and other traditions, it has become acceptable in some Islamic groups for women to travel outside of their family home on only three occasions, when they are born, when they are married and finally when they die. The frustration some women feel with this situation is reflected in a poem called *The Journey* by Atiya Dawood, a modern Sindhi poet living in Pakistan:

> The journey of my life
> begins from home,
> ends at the graveyard.
> My life is spent
> like a corpse,
> carried on the shoulders
> of my father and brother,
> husband and son.
> Bathed in religion
> attired in customs,
> and buried in a grave
> of ignorance.

In some Muslim countries it is normal for a women who wishes to travel any distance to be accompanied by a *mahram* or guardian who is a close male relative. According to various *Hadiths* it is unlawful for a woman to travel more than one night alone; one day and one night alone, or three days or more without a *mahram*. In Saudi Arabia a woman normally has to ask the permission of her husband if she wants to go out of the house. Written permission is required for her to travel any distance. At all times, however, she is required to be veiled.

Similar travel restrictions can be found throughout the Islamic world. Nevertheless, such strict concepts as noted above for Saudi Arabia do not always work and many societies do not follow it. Nowadays, the visible control placed upon women is shown by what they wear, for instance, by women being veiled or by the wearing of *hijab*. In the past, however, attempts to seclude and isolate women have led to the idea of the 'harem' and '*purdeh*'. Veiling when outside of the house is regarded as a way in which the apparent safety and security of *purdeh* is maintained wherever a woman goes.

Seclusion

Seclusion has developed in many regions of the world among urban upper and middle class groups as signs that women from these groups did not have to work and in order to keep them away from strangers. As an extension of these ideas, there is the time-honoured view that the public world is the domain of men, while the world of women is the home. In due course the concept developed of male/family honour and its relationship with female modesty. In addition, the concept of social differences based on 'class' developed, so that a line was drawn between the roles of slaves who filled menial or sexual roles, women who performed non-domestic and domestic labour, and upper class women who did not have to venture outside of the home.

The idea of gender seclusion is not only found with Islamic beliefs. Proselytes within Christian monasteries and convents, for instance, are traditionally deliberately and strictly separated. Indeed, postulant nuns are often described as 'taking the veil'. Such seclusion should be seen as an attempt to separate the mind and body from outside, admittedly usually sexual, forces, which could act as a distraction to the development of the spiritual aspects of a person.

The harem and purdeh

The form and level of sexual and, more specifically, female seclusion varies from country to country. In some regions it is a question of a woman having to wear a 'modesty covering' of some kind over her head and hair. Until very recently, for instance, there was a tradition in Western Europe and America whereby no 'respectable woman' went outside without her hat, and many female Christians still wear some form of headcovering on a Sunday or in church. In other societies, sexual seclusion has become more rigid, with separate areas of a house for men and women (the traditional harem) fig. 116. In more extreme cases once inside such an area women were not allowed out under normal circumstances (the system of *purdeh*).[57]

Although the perception of the 'harem' belongs to the Middle East, it should be noted that the idea of a women's area in a house is not restricted to this region or indeed to the Muslim world. Such restrictions, for example, are also found in countries such as China and Japan.

The origins of these segregated areas are ancient and examples can be found throughout the Mediterranean region, including ancient Egypt and the Near East. In ancient Greece, especially Athens, for example, it is known from written sources that women were deliberately secluded. A man called Euphiletos, was charged with the murder of his wife's lover. As part of his defence he gave a description of his house and the fact it has separate areas for men and women:

> "My dwelling is on two floors, the upper equal in area to the lower, comprising the women's apartments and the men's apartments" (Lysias I,9).

There is also archaeological evidence from Greece concerning the way in which ancient houses were built (Walker 1983). Ground plans of various excavated buildings show that the men's apartments, especially the *andron* or gathering/dining room, could only be approached from the lower court yard, which left the rest of the house accessible to the female members of the household.[58] A more recent example of gender segregation within a house can be seen in Mali among the Dogan (Bedaux, pers comm.). There is a clearly defined male and female areas of the house, part of which is only accessible though one doorway which was guarded.

In the Middle East the region of the house which is regarded as the women's quarters is known as the *harem*. The word is derived from the Arabic word *haram* meaning 'unlawful', 'protected' or 'forbidden'. The sacred areas in and around the holy cities of Mecca and Medina, for example, are *haram*, forbidden or closed to all but the faithful. Similarly, the eating of pork and the drinking of alcohol is regarded as *haram*.

Nowadays, the term *harem* often applies to the man's wife, as well as women and servants associated with the quarters set aside for her. In some cases the harem will include the wife(s), children, unmarried daughters of the house, male and female servants, as well as temporary female visitors.

Depending upon the economic circumstances of the family, the harem may only be made up of a room with a curtain across it or several rooms plus a courtyard. Within such an area the female members of the family may be expected to carry out various jobs, such as child care, food preparation, cleaning and maintenance of the house and personal possessions, as well as tasks such as spinning, sewing, weaving and embroidery (fig 117).

In larger establishments the harem area can be a large complex, especially if the head of the household tries to keep to the Koranic instruction that every wife has to be treated equally:

> "... marry such women as seem good to you, two, three, four; but if you fear you will not be equitable, then only one" (Sura 4:3).

This statement is generally taken to mean that each wife should have quarters of equal standing and receive objects and gifts of equal worth.

The word *purdah* is to be found in both Urdu and Persian *(pardah)* and means a curtain. It has come to mean a system for secluding women by veiling and physical seclusion and enforcing high standards of female modesty in much of South Asia (Papanek 1973:289). For example, according to the anthropologist, Hanna Papanek, there are various types of *purdah* systems in northern India (Papanek 1973:289; 302). The traditional form of Hindu *purdah* is related to affine relatives, thus women are veiled in their husband's homes, but not in their natal homes. In addition, veiling begins at marriage. On the other hand, Muslim *purdah* is related to males outside the immediate trusted circle of kin. Veiling normally begins at puberty. A woman's modesty is enforced by several methods such as seclusion, for example, the physical segregation of the living space; by covering her face and body, and by the strict control placed upon a woman's movements.

As noted previously in this chapter, according to Islamic traditions a woman has to ask for permission in order to leave the harem or home, even if it is to visit her own family. Normally, permission is granted as long as the woman is discreet and dresses correctly (Papanek 1973:310). Nevertheless, due to various reasons, permission may be refused and in some long-term cases this means that a woman becomes mentally and physically isolated (see Chapter 11). But it should be stressed that this is not always the case, especially if the extended family is both large and supportive, in which case the system of seclusion provides the necessary companionship and strength.

It was noted by Satareh Farman Farmaian in her autobiography, *Daughter of Persia*, that the Iranian compound which was her home was about one kilometre long and contained nearly one thousand people (Farmaian 1992:18-20). Within the compound there were various subcompounds which were closely guarded and only men who were near relatives were allowed in. Nevertheless, these areas included kitchens, laundries, gardens and outdoor pools. Her family not only consisted of:

> "... our father and mothers and brothers and sisters and other relatives who lived in and around the compound, but all the other peoples inside our walls: our nannies, our *lalehs* or male caretakers, the cooks,

guards, porters, stewards, secretaries, artisans, old military pensioners, and everyone else my father supported" (Farmaian 1992:20).

As all of the people were part of her extended family, in theory she was able to wonder through the compound without a veil. However, because of the possibility of strangers being present all of the women tended to wear a *chador* of some kind.

In some societies there is considerable, permitted, movement between houses within a street or area, as the women are allowed to visit each other, in other countries the amount of movement is severely restricted. Unni Wikin in her work on a small community in Sohar, Oman, noted that most women were constantly visiting neighbours and friends, albeit in some cases within a comparatively small area (Wikan 1982:120). In addition, itinerant vendors (always old women) were considered welcome visitors, both for the goods they had for sale and the chance to listen to the news.

Ironically, because of the system of extended families which gives women the chance to develop social contacts with other women, the life of these women is often far richer than that of women living in the West. Yet this way of life is all too often portrayed within the cliche of the poor, suppressed, isolated harem female.

Radio and Television

In recent years the introduction of radio and more recently television (including videos, cable and satellite) has meant that an even greater number of films and programmes have become available. In The Netherlands, for example, it is predicted that by the year 2000 there will be over 400 channels available via the cable and satellite. The introduction of these forms of communications into many North African and Near Eastern villages and even nomadic groups has caused a major upheaval in the lives of everybody.

In closed societies where traditional life was the norm, questions were seldom asked about alternative ways of life. The advent of television, however, has meant that real and fictitious lives outside of the local community can be seen and heard. In some cases the division between reality and fiction can be drawn, at other times this is not so simple. It was noted by Carla Makhlouf, for example, that when television was first introduced into Yemen: "some women who were watching television for the first time were caught by surprise by the appearance of the male newscaster and hurriedly veiled" (Makhlouf 1979:61).

The presence of television in Yemen also meant that the women had other subjects to talk about (Makhlouf 1979:161-3). But one of the consequences was that the traditional round of daily life, household work in the morning and formal visiting in the afternoon, was disturbed. Some women simply preferred to watch a particular series on the television. Another result of the

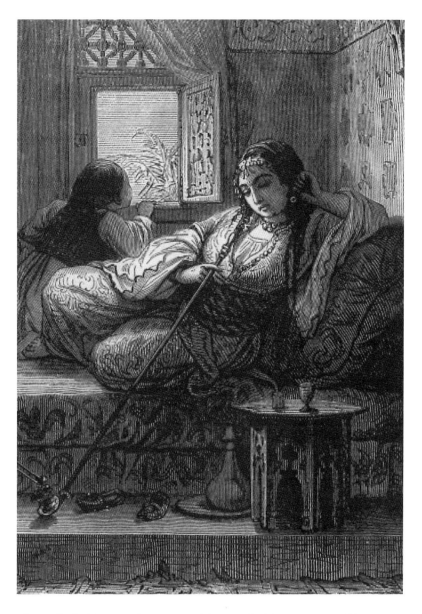

advent of television was that women without a television were placed at a social disadvantage as they could not talk about the latest happenings in a particular soap opera.

With respect to veiling, the introduction of television has meant that a much wider world has become apparent, one in which other women can be seen who are not veiled and who appear to have much greater freedom and happiness. Inevitably comparisons are drawn which lead in some cases to discontent with traditional ways of life.

Some countries, notably Iran, have tried to ban certain videos and the use of satellite dishes in order to prevent the 'Western Invasions'. Nevertheless, the removal of the television or the censorship of programmes will not remove the desire to see the 'forbidden' way of life.

Figure 117. A group of Egyptian women in a harem (from Lane 1895:190).

Notes:

56 See for example, Lerner 1986,15-35; 238-240; Abu-Lughod 1988:78-117.
57 For a discussion on purdeh, see Papanek 1973.
58 Lacey 1980:170; Walker 1983:81.

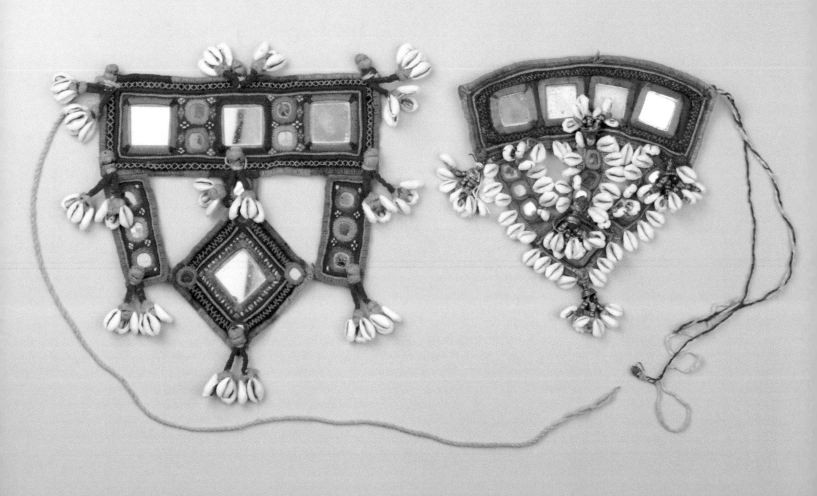

Chapter 9

Identity and anonymity

Earlier chapters of this book included a survey of the various types of veiling which have been developed in various parts of the world. In the last chapter, the concepts of seclusion, chastity, honour and their roles in the concept of veiling have been discussed. In this chapter, an indication will be given about how veiling can be used as a means to identify a person, both physically and emotionally. In order to do this, identity is taken to mean a method which shows who a woman is. This does not simply refer to her name, but also the range of information given by her clothing, especially the veil, about her family and social status.

Anonymity, on the other hand, can be associated with the desire or need to remain as anonymous as possible.

Dress and Identity

"So when the woman saw that the tree was good for food, and that it was a delight to the eyes, and that the tree was to be desired to make one wise, she took of its fruit and ate; and she also gave some to her husband, and he ate. When the eyes of both were opened, and they knew that they were naked; and they sewed fig leaves together and made themselves aprons" (Genesis 3:6-7)

After the 'Fall' of Adam and Eve the first thought of the transgressors seems to have been linked to the realisation that they were naked and that they had to cover themselves. Since this 'event', people's garments and the variations in their dress, have become important signals and symbols which can give considerable information about the wearer.[59]

As may be expected, the range of information available is considered to be greater with respect to traditional and ethnic clothing.[60] Yet, although there is a growing trend to wearing Western style dress (in particular, shirt and tie for men; dress, skirts or trousers with a blouse for a woman), this so-called 'cosmopolitan' clothing still presents hints at the origin of the wearer based on cut, material, combinations and accessories (for example, jewellery and make-up; fig. 118). Such data include clues as to gender, age, status, cultural identity (both geographically and historically), the prevalent climatic conditions (for instance, arctic versus tropical), as well as a person's link with a specific community. Dress is also often used as an indication of the general social position of the person within a particular society. It can indicate a person's past, present and potential future prestige, as well as political or spiritual power. Dress is also capable of serving as a sign that an individual belongs to a specific group, while at the same time slight variations (for example, by the use of lace or embroidery) mean that there is the possibility of differentiating an individual from the group.

Finally, dress, including the materials used, types of garments and accessories, can be seen as a symbol expressing a person's or group's economic position.

Figure 122. North Indian veil (RMV 5868-1,2; photo. by B. Grieshaaver).

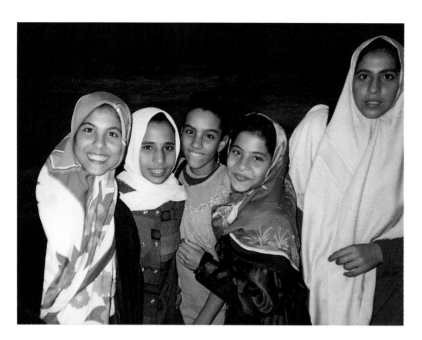

Figure 118.
A group of Egyptian girls wearing various clothing types (photo. by N. Monastra).

Male versus female

As with most societies there are written and unwritten laws about what is regarded as suitable clothing for women and for men. So when Jean Paul Gautier presented men's skirts (as opposed to the very male kilt worn by the Scots), at his spring 1995 fashion show in Paris, there was considerable derision, especially in the press.

Yet, while there have been numerous proscriptions against men wearing women's clothing, there would seem to be much fewer regulations concerning women wearing men's garments. Nevertheless exceptions do exist. Within fiction, for example, there are numerous stories whereby men dress up as women in order to enter forbidden places and to have clandestine meetings with their beloved ones. But these are usually accounts of love, so some adventure and (temporary) disguise is permitted.

It would also seem that desiring to belong to a higher status (namely male) can be acceptable, especially by a foreign woman. For this reason, when the Swiss adventurer Isabelle Eberhardt (1877-1904) dressed up as a man, called herself Si Mahmoud and frequented the male world it was tolerated, although sometimes only just (Eberhardt 1992 ed.). Indeed, she was not allowed to enter the company of Arabic women, although everyone recognised the fact that she was female.

In some Muslim communities where women are expected to be veiled and where homosexuality is tolerated, it is not unknown for homosexual men to follow a different set of clothing rules. In the region of Sohar in Oman, for example, there is a group, locally called the *khanith*, who are regarded as neither male nor female. Instead they are seen as a "third gender" (Wikan 1982:168). The word *khanith* apparently carries: "a sense of effeminate, impotent, soft ... (and that they are) ... socially classified with women with respect to the strict rules of segregation" (ibid 24). As a result of this classification, the life of the *khaniths* can be seen as a compromise between being male and female. They have the legal rights and duties of a man, but they can also talk with women on the street, go to weddings and partake in female festivals. According to Unni Wikan, she even saw one *khanith* lifting the veil of a bride:

> "I was witness to a man casually making his way into the bride's seclusion chamber and peeping behind her veil! But no one in the audience took offense. Later that night, the same man ate with the women at he wedding meal, where men and women are strictly segregated" (Wikan 1982:168).

Khaniths are often recognisable by the clothes they wear, which again is a compromise between male and female clothing. In general, men in the area around Sohar wear a white *dishdashas* (an ankle-length 'shirt'). The female version of the *dishdashas* has a low waist line and is made from brightly patterned cloth. *Khaniths*, however, tend to wear the *dishdashas* of a man, but with a 'female' waist line. The cloth used for this garment is unpatterned, but pastel coloured.

Although *khanith's* may be allowed to wear many elements of female clothing in public, they are not allowed to wear totally female garments, nor are they allowed to assume a woman's face veil. One of the reasons given for this by Wikan is that many *Khaniths* are also prostitutes, and to allow a prostitute (male or female) to wear in public full female clothing would be to dishonour the concept of womanhood (Wikan 1982:178).

Thus at a very simple level the wearing of some form of headscarf, mantle and more especially a veil is used in many Middle Eastern societies to indicate that the wearer is female. This concept is sometimes taken one step further to mean that she was or is nubile.

Cultural identity

It was noted by Andrea Rugh in her book about Egyptian clothing called *Reveal and Conceal* (1986), that the traditional garments worn by a woman indicate that others can identify her with a specific village, economic position and even religion (Rugh 1986:vii-viii). Unfortunately, it is not possible in this chapter to describe this part with regard to veiling. Nevertheless, some comments should be made about various aspects of the concept of cultural identity.

As was shown in previous chapters there are considerable variations in the forms of head coverings, face veils and overwraps. The use of different types of veiling as a cultural identification can also be found in modern (Western) cartoons.

The first example is a political cartoon drawn just after Margaret Thatcher's, the then Prime Minister of Britain, whirlwind visit to the Near East in 1985 (fig. 119). She is shown after her return to London sleep walking while wearing an 'Arabian' style costume complete with face veil.

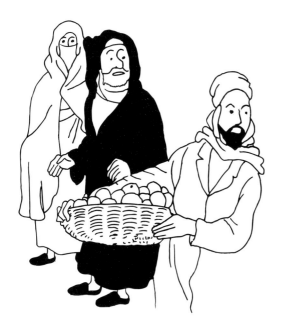

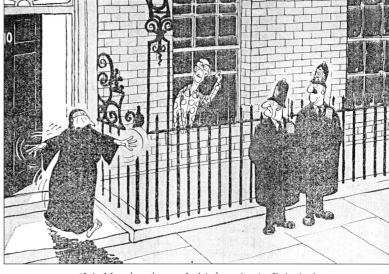

'It's Monday dear – I think we're in Britain.'

The next two examples come from strip cartoons, namely, a story about Tin-Tin (Kuifje) and one about Elno. In the *Crab with the Golden Claws*, the hero, Tin-Tin, is in North Africa. The veiled women who appear as incidental figures in the background are accurately dressed in order to give an air of authenticity (fig. 120). In another, more recent cartoon called *The Mechanical Camel (De Mechanische Kameel)*, the heroine is a left-wing Palestinian whose family has moved to Saudi Arabia. She is normally unveiled, except when she visits her father (fig. 121). The villein of the plot, on the other hand, is a veiled woman from Saudi Arabia who wears a black face-mask and *abaya* while carrying a gun with sleeping gas (Vervoort 1991).

The basic types of traditional veiling (not including *hijab*) to be found in North Africa and the Near East can be seen in Map 2. The wearing of veils during the nineteenth and twentieth centuries is contained within a wide band which does not reflect the extend of the Islamic world. It is also noticeable that in countries where leather clothing is common, such as North America and the Sub-Arctic regions, the veiling of women does not take place, although there are strong patriarchal societies within these regions.

In North Africa the *lithma* is the most common type of face veil, which is usually worn with an *izar* or *huik* of some form. In Syria, Palestine and Egypt, there are considerable variations on the theme of the *burqa`* and *niqab*. As a generalisation, those worn in urban areas tend to be of a mono-coloured material. On the other hand those worn by Bedouin women are usually decorated with coins, beads and chains.

There is a marked change in the veils worn in the Arabian peninsula. In general those worn by urban women are more enveloping and often opaque. The veils worn by nomadic women reflect their more active life and

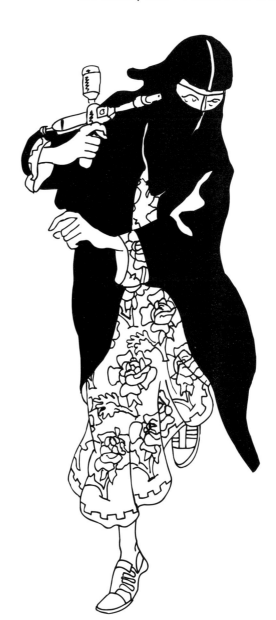

Figure 120.
A cartoon figure based on the Tin-Tin (Kuifje) strip cartoon Crab with Golden Claws.

Figure 119.
A cartoon showing the then British Prime Minister dressed in 'Arab' clothing (Daily Mail Monday, April 15, 1985).

Figure 121.
A cartoon figure based on the strip cartoon book De Mechanische Kameel (Vervoort 1991).

tend to be short, with greater emphasis on the need for visibility by the wearer.

By the time veiling reaches eastern Iran and Afghanistan it has changed dramatically. The combination of veil and chador has produced the all enveloping *chadri*. In areas of northern India, however, where there is a strong preference for colourful, outside ornament and decoration, the masks worn by many Muslim women are more reminiscent of those worn in Palestine than in Afghanistan. The veils from the Kutch region of north India, for example, are heavily decorated with embroidery, shells, and even mirrors which reflect light and colour (fig. 122).

The migration of an ethnic group to another region can have an effect on the type of veiling worn. For instance, there have been strong links between the Arab Batinah coast and the eastern part of the Arabian peninsula with southern Persia, the Makran coast and hinterland. Many of the inhabitants of the southern shores of the Gulf are of Persian and Baluch origin. According to the Norwegian anthropologist, Unni Wilkan, about thirty percent of the population in Sohar can trace their descent from Persia and Baluchistan (Wikan 1982:108).

The type of veil worn in southern Persia until comparatively recently is very similar to that worn in Oman. Whether the *batalu* type of veil (see page 60) went from the Gulf states to Persia or the other way around is uncertain, but it would seem more likely that the movement was from Persia southwards.

Nowadays with the influx of immigrant workers in the Gulf, a woman with a *burqa* is instantly recognisable as a native of some part of the Gulf, and thus a woman of tradition.

Social status
There are various parallels between social status and the type of veiling. These parallels have been discussed in great detail by a number of authors, but certain aspects need to be highlighted here. Namely, the use of veiling in urban regions; differences between nomadic and settled peoples, and finally, the use of veils by slaves and ex-slaves.

Veiling in urban settings
As a generalisation, the veiling of urban women is determined by three main elements: firstly, a settled urban community, secondly, sufficient income within a family to support non-earning members; thirdly, that there was an available labour force large enough so that servants were available for non-working veiled women (Papanek 1973). It should also be noted that in many Islamic countries there are various social levels within which veiling does not normally take place. Lower class women, for example, do not normally veil, nor do upper class women. Instead it is the various levels of middle class women who are normally veiled.

In nineteenth century Egypt, for example, female members of the ruling family were expected to be veiled in public, but not in private. On the other hand it was normal for the *fellaheen* women (the peasants) to be unveiled in both public and private. The women in between were normally veiled.

Similarly, in Oman it would seem that the highest and lowest women on the "ladder of social esteem" were not expected to be veiled. In this case, the highest are represented by members of the Sultan's family (Wikan 1982:96). They represented about six families in Sohar. In addition, the women of several Sohar families who aspired to higher office and those who were of Muscat origin were not veiled.

As will be seen in Chapter 12, the historic movement towards unveiling in the east was usually organised by the government of the day. Members of either the royal family (as in Iran) or that of the presidents (as in the case of Turkey) were expected to be the first to go unveiled in public.

In many families there is a desire by lower middle class groups to move upwards. Nowadays opportunities for education and better jobs, usually within the government, mean that this is possible for women. One of the signs of this upward movement is that women are prepared to be veiled as a public sign of their growing family's position:

"Because this dress [hijab] does not reduplicate the outfits of traditional urban women, but forms a new style, it allies women with modest middle-class women and further differentiates them from lower-class women ... Further, dressing in Islamic clothes tends to dissolve the more obvious differences in dress between upper-middle-class and lower-middle-class women" (Macleod 1991:134).

However, because upper class women tend not to be veiled and can afford expensive materials, the gap between middle and upper class remains too large for most women.

Finally, it was noted by C. Makhlouf in her book about the changing role of women in Yemen, that the outdoor clothing of the women living in the Yemeni city of San`a reflects their social position (Makhlouf 1979:30-1). There are two outdoor garments worn in this region, the *sitara* which is a large piece of cotton printed in red, blue and green (see fig. 54) and the *sharshaf* which consists of a black skirt, cape and face veil (see fig. 56). Normally women of the lower social classes wore the *sitara*. On the other hand, women from more wealthy families wore the *sharshaf*. Women in the middle groups, however, tend to wear the *sitara* on informal occasions, but the *sharshaf* on more formal visits.

Nomadic versus settlement veiling
In addition to the points made above about veiling in urban settings, it is necessary to note whether the veil is

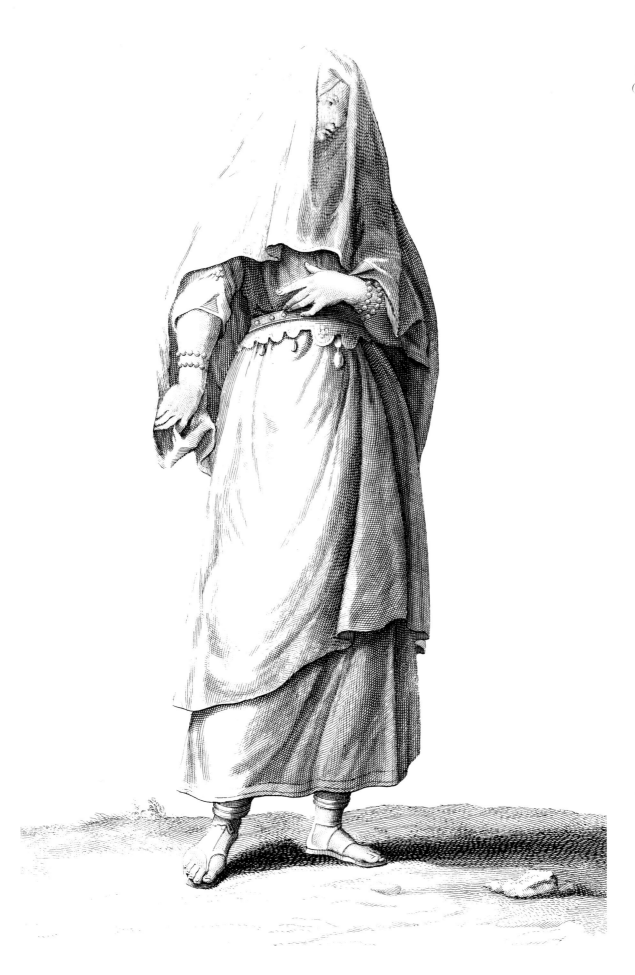

Figure 123.
Jewish woman by
De Bruin c. 1700
(private collection).

A group of Armenian
nuns wearing veils
across their lower
faces, c. 1885
(Hotz collection,
11:59; courtesy of
the Library, the
University of
Leiden).

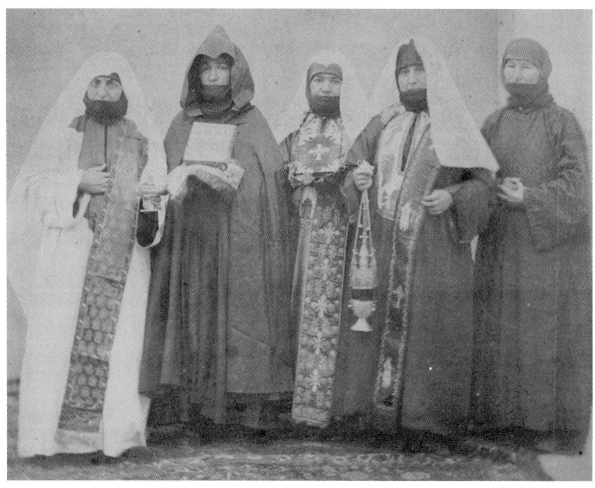

solely regarded as a method of secluding a woman or whether it is used as a means of beautification as well. This point is also relevant when looking at the veils worn by nomadic women as opposed to peasant or lower class women who tend to be unveiled. In Saudi Arabia, for instance, the veils have large mask forms which cover the face while leaving the eyes free so that work can be continued. The veils (*niqab* and *burqa`* forms), are plain in appearance and act as a defence. On the other hand, Bedouin women living in the Eastern Mediterranean and eastern Egypt, have a very different form of veil which emphasises their personal and family wealth. It is not uncommon to find the complete dowry of a woman literally on the woman's face (see fig. 2). These 'veils' thus show the fact that the wearers are respectable, married and financially independent, all at the same time. It is worth noting that cheaper copies of these veils use false coins, sometimes of Turkish forms or English sovereigns, as a means of decoration.

Slave versus free person

As early as the mid-second millennium BC a difference was made between those who could and could not be veiled. In Chapter Two ancient Mesopotamian laws were cited which stipulated that slaves were expected to be unveiled while their mistresses had to be veiled in some manner. A slave who wore a veil could be severely punished. This division between slave and free person and what they may wear continues to this day. Within the Gulf region, for instance, slavery was only officially declared illegal in the 1950's and there are still a large number of ex-slaves alive.

While Patricia Holton was staying with female friends in the United Arab Emirates, she asked them why they wore veils (Holton 1991:250). They were quick to point out that it was not in the Koran. To the contrary: "good and faithful women walk with their face uncovered". However, they did not follow this injunction and wore a veil. When asked why, Holton was told that there were numerous stories and she was given various versions. One story was that there was once a king who was constantly looking for beautiful girls whom he took back to his castle where they were raped and kept as slaves. In order to protect their womenfolk, the men said they had to wear the *burqa`*. In this way the king did not know who was beautiful and who was ugly. It was also suggested that the king was "Allesander", meaning Alexander the Great. Another reason given for the wearing of the *burqa`* was that it separated slaves from free women. "The slave always had a naked face for all to see and sometimes a naked body when selling [sic]. Wives and daughters must separate themselves from this" (Holton 1991:251).

In Oman, slaves were traditionally forbidden to wear any form of face veil, as the *burqa`* was seen as the prerogative of free women. Slavery was banned in the country a generation ago, and nowadays ex-slaves may wear a veil if they wish to. Yet according to Wikan very few of these women now wear a veil (Wikan 1982:96).

Wikan further noted that in the Omani town of Higra it was not the custom to wear a face-veil (Wikan 1982:96). It would appear that this situation developed because prior to the 1950's the Sultan's family representing him in Sohar lived at Higra, with a large number of slaves. Nowadays, there is a large number of high ranking men and women in the town, as well as a large ex-slave population. As a result, the majority of Higra women go unveiled. Nevertheless, when one of these women visits another town or region, then, for politeness sake, they tend to be veiled.

Finally, it is worth noting that among the Touaregs of North Africa, male slaves and members of slave families are not veiled. The only exception would appear to be freed slaves who sometimes wear veils. However, according to Richard Murphey in his article about the use of veiling by the Touaregs, the veil of a free man is normally worn covering the mouth and nose when in the presence of a man of higher social status, including his parents-in-law (Murphey 1964:1267). The veils worn by slaves, however, are placed over the chin and mouth indicating their lower social position.

Christians and Jews

One factor which is often forgotten about women in Muslim lands, is that non-Muslims are also often veiled in public (fig. 123).[61] Indeed, there are Egyptian laws dating back to the medieval period which make it clear that women had not only to be well covered when in public, but that they also had to wear specific colours. Muslim women, for example, were expected to wear white garments, Jewish women had yellow ones, while Christians used blue and Samaritans red garments.[62]

At the beginning of the twentieth century, it was normal in Baghdad, Iraq, for both Christian and Jewish women to be veiled and wear face veils and *izars* when in public (Marmorstein 1954:1). In addition, above their eyes they would wear a projection stuffed with hemp which sloped downwards to cover the eyes and the face. This vizor-like object was called a *hailiya* (probably from the word *hayal*, shadow), and was intended to offer further 'protection' for the wearer.

It is also worth noting that during the late nineteenth century, Armenian nuns living in northern Iran also wore face veils as part of their habit (fig. 124).

Finally, in many traditional Near Eastern countries, such as Iran, Iraq and Saudi Arabia, all women have to be covered when in public. The religions of women either living in these countries or even just visiting them is not taken into account, they have to be veiled on entering the country.

The language of the veil

There is considerable personal information which can be obtained by looking at the different sorts of veiling. At one level the type of veil can say something about where a woman comes from within one country. It may also be used to indicate a woman's mood at a particular time.

It was noted by Sir Flinders Petrie (1853-1942), for example, that the women of the Egyptian Delta wore different types of clothing:

> "In the west, the women wore a long robe and no face veils; in the middle region they had a short tunic and very baggy blue or bright red trousers to the ankle, visible a mile away, and face veils varied; in the east the robe is like the west, but they all have yellow face veils" (Petrie 1931:65).

Petrie was not known for his like of women or interest in textiles, so for him to have noticed these differences means that they were apparent. Sadly, nobody at this time seems to have recorded the smaller variations in dress within the Delta region. In a recent discussion about the garments from the Delta, however, A. Rugh in her book on Egyptian dress, described how the form of the dress, the method of working the yoke, even the way in which the sleeve of a traditional dress is decorated can say something about which village a woman comes from (fig. 125; Rugh 1986:44-5). In addition, she notes that variations in veil types and how they are worn can tell

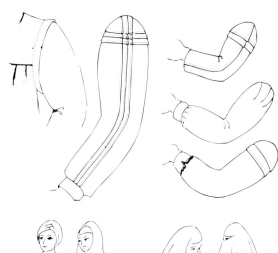

Figure 125. Different forms of sleeve constructions from traditional Egyptian dresses (after Rugh 1987:45).

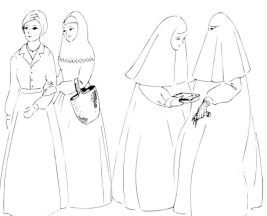

Figure 126. Different forms of modern dress in Egypt (after Rugh 1987:150).

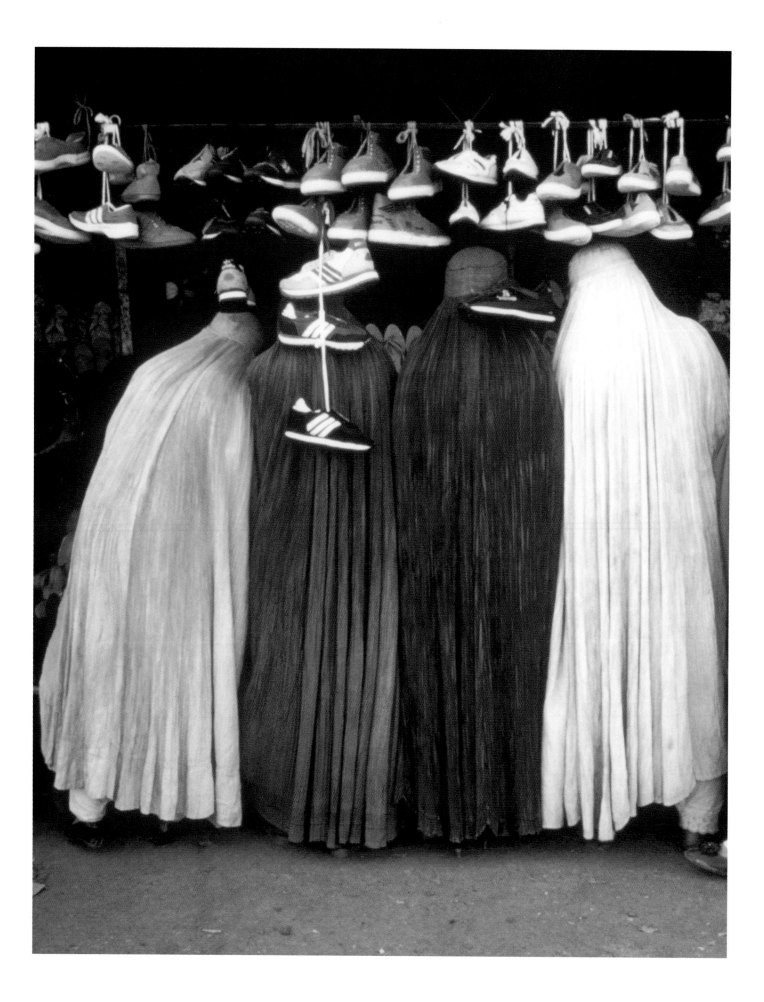

something of the religious beliefs of a person. With respect to *hijab*, for example, there is a difference between a fashionable form, that worn by a fundamentalist and the *hijab* of a pious woman (fig. 126). Thus, the combination of veil type plus traditional dress starts to give a much clearer picture of where a woman comes from and says something about her religious beliefs.

In addition to being a signal for modesty and respectability, veiling can be used in combination with body language to indicate a woman's mood, approval or even disapproval. Wikan noted that the women of Sohar in Oman adapted their face mask or *burqa`* (*batalu* form) to fulfil their own needs:

"They [Sohar women] wear it in all-female gatherings, whether in the role of hostess, guest, or informal friend. But I was rarely able to predict what a given woman would choose to do, thereby singling out the factors that determine this behaviour. One day, in the company of her best friends, chatting or embroidering, a woman may sit unveiled; the next day, she may let her *burqa* cover her face. Her choice of behaviour seems to depend solely upon the way she feels at a given moment - and Sohari women acknowledge the force of such feelings in influencing a person's behaviour. One day, a woman may feel relaxed and secure, happy to expose herself to the world; the next day, she may be uneasy and shy, desiring to keep the world at a distance. The *burqa* gives her welcome assistance" (Wikan 1982:95).

Another writer, Veronica Doubleday, agreed to be veiled while she was living in Herat, Afghanistan:

"Wearing a veil in public initiated an important and subtle change in me, cultivating an aura of modesty and self-containment. It masked my foreignness, enabling me to join many women's outings where I would otherwise have attracted undue attention, and it brought a welcome privacy. It was also fascinating and salutary to discover that being invisible is addictive" (Doubleday 1988:10).

She started veiling at the suggestion of some (female) Afghan friends in order to give herself some privacy when she was out walking in the city. She bought some Iranian cotton with a small flower print and had a *chador* made for herself:

"A few days later the veil was ready. I tried it on, putting the straight edge of the semi-circular cloth on to my head and letting it fall around my shoulders and body ... The women smiled in approval, admiring my new elegance."

"I forced myself to wear it the following day on my quiet ten-minute walk through uncrowded residential suburbs ... I knew the awkward moment would come when I

reached the bottom of Shirin's alley, where unruly children gathered. Surely I would be an object of ridicule, a foreigner dressed as an Iranian! As I approached, I steeled myself for the usual taunts and cries."

"Look! The foreigner's wearing a veil", the call went up. "Here she comes."

"I gave the boys a withering look which Heratis call 'a sour forehead' and uttered a curse, which shocked them into silence. My veil seemed to win me respect."

"*Wah, wah*! Congratulations!' said Shirin. "It looks good, and now you'll be freer. People won't bother you so much."

"Ironically this symbol of oppression had liberating aspects for me, since it minimised the difference between me and the Afghan people. I was freer, less bothered in crowds. If men stared I had only to pull the side of my veil around my face, indicating displeasure, and they had to respect my wish to be left along" (Doubleday 1988:64-5).

In addition to showing disapproval in the street, it was recorded by Makhlouf how the use of a veil could provide a certain degree of distance between two people. She cites the example of a woman whose maternal cousin wanted to marry her. In order to discourage a relationship she did not desire, the woman started to wear a veil in his presence, although this was not strictly necessary as he was a close relative (Makhlouf 1979:35).

A number of other Western women have adopted the veil, not out of religious conviction, but out of necessity. Later when they were in a position to go unveiled they described their feeling of nakedness when not wearing a veil of some kind. Zana Muhsen, who was living in Yemen at the time, described her feelings as follows:

"I was still wearing the headscarf, I couldn't quite pluck up the courage to take it off. I would have felt naked without it" (Muhsen and Crofts 1994:210).

Similarly, Betty Mahmoody wrote:

"My reaction to shedding my hated *chador*, the black fabric designed to cloak Iranian women from head to toe was bizarre ... I felt strange going bareheaded. It was as awkward for me to uncover in Michigan as it had been to cover in Iran" (Mahmoody and Dunchock 1992:19).

It should be noted, however, that the use of veil language is not restricted to women. As noted above, Murphy has described the use of the face veil by free and 'slave' male Touaregs in North Africa (Murphy 1964:1263-9). He further wrote, that the veil was worn once a boy reached

Figure 129. An 'anonymous' group of women shopping in Afghanistan (photograph by S. McCurry; courtesy of the National Geographic Image Collection).

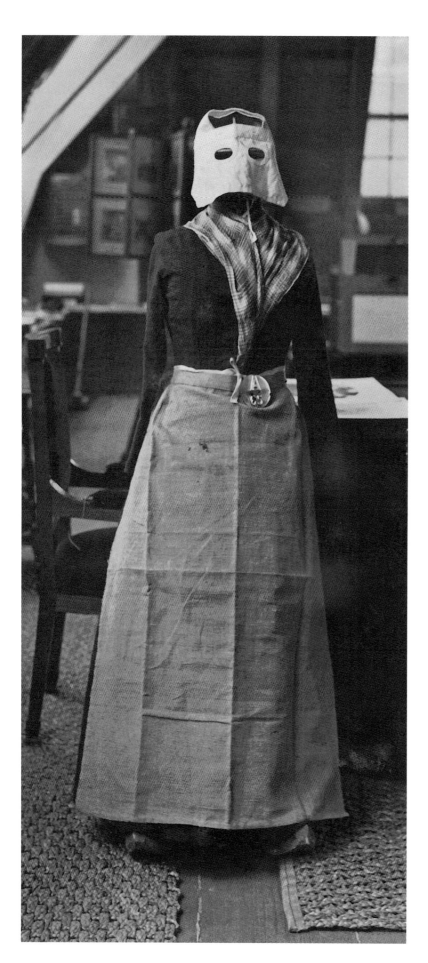

the age of puberty and as a sign of male honour. These veils are worn all the time, even while sleeping and eating (Murphey 1964:1263). Part of the face covering is only allowed to 'slip' down the face, leaving the nose and mouth uncovered, when talking to someone of a lower status. When with friends, even close acquaintances, the veil remained in place.

Anonymity

The desire or need for anonymity is to be found in many societies and for many different reasons. At a superficial level the wearing of masks by such groups as the Klu Klux Klan of North America is one of the best known examples of the use of cloth or garments to provide anonymity. During the late nineteenth century in The Netherlands, for example, both male and female convicts were expected to wear a veil or mask (celkap) across their faces, especially when in public or having their photograph taken (fig. 127; Lissenberg 1991). Similarly, there were special areas in Dutch churches for prisoners who were screened off from the rest of the congregation. Whether, however, this was to protect the convicts or the congregation is not clear.

In many countries not even the name of a wife may be spoken in public, in order that no man may say her name and thus claim a relationship with her of any form. An example of this desire to protect a woman's name, and thus her and the family's honour, can be seen in a recent article about a fashion show in Oman, whereby the lady who opened the show was simply called: "the wife of His Highness Sayyid Fahd bin Mahmood al-Said" (Anon. 1993:30).

The concept that a woman should not be made into a public figure by portraying her caused many problems when the use of photographs in passports became essential. One way around this was to have someone else pose for the photographer. This solution was adapted by Hassan Mazloumi Barjesteh when it became necessary in the 1930's for his wife to be photographed. Although the figure in the photograph is wearing a chador, it is not his wife who posed for the picture, but a female servant (fig. 128).

At first glance many veiled women from the Near East appear to be totally anonymous with no indication of who is present under the cloth (fig. 129).[63] As a result, there are numerous (Western) comments about a veiled woman being so heavily veiled that even her husband would not be able to recognise her.

> " The women wear the universal loose, baggy gown, of white or dark blue cotton, and over the face a white mask in which is a small openwork space for the eyes. The disguise is so complete, that one might pass his own wife or sister in the street without recognising her" (Fogg nd:172).

The idea of total anonymity and indeed humility of movement to the point where the woman becomes virtually invisible has also been noted by a number of authors. When the Rev. E.W.L. Davies, for instance, wrote about the women of Algeria, he described them as ghosts:

"and, lastly, fair Mauresques, enveloped in snowy attire, who, were it not for the beautiful eyes whose sparkle cannot be veiled, might be mistaken for ghosts passing to and fro silently and mysteriously among the human crowd, but taking no part in its affairs" (Davies 1858:77-8).

In another example, written at the beginning of the twentieth century, echoes the same thoughts as those of the Rev. Davies. This time, however, the description is about some Persian women. Two travellers, Eustache de Lorey and Douglas Sladen wrote:

"To complete the gloominess of the picture, the women, who are the flowers of our crowds, are in Persia black, shapeless phantoms stealing silently along in the shadow of the walls ..."
"In the crowd were a number of the black phantoms; they were true daughters of Eve, some of them, for they lifted the white veils, which hung over their faces a little, to watch. But no torturing of my imagination could poetise creatures as void of form as the earth on the day of its creation" (de Lorey and Sladen 1907:2,3)

Yet are such women actually as anonymous as indicated in the quotations given above? Or is it ignorance of the local dress codes which makes the 'ghosts' appear anonymous? C. Makhlouf discussed this point in her study of a group of women from Yemen:

"The veil does not prevent women from recognising friends and relatives in the street or from chatting together when they meet. Women can identify one another through various signs such as differences in stature and particular mannerisms. By moving around the women, I began gradually to learn how to recognise people without seeing their faces. Moreover, for someone acquainted with the culture, the veil itself can express subtle differences, such as those between the various social categories, especially with respect to wearing the *sharshaf* or the *sitara*. There are other outward indicators of status, such as the very material used for the veil. Even though the *sharshaf* is always black, the material can be of good or bad quality and it can be plain or embroidered with black flowers. Also the black skirt can be made to appear more or less fashionable; one young woman had it cut slightly differently (a little tighter and longer) so that it looks, as she said, like a fashionable 'maxi' skirt" (Makhlouf 1979:32).

A similar observation was made by Veronica Doubleday in her book about the lives of three women in the Afghan city of Herat:

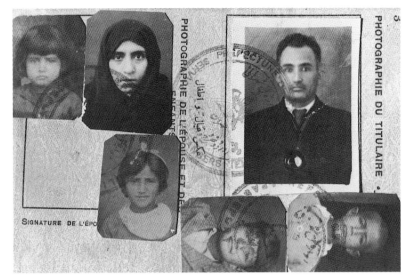

"Herati men claimed they could tell a great deal from seeing a woman dressed in her veil, and later I became attuned to these subtleties. One noticed the style of shoe and the cut and cloth of the trousers that showed beneath the *burqa* hem, and one could appreciate a woman's posture and gait and judge her figure, especially if the veil was smart and tightly pleated. A woman's opulence and sense of fashion were revealed by the quality of her clothes, especially the veil itself" (Doubleday 1988:3).

However, as noted by Makhlouf, if a woman wants to remain anonymous then the veil can be used as an effective disguise, especially if the wearer deliberately alters her normal pattern of behaviour and clothing (Makhlouf 1979:33).

Figure 128.
A group of photographs from an Iranian's passport (courtesy of L.A.F. Barjesteh van Waalwijk van Doorn).

Figure 127.
Clothing worn by a female Dutch convict, c. 1914 (courtesy of the Stichting Nederlands Foto- and Grafisch Centrum).

Notes:

59 For a general introduction to the subject of dress and gender, see Barnes and Eicher 1992. The problems associated with defining dress can be found in Eicher and Roach-Higgins 1992. For the viewpoint that clothes should not be approached as a 'language', see McCracken 1987.

60 For a discussion concerning the differences between traditional and ethnic clothing, see Eicher 1995.

61 There are various articles about the garments worn by Jewish women in Islamic societies. See Stillman and Micklewright 1992 for a review of such works.

62 The use of red for various items of clothing, including the face veil, may also have the connotation of prostitution at this time, so the choice of red for Samaritan women may have been deliberately insulting (Mayer 1943:302).

63 The other side of the coin is that should a veiled woman decide to have an illicit friendship then she would be freer to move around when totally veiled. Nevertheless, this is also one of the reasons why a woman's freedom of movement is severely restricted in some countries.

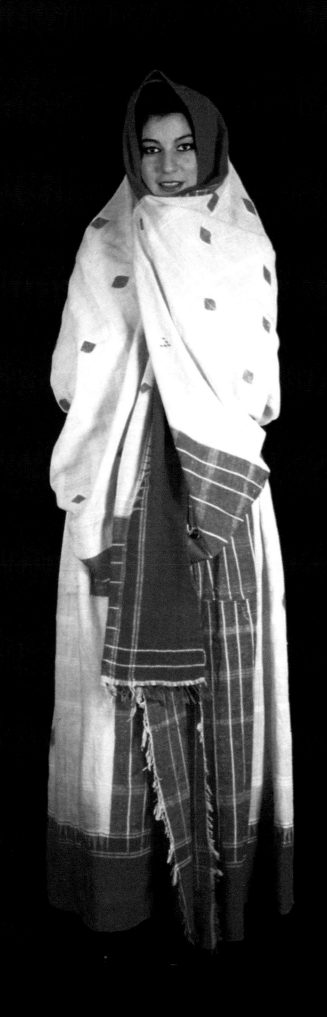

Chapter 10

Figure 134.
A Turkish outerwrap
or carsaf (from
Anon, 1986:31).

Rites of passage

A rite of passage is the term given to significant steps in a person's life. In Europe these are often seen as reflections of working life, for instance, passing the final exams at school, entering and finishing university, getting a job, retirement. There are also more fundamental and deeply engrained rites of passage which are shared by most societies. These rites are based on physical and mental changes. With respect to women these changes include, first menstruation, engagement, marriage, giving birth, menopause and finally, death.

In addition to the rites mentioned above which are basically of a physical nature, there are also certain rites which involve a change in the spiritual well-being of a person. The most important one of these with respect to veiling in Islamic countries is the *hajj* or pilgrimage.

Various ways are used to celebrate the various states in a girl's life. In south Tunisia, for example, a single length of material is dyed various colours and is used to indicate her passage through life. A head covering is called a *bukhnuq* and is woven by unmarried girls as part of their dowry (Buitelaar 1993:160). The cloth is woven to show their weaving skills (fig. 130). The main body of the material is woven in undyed wool, while there are border patterns in undyed cotton. As the cloth is woven in reverse it means that the weaver will not be able to see the results as she is working. After the girl was married the cloth was dyed red. The intention is that the wool will take up the dye while the cotton will resist it, so

leaving a white design on a red ground. Later in life the headcovering is dyed again, but this time in a more sober

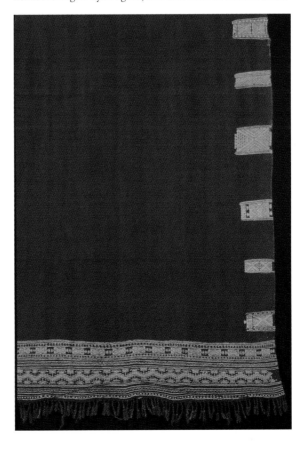

Figure 130.
A section of a cloth (bukhnaq) woven by an unmarried Tunisian girl. When it was woven the cloth was white, it was dyed red when she married and then blue as she had children (Volkenkunde Museum, Rotterdam, 69215).

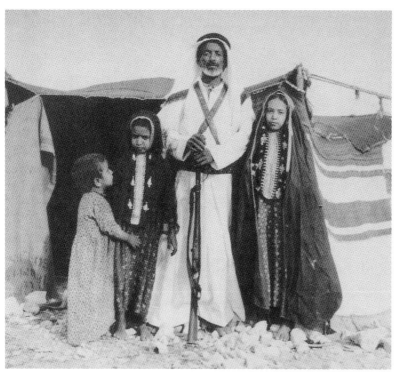

Figure 131.
A group of nomadic girls, the youngest is wearing a long dress, her sister has a long dress and bukhnaq, while her eldest sister is wearing a long dress, bukhnaq and abaya (from Ferdinand, 1993, fig. 8,30).

blue colour. In this way one length of material, used as a head covering, can reflect the different stages in a woman's life.

In other countries, marked changes in the garments worn by a female can be seen. These differences can be looked at according to the main rites of passage in a woman's life.

Babies and childhood

The veiling of a child does not commonly take place. In most countries the infant's head is usually covered, and its body may be wrapped or even swaddled, but the face is normally left uncovered.

The situation changes somewhat as the child grows and can take part in social activities. In some societies the stages of a girl's development can be seen in the garments which she wears. A young girl amongst some tribes of *bedouin* in Arabia, for example, wears a small cap or *quba`a*. When a girl is about eight or nine years old she is expected to wear the *bukhnuq* (this is not the same garment as the Tunisian item mentioned above), which is a large hood like garment made from a rectangle of material folded in half vertically and then sewn along the upper short edge (fig. 131). The wide end of the *bukhnuq* covers the head and hair and is usually worn to waist height. At the age of twelve or thirteen a second garment is assumed, which is *abaya* or sleeveless coat which is worn over the *bukhnuq*. At the onset of puberty these garments are changed for the adult woman's face veil and *abaya*.

Puberty

The moment when a girl actually starts to be veiled varies from one country to another. Normally, however, the onset of physical maturity, namely the first menses, is

marked by a change in both the conduct of a girl and what she wears. In ancient Greece, for instance, a girl was allowed to wear her first girdle at puberty (King 1983:120). The girdle was then dedicated to the goddess Artemis as part of the marriage ceremony. A similar usage of belts to indicate stages in a woman's life cycle can be seen amongst the *bedouin* women of northern Egypt who wear a belt or colourful kerchief when unmarried, which is changed to a red belt after marriage (fig. 132; Abu-Lughod 1986:145).

Another form of change in clothing during female puberty is more widespread, namely that of veiling. It should be stressed that the veiling of prepubescent girls is not required in all traditional muslim societies. Nevertheless, in some countries, especially where fundamentalism is strong, it is not unknown for girls as young as five to be veiled in some form. In Iran, for example, girls are legally required to start wearing a *chador* at the age of nine, although many are wearing it long before this age (fig. 133; Goodwin 1995:107). This age was considered by the Ayotalla Khomeini, when he was religious leader of Iran, as the time when girls were mature enough to be married. This choice of nine years old is based on the age of A'isha bint Abi Bakr (d. AD 678) when she became the Prophet's wife (Spellberg 1991; Goodwin 1995:36-8). A'isha was married to the Prophet when she was six years old, although she stayed at home with her parents for a few years. Her marriage was consummated when A'isha was nine or ten years old (her exact age is open to dispute).

In other parts of southwest Asia a girl is expected to start being veiled during or following the first menses. There are numerous official and unofficial ceremonies following the moment of veiling. In nineteenth century Turkey, the "Passing of the Veil" was the name traditionally given to the ritual when a (urban) girl first menstruated and from that day onwards her face was veiled and her hands gloved when in public (Croutier 1989:77).

In Saudi Arabia the onset of the first menses is also taken as the time when a girl/woman needs to be veiled as she has now become sexually mature.

"I had hidden the passing of my first blood from my father, since I was in no rush to swathe myself in the black garb of our women. Unfortunately, Nura and Ahmed decided that I had postponed the inevitable long enough. Nura told me that if I did not tell my father immediately, she would. So I gathered my friends around me, including Randa, and we made the mission to purchase my new 'life's uniform', black scarf on black veil on black *abaaya*.
Omar drove us to the entrance of the souq area, and we four young women disembarked, agreeing to meet him in two hours at the same spot....
We milled about the shops, hands examining the various scarves, veils and *abaayas*. I wanted something

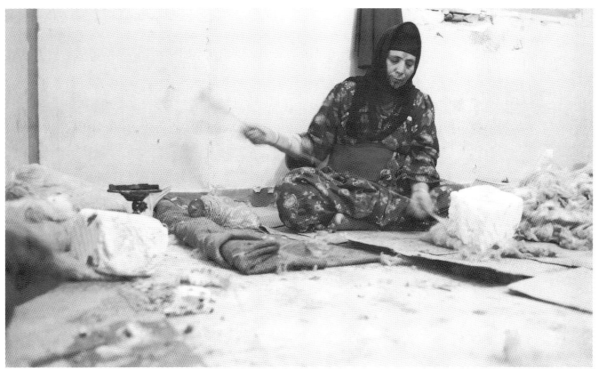

Figure 132.
*A bedouin woman
from Matruh,
Egypt, wearing the
red belt of a married
woman (courtesy of
N. Monastra).*

special, a way of being an original in the ocean of blacked-garbed women. I cursed myself for not having an *abaaya* made in Italy, from the finest Italian silk, with an artist's intricate designs, so that, when I breezed past, people would known there was an individual under the black covering, a woman with style and class ...
Life changed quickly. I entered the *souq* area as an individual bursting with life, my face expressing my emotions to the world. I left the shopping area covered from head to toe, a faceless creature in black" (Sasson 1993:107-8).

Girls in other regions of the Arabian peninsular also start to wear a veil before they are married. In Oman, for instance, girls may start wearing a *burqa`* before they get married if there is a significant amount of time (more than one year) before their first menses and their weddings (see below). The instance that a girl should wear a *burqa`* is usually done at the insistence of the parents who may feel that it would be shameful for her to be seen with "fully matured cheeks" (Wikan 1982:94).

Similarly, in other parts of Asia (notably northern India), it is normal for a girl to start wearing the *burqa`* when she is married. However, in some families there is family pressure to wear it earlier:

"When I was about 12, I became very tall, and my mother wouldn't let me go without a burqa. But I refused! For two years I never left our house ... In the end, I thought there was no point in carrying on like this any more. Staying at home makes people go mad - so I decided to wear a burqa only so that I'd be allowed to go out at all" (Jeffery 1979:156).

Sometimes, girls choose to wear the *burqa`* so that they feel more adult. In P. Jeffery's book, *Frogs in a Well*, there is a description of how one girl, in her late teens, lamented that she had started to wear the *burqa`* earlier and that she was now 'forced' to wear it:

"Then one day, I began to go out without my burqa, and my mother called me back. She was furious! How could I dare go out 'naked' like that! It was only then I realized what a silly mistake I'd made in ever wearing the burqa at all" (Jeffery 1979:156).

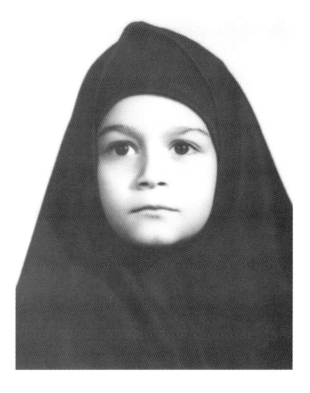

Figure 133.
*Iranian child
(Mariam Barjesteh,
6 years old)
wearing a chador
(courtesy of L.A.F.
Barjesteh van
Waalwijk van
Doorn).*

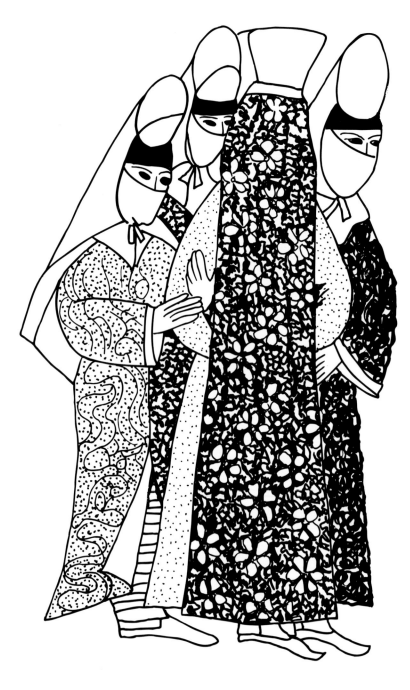

a similarly coloured headscarf was worn under the mantle in order to cover the head and hair.

A similar, shirred garment was worn by women in the Adana-Kadirli region of Turkey in what is now southern Anatolia (Gunay 1986:22). In this case, however, the outerwrap is also tied under the chin. Traditionally, this garment was given by a young man to his fiancee, and any woman seen wearing this garment was left alone as she was regarded as having been "spoken for".

Marriage

The tradition of a bride's face being hidden by one or more veils can be found in many societies. In some cases the veil is simply one thin layer of netting which can easily be seen through. In other cases, however, so much cloth is used that the bride has to be physically escorted to the wedding ceremony (fig. 135).

One of the most familiar aspects of a western style wedding is the long veil which covers the bride's face as she arrives in the church. Once married the veil is lifted and the wife's face is revealed. The tradition of veiling at a western wedding can be traced back to at least ancient Rome when the bride wore a bright yellow veil called the *flammeum* (La Follette 1994:55-7).

In medieval Europe no specific colour was reserved for bridal wear. Indeed the status of the bride and groom were expressed through the richness of their clothing. During the sixteenth and seventeenth centuries, the wearing of white was gradually becoming popular as the colour for a bride, as it was seen as a symbol of purity and virginity. However, it was not until the nineteenth century in Northern Europe that white was generally accepted as the ideal colour for wedding dresses. The wearing of a wedding veil only became common during the nineteenth century. These veils varied in size and shape, with the more familiar form of the long, trailing veil made of transparent net or tulle coming into fashion in the 1870's (fig. 136).

In the Near East the tradition of veiling a bride during the wedding ceremony can be traced back to at least 1300 BC. There are various indirect references in Hittite period (1400-1200 BC) literature which suggests that a full wedding lasted six or seven days and the veiling and unveiling of the bride took place at the opening and concluding celebrations (Stol 1995:125-127). It would appear that at the beginning of the wedding ceremony the bride was covered with a blue veil, presumably by her father or some other close male relative, with a (blue) veil. At the end of the celebrations the veil was taken off by her husband (Stol 1995:124). There are also two Hittite laws (nos. 197-8), which include a description of "the husband veiling the wife" which relate to the veiling of women and the role of a veil for the confirmation of a marriage after an accusation of adultery (Tsevat 1975). Again this stresses the importance of veiling as a confirmation of marital status for a woman.

Figure 135. An 18th century Turkish bride being escorted to her wedding ceremony.

Figure 136. A modern European wedding dress worn by Jacqueline Kanters-Plazier (courtesy of V. Kanters).

As can be seen from the above, when actually the wearing of a face veil is assumed can vary considerably from one community to another. In general, however, all women from veiling societies will have started to wear a veil by or at the time of their marriage.

Engagement

In some regions the wearing of veils and long outerwraps starts when a girl becomes engaged and thus associated with a specific man. In Amasya in northern Turkey, for example, it was traditional for middle aged women looking for a suitable bride, to wear a long length of material as an outerwrap (*corsaf*; fig. 134; Gunay 1986:31). In the centre (horizontally placed) of the cloth was a drawstring which was tied around the waist. Often

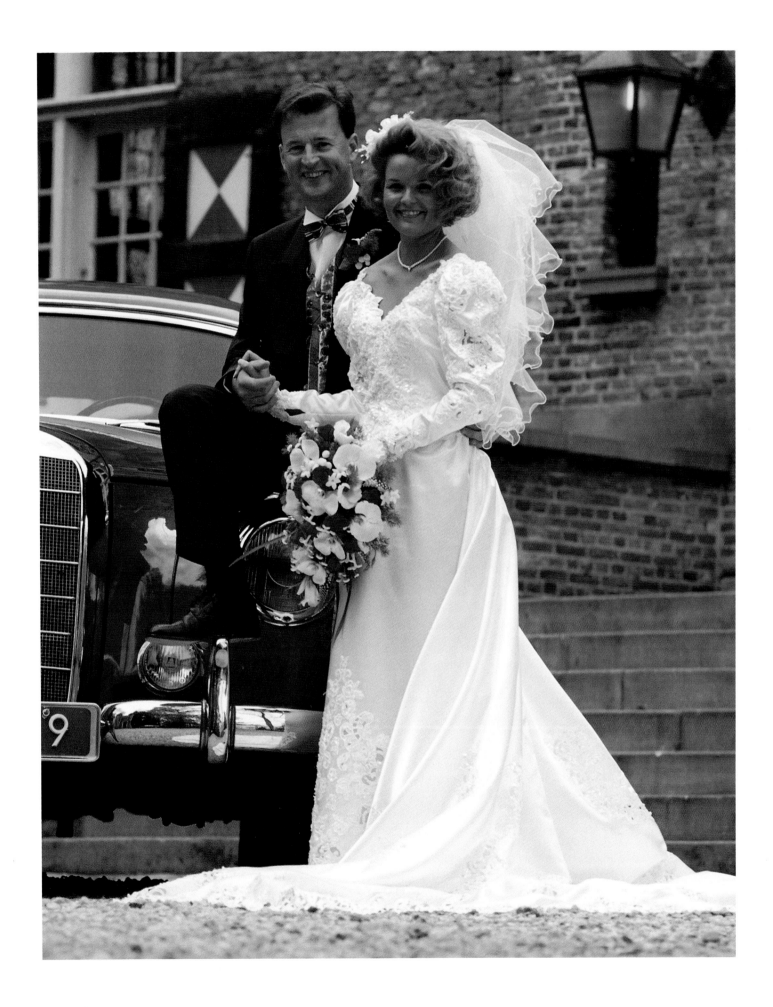

Figure 138. An outfit for a married woman from West Turkestan.

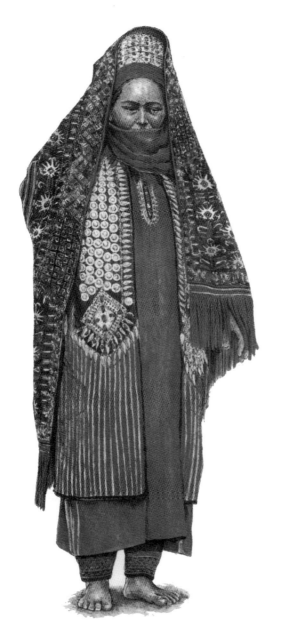

In some Middle Assyrian laws from Syria, a respectable, married woman is favourably compared with one who "wears no veil and has no shame", thus indicating that married women were veiled (Stol 1995:124).

Nowadays, there is a great variety of clothing designed for traditional Islamic weddings. Often brides wear ordinary style clothing, but made from new and expensive materials. In some countries such as Oman and Afghanistan, a green marriage shawl will be placed over her head (Wikan 1982:217). In parts of Oman, such as Sohar, a bride goes to her wedding wearing a formal *abba* (long mantle), a green shawl, as well as her normal dress, headscarf and long pantaloons (Wikan 1982:220). The bride and groom are kept in seclusion for a week. The bride is not expected to start wearing the *burqa`* or face mask until after the seventh day of her marriage (Wikan

1982:94). However, many women start wearing this garment by the third day. This is done as a sign of the fundamental change in status of the bride, namely, from girl to woman. In other areas the bride is expected to wear so many layers of cloth at the wedding that she needs to be physically helped because of both her inability to see and the sheer weight of material involved (fig. 137). Such is the case in Eastern Turkistan where a bride will wear an elaborate headdress (*bogmaq*), covered by a cloth (*chuba*; fig. 127; Stucki 1978:146). Traditionally it was worn for one year after her marriage, although nowadays it is usually worn for two months. In some tribal areas a beaded veil (*shärmenjä*; see page 54 fig. 63) is worn by newly married women (Stucki 1978:146).

There is a growing tradition in Near Eastern countries for brides to wear Western style gowns with net veils. These gowns are usually modified to fit Islamic concepts of modesty, for example, they have fitting, high necklines and long sleeves. In some areas of the Near East these gowns are now known as "Egyptian Dress", to separate them from their Western origins.

Finally, the way in which garments are worn can send out important messages which, if misunderstood, can lead to difficulties. Within the Shi`ite tradition of Islam, for example, it is possible to have a temporary marriage called a *sigheh* or *muta*. G. Brooks recalled how one day she was waiting for a female friend when she became aware of a young man following her and asking her something in Farsi (Brooks 1995:43). Later she learnt that the man had been asking her to marry him. It was explained that she had probably put her *chador* on the wrong way around, which is a signal used by Iranian women that they are looking for *sigheh*.

Married life

The clothes worn by married women can be dramatically different from those of either an unmarried girl or an 'older' woman. Among the Turkmen peoples for example, a married woman wears a coat (*brenjäk*) over her head which is made out of coloured material (fig. 138 see also figs. 95a-b).

Among the Awlad `Ali Bedouin tribe who live in northern Egypt there is a dramatic change in the garments worn prior to marriage and afterwards. The costume of an unmarried girl is made up of a long colourful dress with coloured kerchiefs around the heads and waists (Abu-Lughod 1988:17). During her wedding she wears a man's white robe (*jard*); after the wedding she wears a married woman's costume, made up of a long dress with two essential items, namely a black headcloth that doubles as a face veil and a red (the colour of fertility) woollen belt. The importance of these garments was stressed by Lila Abu-Lughod, who was living with this tribe for a while and was often told to: "wear a veil and a belt and you'll be a real Bedouin woman" (Abu-Lughod 1988:136).

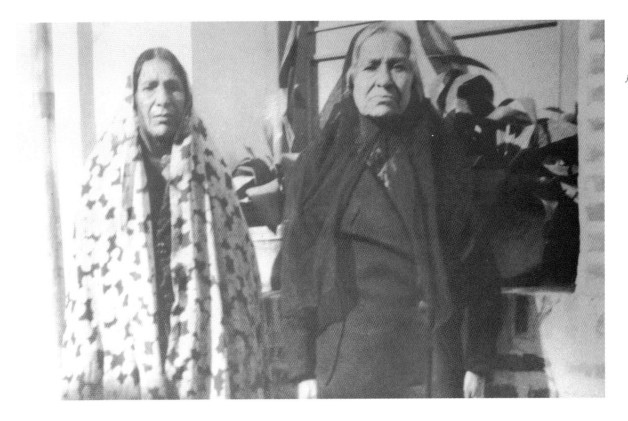

The use of a veil of some kind by married women is prevalent throughout traditional Near Eastern and south east Asian societies. Many rules and rituals concerning the persons to whom she may appear unveiled have developed throughout these regions (see Chapter 8). Thus even when standing in the house or taking a few steps down a path many women will wear their veils in order to show that here is a modest woman. It is also common for women to wear some form of veil ready for potential use, so should a male friend of the husband unexpectedly enter, the veil can instantly be in place.

Despite such restrictions and practices there are two consistent occasions when a married woman is expected to remove her veil, namely, when she is in front of God, for instance when she is praying, and when she is alone with her husband.

Inevitably, however, there are exceptions to these two occasions. If prayers take place while a woman is travelling, she may be excused from removing her veil if strange males are present and she is unable to pray in private. Exceptions to a woman unveiling before her husband may also take place if there is a conflict between husband and wife. Thus a woman can signal her strong disapproval in a particular situation by remaining veiled in her husband's presence.

Menopause

The menopause is an important time for many women and one which is not always looked forward to. In addition to the physical discomfort which its onset brings, the menopause also means that a woman's so-called productive life is now over. As a form of recompense, however, women are often looked upon as being less threatening and almost (but not quite) accepted as a male. As such, an older woman is often allowed to carry out more activities and given more freedoms.

With respect to clothing and veiling in particular, it is stated in the Koran that women who are passed childbearing age, can go with special outer clothing:

> "Such women as are past child-bearing and have no hope of marriage - there is no fault in them that they put off their [outer]clothes, so be it that they flaunt no ornament; but to abstain is better for them (24:60)

In societies where veiling is the norm, however, women continue to wear some kind of veil long after menopause, even though they are now regarded as 'safe' (fig. 139). Often, after wearing veils for much of their lives, women do not want to remove the veil when outside, as the veil becomes an integral part of their life. The wearing of a veil by older women can be seen, therefore, as a reflection of their own self-esteem.

Burial

There has long been a tradition in the eastern Mediterranean of burying the dead in their ordinary clothes and in some cases of covering their faces. Within eastern medieval Christian tradition a veil was sometimes placed over the face of the deceased. Such a cloth was found in the grave of Bishop Timothea who died in about

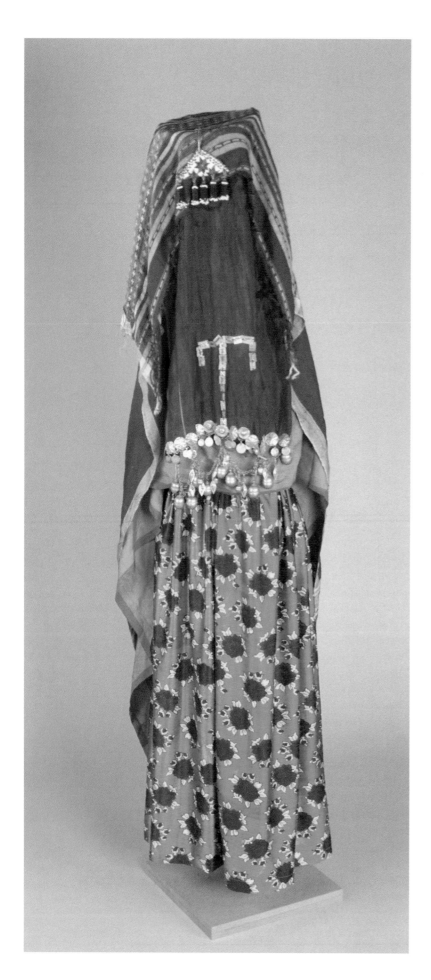

AD 1372 and was buried in the cathedral at the southern Egyptian site of Qasr Ibrim (Crowfoot 1977). A pale blue cotton veil was wrapped around the bishop's head and over his face. In addition, a cloth called a *mappa* was tucked into the line of the neck.

In some early Chinese communities, especially in the eastern regions, the deceased were provided with many grave goods, including clothes, and a special veil or mask with eye holes cut out of them. However, this custom was not widespread.

In Muslim societies there is another tradition whereby the deceased is covered or shrouded in one or more long lengths of white cloth, without other clothing (including veils) of any kind. After being placed in the grave it is believed that two Angels of Death (Moenkar and Nakir) come to the dead person, who should have his or her face uncovered so that they should immediately see and recognise these emissaries from Allah.

Mourning

Veiling and death come together when veils are used as an aspect of mourning and grief. It is common in many societies for relatives and friends of the dead to wear special clothing. There are numerous gradations of mourning, ranging from a set of clothing to a narrow arm-band in black. It is noticeable that in many societies women are expected to wear a wider range of mourning clothing than men and that these garments are worn for a much longer time.

In Victorian England, for example, there were elaborate rules and regulations concerning the type of mourning outfit to be worn and for how long. The type usually depended upon the relationship of the woman to the deceased, for instance, wife, daughter, cousin. The closer the relationship, the longer mourning lasted. Black has been the most usual colour for mourning in the West since Classical times. In other counties, such as Japan, white predominates.

The dress of a Western widow has traditionally expressed her loss and sadness, while the wearing of a veil over her face gave seclusion in grief and prevented her emotions from being seen. In addition, it meant that those attending the funeral would immediately recognise her as the bereaved and give special attention to her. In many Muslim countries, however, it is believed that the dead should be buried quickly and with a degree of joy because if they had been true believers they will speedily enter Paradise. In countries such as Saudi Arabia and Afghanistan women are not allowed to attend funerals, even those of other women. One of the reasons given for this exclusion is that the emotional state of the women would be a distraction to the (male) mourners and a discourtesy to the dead.

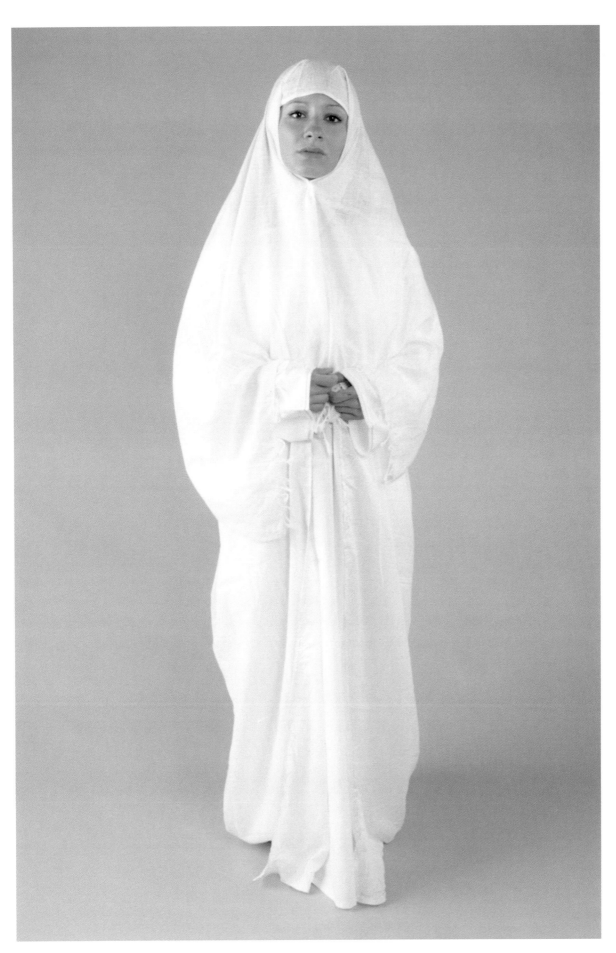

Figure 140. *Modern pilgrim's clothing from Egypt (RMV 5863-10,11; photo by B. Grishaaver).*

Figure 137. *A Turkeman's bride's outfit (RMV 5000-132; photo. by B. Grishaaver).*

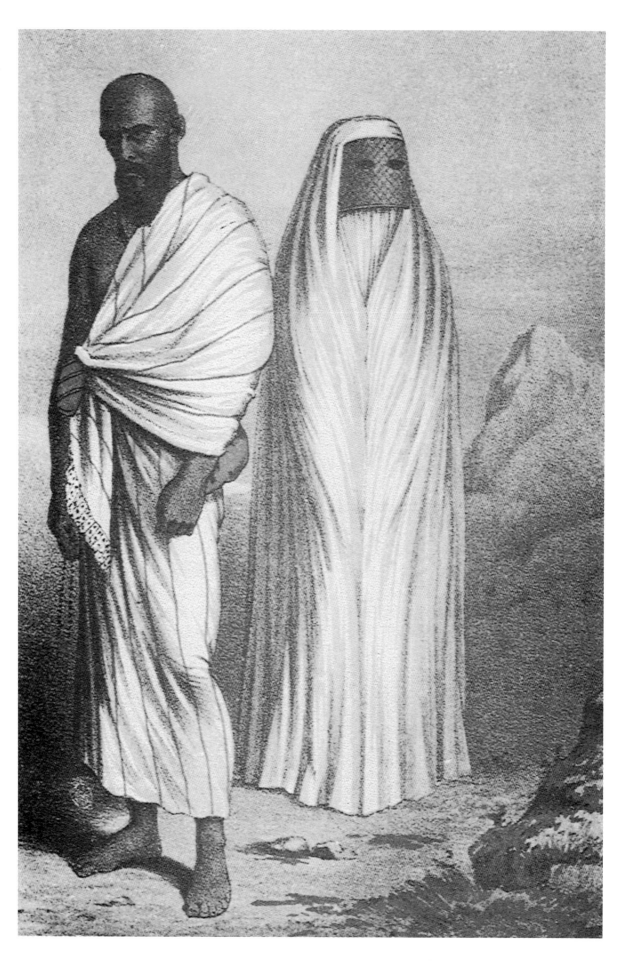

Figure 141.
Burton's pilgrim's clothing (after Burton 1893, II, fig. opp. page 139).

In other areas of the Middle East, however, women do attend funerals and there is the tradition of tear or renting their clothing as a sign of mourning. In some areas, including Egypt, women in mourning, especially a wife, are expected to wear black or dark coloured clothing, remove all jewellery and wear no make-up for a period of time, after which they may resume normal life (Abu-Lughod 1988:137).

The Hajj

Finally, it is necessary to look at veiling and a spiritual rite of passage, namely the Pilgrimage to Mecca or the *Hajj*.

The basic tenets which govern Muslim life are called the "Five Pillars of Islam". These are made up of five acts which confirm the faith of the believer. The first pillar is the public declaration that: "There is no God but Allah and that Muhammad is His Messenger". Secondly, Muslims must face Mecca five times daily and pray. Thirdly, they must pay tithes. Fourthly, they should fast throughout the daylight hours during the month of Ramadan, and fifthly, if possible, every Muslim must make at least one pilgrimage (*al-Hajj*) to Mecca, the holiest city of the Muslim faith.

The pilgrimage takes place during the month of Dhu al-Hajjah, and rigid rites govern both the trip itself and its religious climax. At the shrine, the devout circle the "Black Stone" or Ka'abah[64] seven times; they run seven times between two hills near the ancient springs, and they spend the ninth day of the month on the plains of Mount Arafat. The tenth day of Dhu al-Hijjah is called the Id al-Adha. It is celebrated throughout the Islamic world with sacrifice, prayer and feasting in memory of the prophet Ibrahim (Abraham). Al-Hajj is the greatest proclamation of faith a Muslim can make.

In addition to instructions governing the movements of a pilgrim's behaviour during the pilgrimage, there are detailed instructions concerning the type of clothing to be worn. Men are expected to wear the *ihram*, which consists of two simple pieces of cotton, linen or woollen cloth, without seams or ornaments. One of the lengths is wrapped around the loins (*izar*), while the other is thrown over the shoulders (*ridda'*). The head and feet should be bare. The rules governing what women wear are not quite as strict and in most cases they are allowed to wear their own clothing (fig. 140). However, it is required that their faces and hands should be uncovered. Although it is expected that the face will be uncovered, various methods have been found in the past around this rule.

In one set of instructions for pilgrims written during the nineteenth century it was stated that:

> "A woman may wear sewn clothes, white or light blue (not black), but her face-veil should be kept at a distance from her face" (Burton, 1893:II, 284).

In the 1850's Sir Richard Burton travelled to Mecca dressed as a Muslim. During his journey he noted that the wife and daughters of a Turkish pilgrim had changed from their normal clothing into special garments once they were officially on the pilgrimage:

> "They appeared dressed in white garments; and they had exchanged the Lisam [lithma], that coquettish fold of muslin which veils without concealing the lower part of the face, for a hideous mask, made of split, dried, and plaited palm-leaves, with two "bulls'-eyes" for light" (Burton 1893:II, 141).

Burton then went on to explain that the "ugly" (the mask) must be worn, because a woman's veil was not allowed to touch her face during the pilgrimage ceremonies (fig. 141).

Similar masks were noted by Th. W. Juynboll, in *Handleiding tot de Kennis van de Mohammedaansche Wet* (1930):

> "Toch plegen vrouwen zich ook bij de bedevaart meestal te sluieren. Dit is, volgens de wetgeleerden, strikt genomen niet ongeoorloofd te achten, mits zij haren sluier dan (door middel van eene soort van gevlochten masker) althans op eenigen afstand van het gelaat dragen, zoodat niet in eigenlijken zin kan worden gezegd, dat de sluier haar gelaat bedekt" (Juynboll 1930:134).

Another form of a pilgrim's veil includes a bent stick which goes over the head and projects in front of the face. This stick is used like a curtain rod from which a long white veil is hung. In this way no material touches the woman's face. One such example of a pilgrim's veil is now in the National Museum of Ethnology, Leiden (RMV 370.2992) and has a long veil which is decorated with metal thread (fig. 142a-b). The veil was purchased at the 1883 Colonial exhibition, and originated from the Aceh reigon of Indonesia.

Nowadays, it is regarded as totally unnecessary for a woman to be veiled when she goes on a pilgrimage, especially the main *hajj* to Mecca. There is a prevailing view that because both men and women have to be chaste and in a state of purity with their thoughts only on Allah, it should be unnecessary for women's faces to be veiled. Nevertheless, many female pilgrims still prefer to wear a headveil of some kind. Similarly, female pilgrims visiting less important Muslim shrines also tend to be veiled.

Notes:

64 The Ka'abah is covered in a large cloth called the *kiswah*. During the nineteenth century, the covering used for the door to the Ka'abah was called the *Burka al-Ka'abah* (the Ka'abah's face-veil). It also had the nickname of the *Burka Fatimah* (Fatima's face-veil) after the Prophet's daughter (Burton 1893:II, 212).

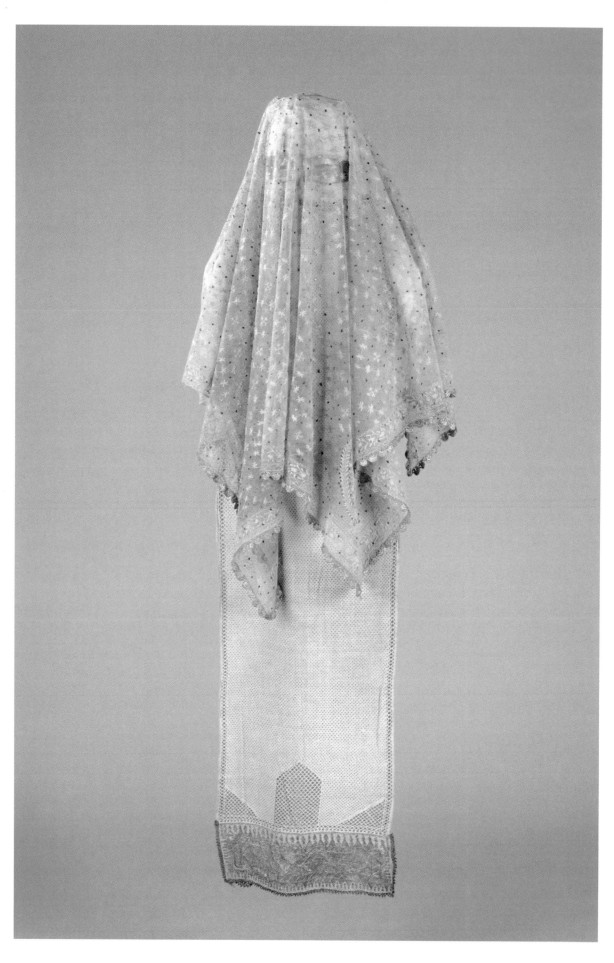

Figure 142a-b.
A pilgrim's face and
headveil worn by
Aceh women in
c. 1880 (RMV
370-2991; photo.
by B. Grishaaver).

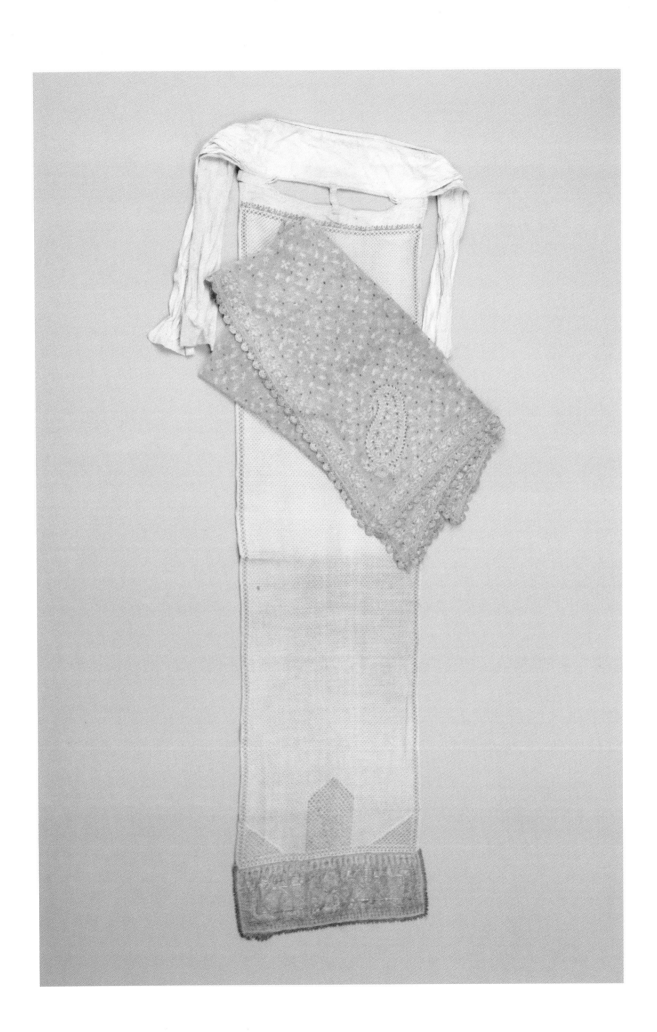

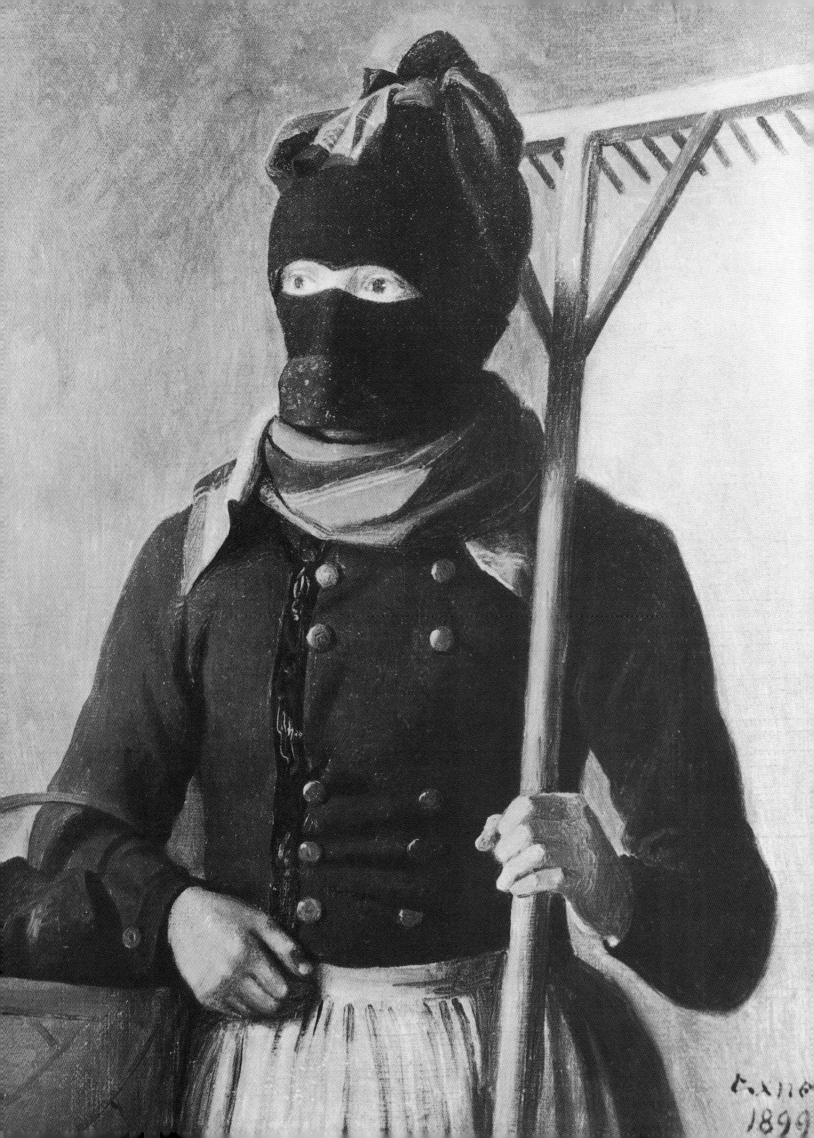

Chapter 11

Beauty, fashion and health

The image of the black veil and the subjugation of women are themes which are frequently combined during discussions about the use of veiling. Yet when veils are looked at as an item of clothing, they can be seen as representing an important element in the traditional and modern appearance of women. They are used to enhance a woman's appearance, to accentuate certain details (for instance, the way in which a woman moves), as well as to show the wearer's interest in and knowledge of the world around her. In many cases, far from showing a woman's closed world, they indicate an increasingly open world.

At first glance it may seem strange to link beauty and fashion with health. Yet there is a close connection between these forces. The wearing of a veil, for example, can protect the skin from the elements, especially dust and wind. It can also have profound effects (both negative and positive) on the physical and physiological health of a woman.

Beauty

Although the wearing of a veil is, in general, intended to prevent men from becoming sexually attracted to a woman, in some cases the effect seems to be the opposite. It is a classic case of what cannot be had, becomes more desirable.

"I must admit the first few moments of veiling were exciting. I found the veil a novelty and looked back with interest as Saudi teenage boys stared at me, now a mysterious figure in black. I knew they were wishing for a bit of breeze to blow the veil away from my face so that they might catch a glimpse of my forbidden skin. For a moment, I felt myself a thing of beauty, a work so lovely that I must be covered to protect men from their uncontrollable desires" (Sasson 1993:108).

Ironically, the concealment of the female face and body often makes the wearer seem more attractive and, in some case, seductive.

The wearing of a veil with the deliberate intention of beautification appears to be divided into three forms. Firstly, the desire for a light coloured skin created by protecting the body from the elements. Secondly, the importance of highlighting parts of the face, notably the eyes, by wearing a face veil. Thirdly, the veil is regarded as a facial decoration which enhances the whole face.

Until very recently it was fashionable in the West for a woman to have a light, if not white, coloured skin. Great care was taken to protect the skin from the sun. Parasols and sunshades were used since antiquity, indeed the Latin *umbraculum*, from which the word umbrella is derived, denotes a shady place or bower.

An important element in this desire for a fair skin was the wish to show the social difference between those who had to go in the sun, such as field hands, and those who did not work and could remain indoors. In some

Figure 148. A Danish woman from the Island of Fano woman wearing a mask, c. 1900.

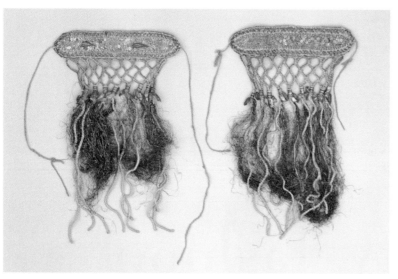

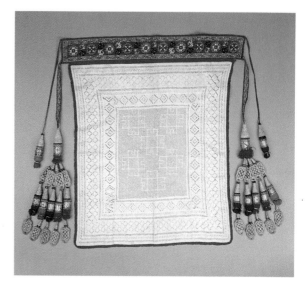

societies this difference was extended to the idea that women who do not work usually live in an urban setting, wear veils, while 'peasant' women are unveiled.

An important change in the desire for a fair skin came during the mid-twentieth century, when many Westerners tried to become brown by getting a sun tan. The presence of such a tan indicated that they had both the time and money to "chase the sun". Thus brown became beautiful. Ironically, a radical change in attitudes towards the sun is also being detected in Western societies, due to the effects of the depleted ozone layer, and because too many people have sun tans. Fair is becoming beautiful again!

People who live in more traditional communities where sunshine is regarded as a constant factor in life, have never had such doubts. A fair skin was and remains beautiful!

Another aspect of wearing veils is that the garment can be used to highlight specific features of the face. In Oman, for instance, urban women tend to wear a veil called the *Sohari burqa* (see fig. 77). It is made from black cotton which has an emulsion of gold, purple or red dye applied to it giving it a black colour with a golden, reddish or bluish sheen (Wikan 1982:88-89). It covers the upper lip, central part of the checks above a line extending from the corner of the mouth, the front part of the nose and the lower third of the forehead, including the eyebrows. The eyes, the upper and lower parts of the cheeks the sides of the nose, the upper part of the forehead, and all the chin are left uncovered.

The use of the urban *burqa`* has the effect of throwing the eyes into relief and is regarded as a garment which beautifies the wearer both spiritually because it stresses her modesty, and visually as it highlights certain features of the face, as was noted by U. Wikan:

"Time and again I was struck by the marvellous ingenuity of this cloaking device in beautifying not so beautiful women. I remember one case in particular, a Baluch woman of striking beauty. She seemed to have the most superbly balanced facial features, and eyes of enrapturing, magnetic beauty - when wearing the *burqa*. I was struck with surprise and disappointment when, one day, she presented herself without the *burqa* to have her photograph taken. Gone was the wonder. She had been transformed into a woman of only ordinary good looks - her face too square, her features too coarse; but, most importantly, without the *burqa* her eyes were not longer in focus, and their radiant magnetism was gone" (Wikan 1982:98).

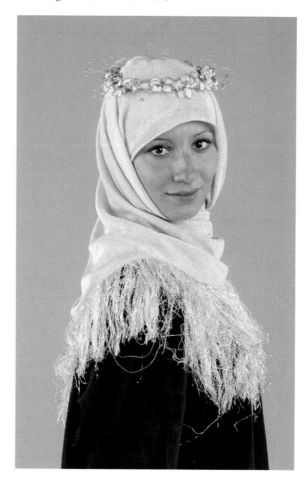

In order to make sure that the veil fits the face correctly, and so emphasises its form, the veils are closely tailored to the shape of the individual's face. In Oman there are also itinerant female makers and sellers of these veils who have stocks which can be tried, or special examples can be ordered.

In other societies the wearing of a veil is regarded as an enhancement of a woman's beauty while, giving her the protection of a garment signalling respectability and modesty (figs. 143 and 144). As a result of this dual nature various types of veils can be found in one region.

Married Bedouin women in the Palestine region, for instance, have similar views towards wearing veils as expressed by the Omani women. The Bedouin women of southern Palestine (especially those of the Negev desert and Gaza strip) have two main types of veils, one which covers the face completely, the other which covers the forehead, nose, parts of the cheeks and mouth (see fig. 2; Weir 1989:188-191). However, the difference lies in the fact that these garments are basically made of coins, beads, stones and chains on a cloth foundation. Such garments not only highlight the woman's eyes, but the presence of the coins and jewellery signifies her family's social status.

Fashion

Traditionally, most regions or even cities, towns and villages have their own way of tying a headscarf or wearing a particular sort of veil. In recent years, however, the range and form of veils (of all types) has decreased considerably.

Such changes are partly due to an increased awareness of Islamic beliefs and traditions, but also to a growing affluence. This affluence has meant that more people have the chance to travel; there are more foreigners (of all nationalities, not just Western) in their countries. In addition, different ways of life on television and in magazines. But perhaps of equal importance is the fact that many textile production centres have been growing, especially in the Far East. As a result, a far wider range of textiles are now available and people are no longer dependent upon the produce of their local manufacture. Instead, they can easily buy a wide variety of cloth woven in Korea, Japan and China.

There are various sources of fashions changes, not only from the West, but also from countries such as Saudi Arabia. The wearing of the *abaya*, for example, is spreading among Islamic women and there are now a number of different variations. In fashion shops in Cairo, for example, it is possible to buy long or short *abayas* made from heavy or light-weight materials. Some are also decorated with embroidery.

It was noted by U. Wikan that in 1974 there was a new fashion in parts of Oman for wearing the *ghashwa*, or black, transparent veil attached to the woman's black cloak (*abaya*):

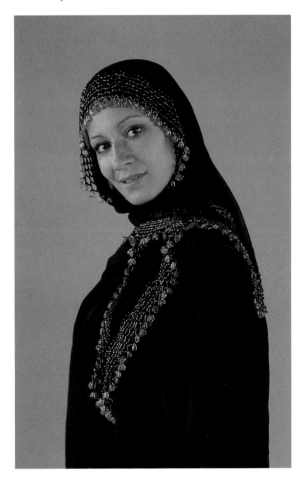

Figuge 145a-c. Three headcoverings from Cairo, Egypt. The white and silver example would be worn to a festival, while the red example with cap would be worn on a special occassion. The the black example with beads can be seen on an everyday basis worn by women in Cairo (RMV 5825-5a,b, 16a,b, 5828-15; photo. by B. Grishaaver).

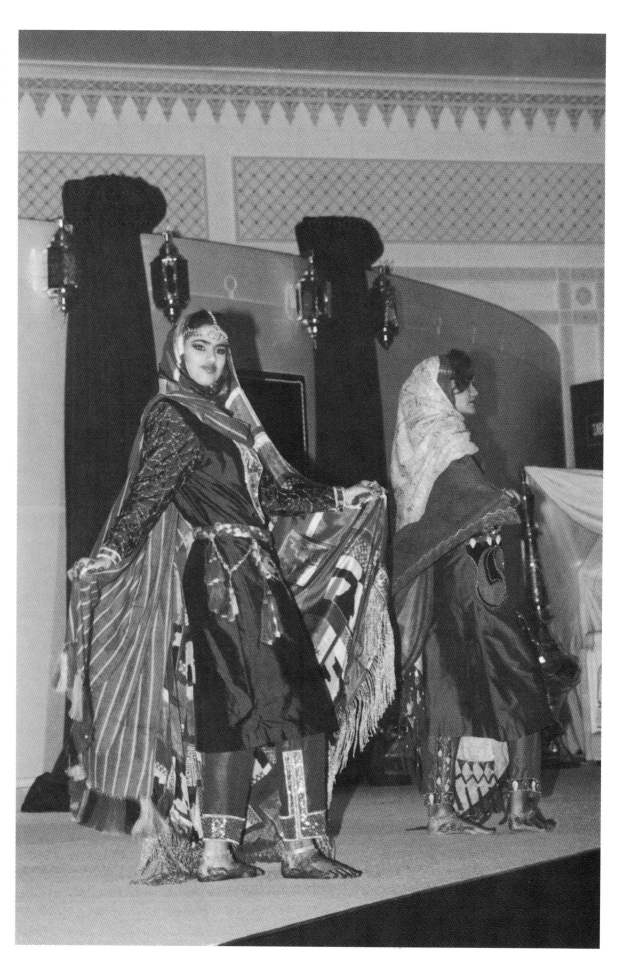

Figure 147*a.*
Modern Omani
clothes by the
fashion designer
Kefah Sadiq
Abduwani, Ruwi,
Oman.

"None praised the new fashion, and the most modern of Sohari women wore a *ghashwa* on top of their *burqa* for more formal visits, thereby doubly protecting and embellishing themselves" (Wikan 1982:107).

There is also a rapidly expanding market in fashionable veiling based on Western fashions. In Egypt, for instance, 'street level' fashions in headscarves and veils are now beginning to change yearly if not with the seasons. In the West at this moment, printed animal skins are popular and it is also possible to buy headcovers in Cairo which are similarly decorated. There is also a wide variety of headcover forms in Cairo. Some are simple squares of materials, others are more intricate forms based on the traditional *torah* or hair veil, but they are now made in a variety of materials (fig. 145a-c).

In the case of Western *haute couture*, several of the major fashion houses have lines for Near Eastern clients. Yves St. Laurent, for example, is producing (by licence) various special veils for Saudi women which are totally black except for his small logo (intertwined YSL) in gold (fig. 146).

There is also a growing number of fashion houses in the Near East which are producing garments based on traditional designs, but with an eye to the future. One such designer in Oman is Kifah Sadiq Abduwani, who has recently had an influential fashion show in Oman (fig. 147a-b). The show was entitled "Modernising Traditional Omani Costumes" (Al Bustan Palace Hotel, May 1993). According to Kafah Sadiq Abduwani, she is trying to: "change the black abaya to coloured ones. I did not want to bring out any drastic changes in the original clothes. All I have attempted to do is modify the present trends by changing the fabric quality, colour combination and so on" (Anon, *PDO News 2*, 1993:30).

One point which becomes clear when looking at the work of these and other designers is that the veil, in all its forms, is not simply a garment used to hide the wearer from the eyes of the world. It is increasingly becoming an item of dress which can have, and indeed does have, a strong element of fashion.

Health

There have been various discussions recently about the role of veiling upon the health of women. In some cases, the use of veils appears to have beneficial aspects. At other times, however, the long term use of total veiling would seem to be detrimental to a woman's physical well-being. Two factors are of importance in this debate. Firstly, how much of the face and body of the woman is covered. Secondly, whether a woman is allowed to go outside the home.

Account also needs to be taken of the prevailing climatic conditions, for instance, whether it is very hot; if there is considerable sunlight, and how much wind there is. The desire to protect the skin from the effects of the sun and wind has led many women to wear veils over their faces. Mostly these cover the face completely leaving only the eyes visible. Such a veil was in use during the late nineteenth century by women living on the Danish island of Fenø (fig. 148). Here women working in the fields near the sea or on the beaches themselves, tended to wear a black 'veil' made out of a tube of material tied at the top with a scarf or a ribbon. Two eye holes were cut out so that the woman could see what she was doing. The aim of this type of veil or mask was purely to protect the face from the damaging effects of the sea winds and the sand.

An example of the protecting effect of veiling was noted by Patricia Holton in her book entitled *Mother without a Mask*:

"Shama was sitting on her bed ... she took off her mask and sat there without it. Her face was startling. From behind that long, old-fashioned mask the full person revealed itself. She sat without her burgah, without her veil, an old woman of perhaps seventy or seventy-five, but her face - what an amazing face, a face of unimaginable fascination. Every feature was still perfect. The skin, protected over the years by the long mask, moistened by its own sweat, was almost unwrinkled" (Holton 1991:252).

The effect of local conditions is not always recognised as a reason for wearing a veil of some kind. A group of women from the United Arab Emirates were asked about the origin of veiling (Holton 1991:250-1). A number of reasons were given, but one which they did not seem to have thought of was that the veil acted as a skin protection from the wind and sun.

"The Sheikha and her mother agreed that this was so, but had never heard of it as a reason. It was plausible. Arabs admire light skin. Their prejudice against dark skin is different from ours {western}. It has nothing to do with the fears of the unknown, the dark fears with which Northerners have burdened themselves from the days when we wore woad. The Arab prejudice is on the basis of beauty. One brother will say of another, 'Look at him. He is too black. Look at this hand', and he will compare his hand to his darker skinned brother, just as two Northern sisters will argue about hair that is too fine or ears that stick out. Yes, they like light skin. Where Western women spend their time baking on the beaches of at least five continents to achieve a fine shade of *café au lait*, Arab women cover up against their common enemy - the sun" (Holton 1991:251).

The problems of wearing a veil in extremely warm conditions is one of the reasons sometimes given for the abandonment of veiling. In the *NRC Handelsblad* (22nd May 1995), there was a report on how the "summer offensive" against women and their clothing was underway in Iran as the weather began to get hotter and

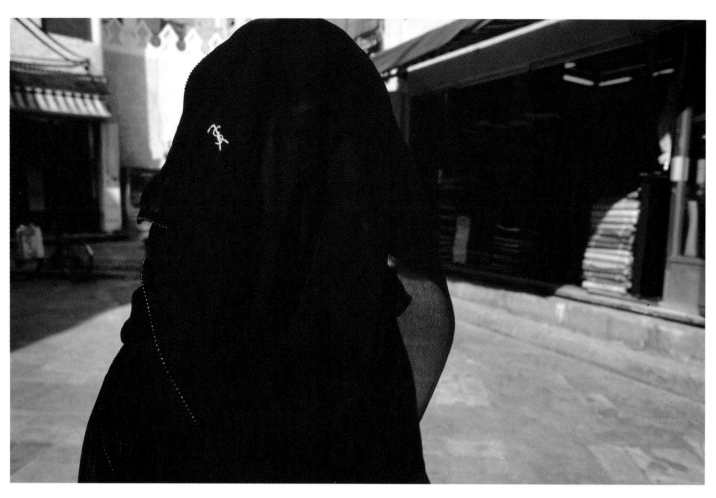

women wanted to wear cooler and lighter clothing. Quoting the Iranian newspaper *Keyhan*, apparently 120 shops in Teheran were closed for selling garments which did not conform to the Islamic criteria.

Another problem related to heat was given in an account by Arlene Macleod in *Accommodating Protest* of how a woman was seated on a bus next to her husband. It was a hot July day in Cairo, he wore a light shirt with Western trousers. His wife, however, was wearing a long dress, with long sleeves and a high neck line. Her head was wrapped in a long scarf. As the trip progressed the bus became hotter, eventually, and not surprisingly, the woman fainted (MacLeod 1991:138; other dangers with public transport and long dress include the problems of actually getting on and off over-crowded buses!).

There are similar tales of exhaustion from the summer heat. For example, in the autobiographical work, *Princess*, the author wrote about her experiences in Saudi Arabia:

"When we walked out of the cool *souq* area into the blazing hot sun, I gasped for breath and sucked furiously through the sheer black fabric. The air tasted stale and dry as it filtered through the thin gauzy cloth. I had purchased the sheerest veil available, yet I felt I was seeing life through a thick screen. How could women see through veils made of a thicker fabric" (Sasson 1993:108).

Reference has already been made to the desirability or otherwise of a tanned skin. In this section mention should also made to some of the physical effects of sunlight on the skin. A moderate amount of sunlight is necessary for the physical and mental health. It is beneficial in healing skin disorders such as eczema and ulcers because sun acts as a drying agent. Without it such problems would take much longer to heal.

Sunlight is also essential for the production of vitamin D. The lack of this vitamin can cause the irregular growth of bones (osteomalacia). In two recent letters in *The Independent* (21st June 1995) two different view points on the relationship between Vitamin D, disorders of the pelvic region and veiling were given:

"All those I had spoken to [health workers from three Middle Eastern countries] believed this to be the result of vitamin D deficiency, which they attributed to the covering of girls from early adolescence. The degree of covering might vary between countries , and between rural and urban situations, but it was coming increasingly common to see total covering, including the wearing of black gloves and socks."

"It does not seem unreasonable to suppose that a sudden limiting of exposure to sunlight following a comparatively sun-filled childhood, and

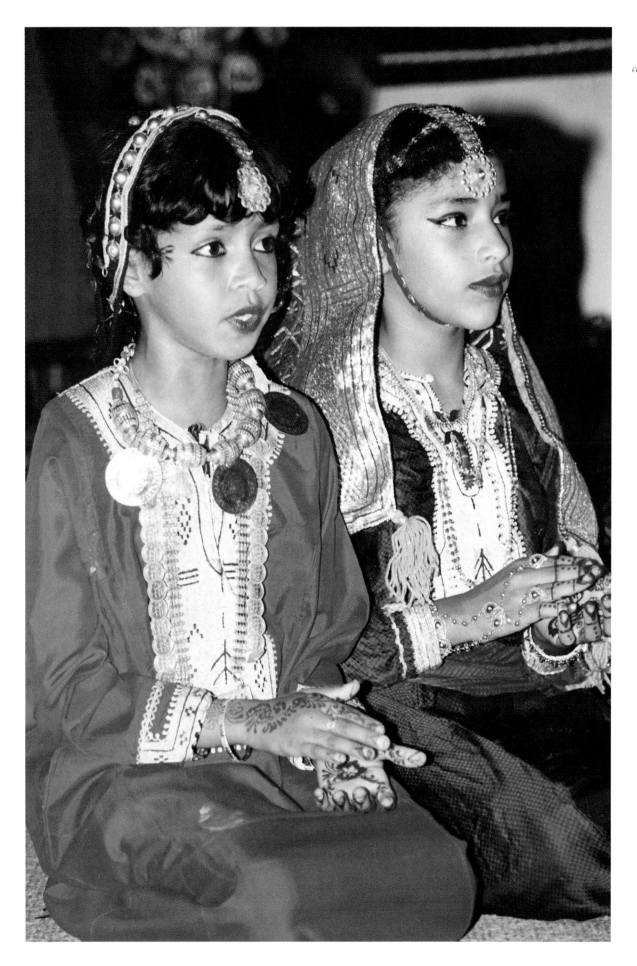

Figure 147*b.*
Modern Omani
clothes by the fashion
designer Kefah
Sadiq Abduwani,
Ruwi, Oman.

unaccompanied by any dietary compensations could have serious effects on a body undergoing the major changes of adolescence" (M.R. Swinbank).

In contrast, Hamzah Baig wrote:

"... *hejab* does not require women to be shrouded from head to foot in black but states that a women [sic] should be modestly dressed and should have her hair covered. This is applicable only when she is in public ... The shrouding in black approach is culturally to do with Arabians and is only loosely connected with Islam ..."

"Since proper *hejab* only requires modest dress when out in public, I can hardly see vitamin D deficiency being more of a problem than wrapping up when it is cold or rainy".

Although there are numerous rainy days in Europe, it is not normal for a woman to be covered every day of the year, nor is hijab clothing solely restricted in many countries to the "modest dress" as envisaged by Mr. Baig.

On the other hand, there are circumstances when veiling may have a beneficial effect on health.[65] For instance, there is an eye problem called pterygium found in countries where there is considerable bright sunlight. Pterygium is the term given for a condition whereby the white of the eye gradually grows over the iris. Although it would appear that wearing sunglasses can help this disease, there seems to be a conflict of views whether the wearing of a veil is beneficial or not.

Throughout the world there is growing concern about the ozone layer and how radiation from the sun can cause skin cancers of various types. As an example of "covering-up" when going in the sun, in Australia it is now required that children should wear some form of headcovering and preferably sunscreens of some kind while out of doors. Melanomen, a malignant form of skin cancer, is caused by a change in the nature of the skin's pigmentation (melanin). Apparently, it is rare amongst Middle Eastern women because they are veiled and thus protected from the effect of the run's radiation.

There is growing concern in the West for the effects on the body due to lack of exercise. Such problems are generally attributed to a sedentary way of life, too much 'junk' food and cars. In the Middle East, the question of the seclusion of women and their lack of exercise should be of equal concern. But it is important to recognise that there are two major elements in the question of veiling and exercises. Firstly, the differences in the amount of exercise (work) carried out by women in nomadic groups versus those women in settlements. Secondly, within settlement societies, the differences in amount of work carried out in normal village and urban life.

There are, however, a number of negative aspects to the concept of veiling and health. In general, nomadic and village women do not experience a lack of exercise. However, the same cannot be said of urban women where the concept of seclusion has caused a major problem, albeit one which is not widely recognised. In addition to the physical effects of veiling and seclusion, there are also a number of psychological effects to its use. The two major psychological problems related to the seclusion of women are isolation and boredom.

The physical and mental problems associated with seclusion were recognised several millennia ago. Xenophon, writing in the fifth/fourth century BC Greece, wrote a narrative in which the Athenian gentleman Ischomachos recounted to his friend Socrates the guided tour he offered to his (unnamed) wife on her arrival at her new home. The house was described as a centre of production in which clothes and food were made. It was also regarded as a nursery for children who would later care for their parents in their old age. Xenephon also wrote that his new wife was expected to guard against the dangers of indolence, ill-health and self-indulgence by helping the servants in household jobs such as shaking out blankets and clothes and making bread (Xenophon *Oeconomicus* 10).

In the Grand Seraglio of the Turkish sultans, the members of the harem used to occupy themselves with prayer, poetry, games, riddles and stories, singing and dancing, shopping, excursions as well as bathing, as well as less acceptable pastimes such as opium smoking, fortune telling, magic and cabalism (Croutier 1989:41ff). Inevitably affairs with the guards, eunuchs and other women must have taken place. Another method of passing the time was simply by sleeping.

Nowadays, education and sport are two methods being used to help combat the boredom and isolation experienced by many women. As may be expected, however, numerous problems have arisen in some countries about education and whether it is acceptable for a girl to attend schools or universities which are co-educational. Often special areas in such institutions are set aside for women and in some cases the women are not allowed to enter the same room where male lecturers and students are seated. However, for many of those participating the fact that women are allowed to go to the lectures in the first place is regarded as more important than their physical exclusion from the classroom.

Although women are sometimes prevented from using the libraries or have access to less well-stocked libraries, it was noted that women in Saudi Arabia often score higher in the examinations than their male counterparts. One woman professor quoted by G. Brooks in *Nine Parts of Desire*, gave an explanation for this difference:

"It's no surprise ... Look at their lives. The boys have their cards, they can spend the evenings cruising the streets with their friends, sitting in cafés, buying black-market alcohol and drinking all night. What do the girls have? Four walls and their books. For them education is everything" (Brooks 1995:150).

As with education, there has and is considerable disagreement as to whether women in strict Islamic households should be encouraged to participate in sports or not. It is noticeable that this argument pertains to urban women, rather than peasant women who have to work and are thus, in general, physically much fitter.

The effects of seclusion upon fitness were noted in the United Arab Emirates when it was decided to admit women to the army. They found that physical fitness of the new recruits was a problem as many of the women had never walked to a local shop let alone completed a forced march (Brooks 1995:113).

In Iran, after a long debate, it was accepted that physical fitness is an important aspect of women health and thus the health of the family. As a result, many sports facilities have a certain number of women's hours each week. In Tehran, for example, the so-called Runner's Park is banned to men for three days a week between eight and four, so women can jog without wearing *hijab* (Brooks 1995:304). In addition there are certain Islamically acceptable sports, including swimming, archery (and the modern equivalent, shooting), as well as horseback riding.

The first Islamic Women's Games were held in the spring of 1993 at the Azadi stadium in Tehran, Iran. Athletes from countries all over the world, including Syria, Pakistan, Bangladesh and Malaysia, as well as representatives from the Muslim republics of the former Soviet Union including Azerbaijan and Kyrgyztstan (Brooks 1995:200-1). In order to allow women even greater 'freedom', a special hijab track suit was developed for these games which enabled female athletes to appear during the opening ceremonies. The garment had a white hood which concealed the hair, and a black, ankle-length tunic worn under a long jumper. The tunic was worn over the trousers of the track suit. It was noted by Brooks that these garments were later discarded in the games when men were banned from being present (Brooks 1995:201).

Driving a car and veiling

Finally, something should be said about driving a car and veiling. Although a section entitled "Health" may seem a strange place to include it, the reasons for allowing a woman to drive or not are often explained in terms of how much they can see and whether they are likely to have an accident or not.

In Kuwait, for example, women are prohibited from wearing veils while driving because it diminishes visibility and presents a danger. The veils may be made up to two or more layers of fabric and as a result they diminish peripheral vision and can literally turn a bright sunny day into night.

On the other hand, for many years it has been the tradition in Saudi Arabia for women to be banned from driving a car. One of the reasons cited for this banning is that women should be veiled in public and if they are veiled they are not safe to drive because their range of vision is limited. If they are not veiled on the other hand, then they should not appear in public and can be arrested under Saudi religious law.

In November 1990 the situation in Saudi Arabia with regard women driving was made official. Sheikh Abdulaziz bin Abdullah bin Abdulrahman bin Mohammad bin Abdulla Aal bin Baz, pronounced that it was illegal for women to drive, thus making Saudi Arabia the only Islamic country with this ban. At the time, Sheikh bin Baz was one of the country's highest religious figures and at that time head of the Committee for the Propagation of Virtue and Prevention of Vice.

The prohibition on women driving came after forty-seven women in Riyadh, the Saudi capital, gathered at a supermarket car park and drove in a fifteen-car convoy to the city centre.[66] All of the women were arrested, along with their male relatives, and accused of renouncing Islam. This offence is regarded as very serious in Saudi Arabia and can be punishable by death.

Following an official investigation, however, it was shown that the women had not broken any religious laws, only tradition. During the time of the Prophet women had often led camels and Bedouin women are still doing so to this day. Nevertheless a *fatwa* or edict was issued stating that "women should not be allowed to drive motor vehicles as the *Shariah* instructs that things that degrade or harm the dignity of women must be prevented" (Goodwin 1995:212).

The ban has led to the strange position whereby it is acceptable for Saudi women to get into a taxi (the back seat only) driven by a man who is a total stranger to her. It has been argued that it would be better to relent on the laws wearing a veil while driving, rather than allow such a prohibited contact from occurring. But so far this has not occurred.

Notes:

65 My thanks to Dr. H. Bernard for his help and comments on the subject of veiling and health.

66 See Goodwin 1995:211-213, Brooks 1995:197-200 and Sasson 1993:281-297, for three different accounts of this event.

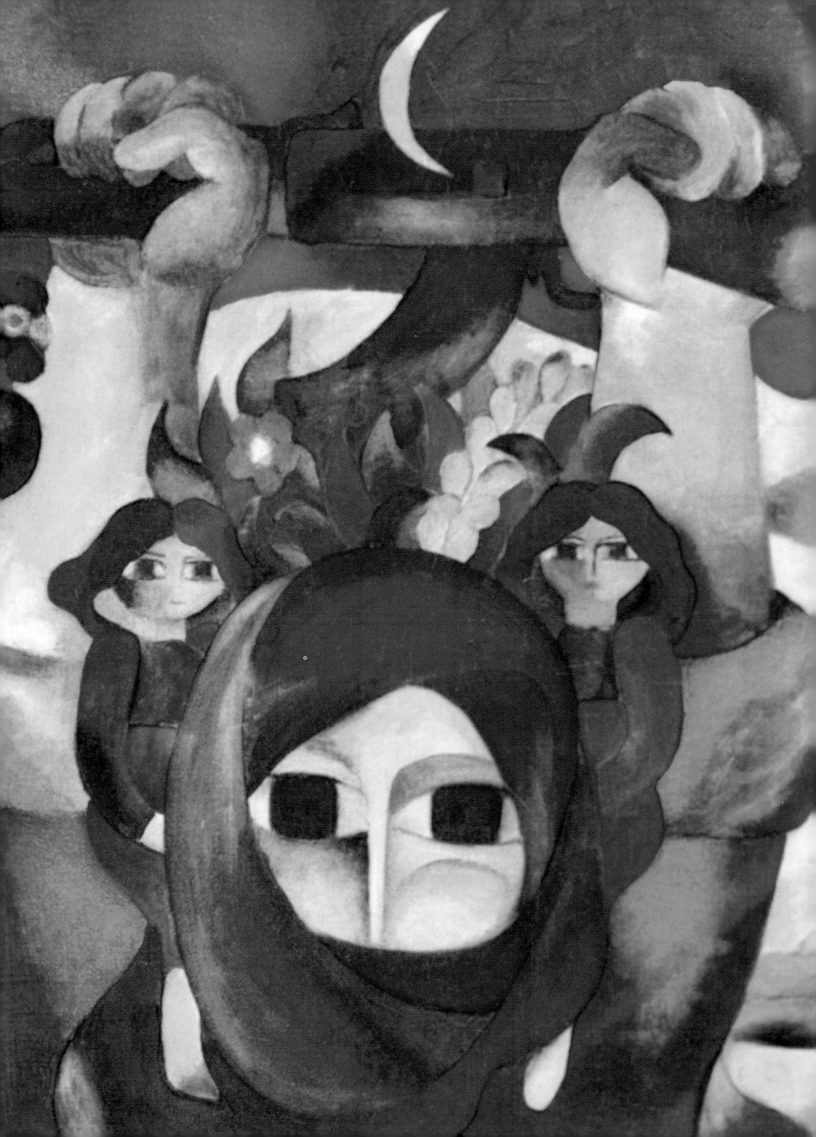

Chapter 12

Veiling and governments

In the late nineteenth and early twentieth century a number of Middle Eastern countries, including Egypt, Turkey and Iran, embarked on programmes to reform and update their social and political infrastructures. In all of these countries the wearing of various types of veils was beginning to be seen as a public symbol of the respective country's backwardness and, to a lesser extent, their oppression of women. As a result of these changing attitudes the subject of veiling became a political issue with considerable religious overtones. In some cases there were demands for the removal of the veil, at other times its return was sought (fig. 149).

The First World War can be seen as a watershed for many political and social changes, especially in the sphere of clothing worn throughout the West and Middle East. In Europe women started to have their hair cut, dresses became shorter and the use of corsets declined. Women throughout the Middle East were encouraged to wear Western, especially Parisian fashions. Even the wearing of the 'fez' or *babush* by men was banned from the ex-Turkish Empire as it was a headcovering worn by officials with its overtones of empire and servitude.

Two countries provide good examples of the demand for the removal and return of veiling, namely Turkey and Iran. Both examples form part of 'modernizations' programmes by their respective governments. In Turkey the removal of veiling was a slow process which occurred without major legal intervention. In Iran the change over came as a very abrupt event for many people.

Turkey and veiling

Turkey has an extremely long tradition of women being veiled going back to at least the Hittite period (1400-1200 BC; see page 21). There are numerous depictions of women from this time wearing long mantles over their heads which reach down to their ankles (see figs. 9-11). The tradition continued into the medieval era.

During the Ottoman empire (AD 1517-1918) veiling took several forms, but one of the most widespread was the *carsaf* (an ankle length garment made out of a rectangle of cloth with a drawstring at the waist), which completely concealed the body and which was often worn with a veil (*yashmak*) over the face. By the 1850's French influence on fashions, especially in Istanbul, was dominant and vast quantities of Western cloth and clothing ideas were imported into the country

In 1863 Sultan Abdul-Aziz ordered the opening of a teacher training school for women as part of a movement towards giving women more education (Abadan-Unat 1981:6-7, 9, 267). His successor, Abdulhamit, prohibited the wearing of the *caraf* in favour of a long coat called a *ferace*. In addition, women, usually of the upper classes began to appear in public without a veil. One particularly noteworthy appearance occurred at a reception at the American Embassy in 1912 (Abadan-Unat 1981:7). A considerable stir was caused by this event both in the press and within court circles. Nevertheless, towards the end of the Ottoman Empire in the 1910's women were still veiled when visiting the court. Writing about her

Figure 149.
A Palestinian painting by Helmi Altouni depicting a revolutionary (veiled) woman (private collection).

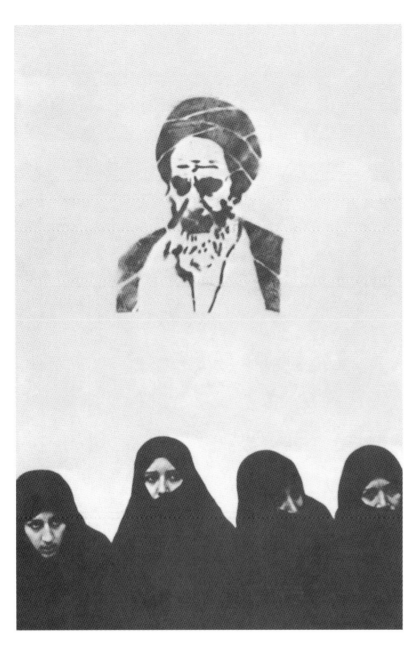

and compromises had to be reached on several occasions. For example, although women were allowed to attend the Faculty of Philosophy at Istanbul University, it was not until 1921 that mixed classrooms were allowed (Abadan-Unat 1981:9). Female students attending these classes were only permitted to lift their veils during the lectures.

In a speech given in August 1925, Mustafa Kemal Atatürk, the president of Turkey, stated that secularisation for men included: "Boots or shoes on our feet, trousers on our legs, shirt and tie, jacket and waistcoat - and of course ... [a] hat" (Hiro 1995:51). The *fez* was totally banned and the wearing of it made a criminal offence. Yet Kamel refrained from totally banning veils for women.

On the 17th February 1926 the government introduced the Turkish Civil Code, which was based on the recently written "Swiss Code" (Abadan-Unat 1991:179). Kemal travelled around the country in order to prepare the people for various changes, including the position of women. On reaching the town of Inebolu he is reported to have read a speech against the use of veiling:

> "I have noticed during this tour, not in villages, but in small towns and cities, that our women were tightly veiled. I can imagine how difficult it must be for them to breathe in warm weather behind such thick covers. Friends, I realise that such customs are the result of our chastity and care, but nevertheless of our selfish nature as well. Our women are not less intelligent and not less reasonable than ourselves, and provided they live up to our moral standards, and are given the knowledge of our national character, there can be no further necessity for such sheer egotism. Let them reveal their faces to the world!" (quoted in Castle 1942:127).

Despite such passionate appeals to the nation, again no action was taken by the legislature against veiling. It would appear that this was due to the expected mass protest against the abandonment of veiling. As a result, the unveiling of women occurred within the upper and educated classes in the large towns and cities, while it made very slow progress elsewhere. Ten years later, in 1935, a ban was proposed at a congress of the People's Party, but again it was not taken further (Lewis 1968:271). Nevertheless, the movement away from veiling continued especially in the urban areas. Women in rural areas, however, remained more conservative and veiling continued for many decades and continues to the present day in the form of headscarves and headveils.

Following the death of Kamel there was a gradual movement towards the restoration of religious institutions. It was, for example, no longer a finable act to recite the prayer call in Arabic (Hiro 1995:54). Religious education was introduced into secondary schools, Quranic schools were opened, charitable associates centred around mosques developed.

Figure 150. An Iranian postcard depicting a group of veiled women under a picture of the Ayatollah Khomeini (private collection).

Bayram festival dress which she wore in 1913, Emine Foat Tugay wrote:

> "On the morning of the first day of Bayram, wearing yashmaks (still the correct thing when going to Court) and light silk cloaks over our dresses, and accompanied by women attendants and an eunuch, we proceeded on board our launch to the Dolma Bagçe Palace" (Foat Tugay 1963:292).

In 1915 an imperial decree (*irade*) was issued which permitted the discarding of the veil during office hours. As may be expected there were numerous protests against such public exhibition of women. Nevertheless, gradually more and more women chose to leave their veils at home. This did not mean that they went bareheaded, but rather they wore Western style hats with long coats. There were still conflicts between the pro- and anti-veiling groups

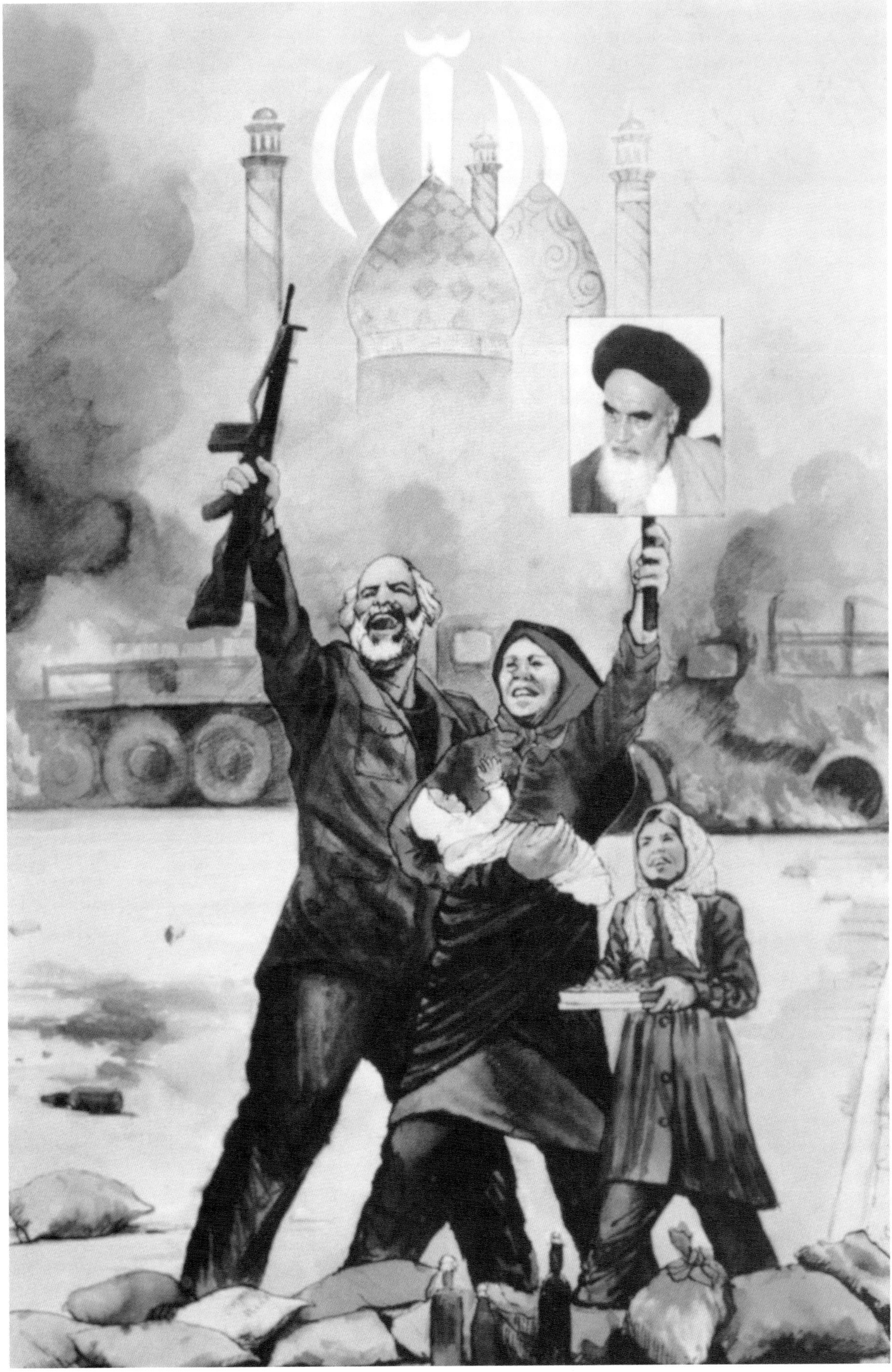

Figure 152.
*A modern Iranian
postcard depicting a
revolutionary family
(private collection).*

In October 1972 the National Salvation Party (NSP) was formed with a rally call against "Western-Christian capitalism" (Hiro 1995:57). Following a coup in 1980 the National Security Council (NSC) was established which encouraged Islamic ideas and education. The reestablishment of Islamic principles within Turkey was re-enforced by the 1983 parliamentary poll in which Evren, the son of a prayer-leader, became president. During his period of leadership the number of mosques increased three-and-a-half fold.

During this period there was also more attention paid to the concept of Islamic dress, especially for women.[69] Every Thursday evening there was a two-hour long programme for women in which the return to the veil was advocated. A sales assistant from Bursa, Emile Serdengenchti, noted that: "Women wear the veil voluntarily, out of fear of leading a sinful life. The idea of sin has come to them from the religious men who preach on the women's television every Thursday evening".[70] The then prime minister, Turgut Ozal, was a conservative man with a firm belief in Islamic principles. Shortly after his visit to Mecca in 1986, the Turkish government became embroiled in a controversy about the wearing of headscarfs by university students. When several students wore headscarfs during classes, the women were ordered to remove them or be expelled. Ozal then had a bill passed in the Grand National Assembly legalizing the headscarf. But President Evren vetoed the bill and asked the Constitutional Corut to pass a judgment on the situation. In February 1989 the court overturned the bill on the grounds that it contravened the secularist articles of the Turkish constitution.

In order to get around the ban on headscarves some students started to wear specially made turbans, which were not initially prohibited. Nevertheless, in the early 1990 the controversy on the headscarf/turban issue was revived when students staged a sit-in at Ankara's Middle Eastern Technical University in protest at the wearing of a headscarf/turban. The Ozal government issued a decree authorizing individual universities to decide whether or not to allow the (banned) headscarf/turban on the campus. Later that year women students at another university where the headscarf had been prohibited took their case to the local court. The court repealed the ban on the ground that it infringed personal human rights. The subject became so charged that the students and teachers involved in the controversy resorted to boycotting classes. This time the government refrained from intervening. The situation seems to be that a woman may now choose whether to be veil or not.

Iran and veiling

A different course of events took place in Iran. As was shown in Chapter 5, page 72 the traditional outdoor clothing for Persian women is the *chador*. The use of outerwraps and *chadors* in this region goes back for at least three thousand years and probably longer. Its role

therefore lies deep within the society at all levels and not only as an essential part of women's clothing.

Iranian women have traditionally worn a large length of material called a *chador*. It covers the head, hair and body, but leaves the face uncovered. Movement towards the "unveiling" of women started during the late nineteenth, early twentieth centuries in Iran following the establishment of the first women's newspapers such as *Danesh* (Knowledge, first published in about 1910)[71], *Shekoofeh* (Blossom, foundation date unknown) and *Zaban Zanan* (Women's Voice; founded in 1919). The latter was very critical about the condition of women in Iran and was greatly influenced by its publisher, Sediqeh Dovlatabady.

Dovlatabady was an active feminist who established, amongst other things, schools and weaving workshops for women (Sanasarian 1985:92). She was critical about the *chador* in her newspaper, which resulted in both herself and the newspaper offices being threatened and, on occasions, attacked. Dovlatabady was later exiled from Tehran, for her vehement comments on the position of women and the role of the Shah. When she died at the age of 80 her last request was that no veiled women should be allowed either to participate in her funeral or to visit her grave.

Several societies were founded at the beginning of the twentieth century including the Patriotic Women's League. It held numerous meetings about veiling (Sanasarian 1985:94). Its leader, Mohtaram Eskandari, frequently lectured against the use of the *chador* and for the introduction of education for women.

It was not only women who agitated against the wearing of veils. One of the most outspoken activists was the poet and writer Mirzadeh Eshqi (1893-1924), who wrote an influential poem called "Women in Shrouds":

"Why the fuss?
Men are God's servants and women are too.
What have women done wrong to feel shame before men?
What are these unbecoming, uncouth, cloaks and veils?
They are winding sheets meant for the dead,
not the living.
I say, "death to the men who bury women alive
in the name of religion!" That is enough to say here.

If two or three poets add their voices to mine,
the people will soon start humming this song
Their hums will uncover the women's fair faces,
the women will proudly throw off their vile masks,
the people will then have some joy in their lives.
But otherwise, what will become of Iran?
With the women in shrouds, half the nation is dead"
(Bambad 1977:135).

During the twentieth century the *chador* was used at least three times as a political and social symbol (fig. 150). The first time the *chador* was used in this way was during the early 1930's, by the ruler of Persia, Reza Shah (reign: 1925-1941; Vatandoust 1985:108-110). He initiated a process of westernization and modernization which included the emancipation of, or appearance of, women by the removal of the *chador*. On January 8th 1936 the shah, the queen and two princesses appeared at the new Normal School, Tehran, to address the female students. All of the women of the royal party were unveiled and wore western style clothing. On the 1st February 1936 regulations designed to encourage the abandonment of the chador came into effect (fig. 151; Hiro 1995:274). As a result of these regulations any officials of the Ministry of Finance, for example, whose wives were found wearing a *chador* were subject to dismissal. Women wearing the *chador* were not permitted in public places such as cinemas and baths, nor were they allowed to use taxis. Bus drivers who accepted veiled women as passengers were liable to fines or even dismissal (Wilber 1975:174).

Fitzroy Maclean recorded in *Eastern Approaches* (written in 1940), the de-veiling of a woman. This occurred in Tabriz in the north west of Iran:

"In the main square of the town I saw a policeman tear the veil from a woman's face and throw it in the mud. The Persians were being modernized, whether they liked it or not" (Maclean 1982:171).

In *Daughter of Persia* Sattareh Farman Farmaian described her mother's reaction to the new law:

"When my mother had learned that she was to lose the age-old modesty of her veil, she was beside

herself. She and all traditional people regarded Reza's order as the worst thing he had yet done - worse than his attacking the rights of the clergy; worse even than his confiscations and murders ... My father resolved that for the sake of his family's safety, his wives would be the very first of the old aristocracy to appear formally in Western dress. He sent to the Avenue Lalezar for hats for all his wives in the compound and told them that the next day they were to put them on and ride with him in the open droshky. To my mother, it was exactly as if he had insisted that she parade naked in the street ... The next day, weeping with rage and humiliation, she sequestered herself in her bedroom with Batul-Khanom to put on the hat ... As she wept she struggled futilely to hide her beautiful masses of waist-length black hair under the inadequate protection of a small French cloche. There was nothing my stepmother could say to console her" (Farmaian 1992:137-8).

Some families went even further and moved to other countries to avoid the ban on veiling and other forms of traditional clothing, in particular the turban:

"We were much upset. Reza Shah Pahlavi wanted to change people by force, make everyone like the Europeans ... Here in Sohar [in Oman], we were free to pursue our own customs. Our customs were like those of Arabs of Sohar already when we lived in Bandar Abbas; *burqa*, turbans, clothes, and so forth. So that's precisely why we moved: Pahlavi banned the

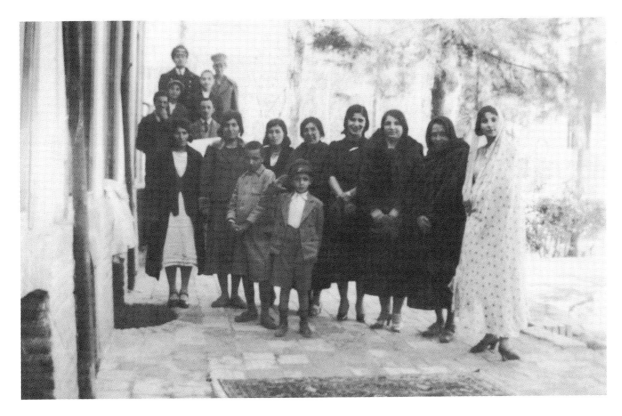

Figure 152. Photograph of a group of Iranian women of the Bolourforoush(an) family from the mid 1930's. Most of the women are wearing modern/Western style dress (courtesy of L.A.F. Barjesteh van Waalwijk van Doorn).

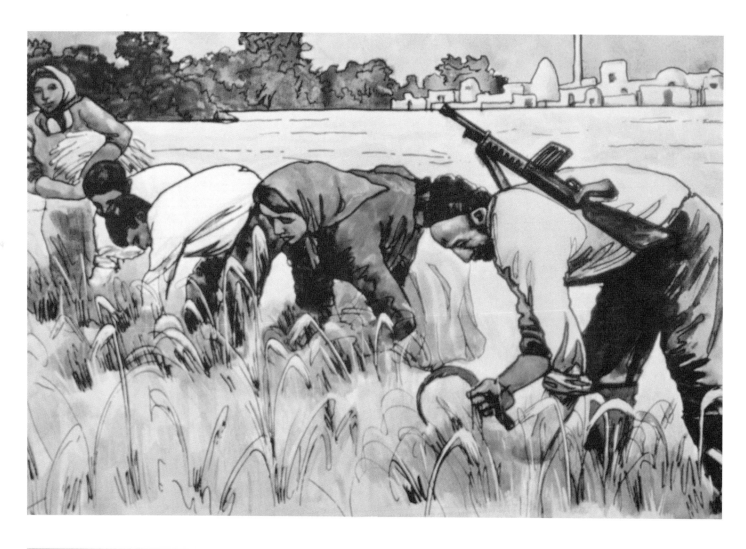

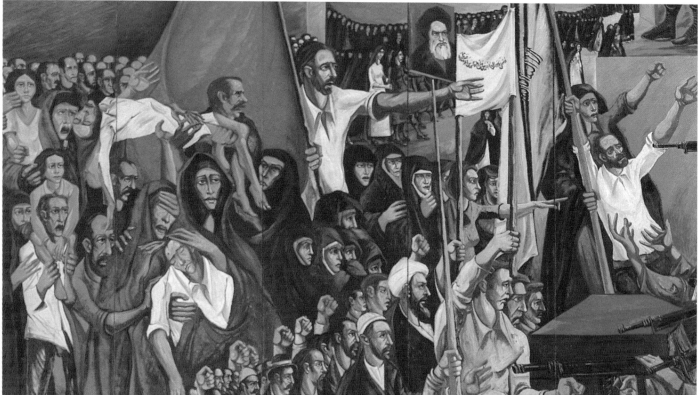

burqa and the turban; we wanted to keep these things. When today some young men want to leave their customs, and go bareheaded instead of wearing the turban, that is voluntary, with changing times, not force" (Wikan 1982:108).

One of the unexpected effects of forbidding the *chador* was that the garments worn underneath became public and the poverty of many women became apparent. This resulted in an Iranian trade commission being hastily sent by the government to Germany and France to buy 500,000 rials worth of ladies ready-to-wear clothing for distribution (Wilber 1975:174). The ban on *chadors* was strictly enforced from 1935 to 1941 when the law was eased following the death of the shah.

The second time the *chador* was used as a political and social symbol was during the 1970's as dissatisfaction increased with Reza Shah's successor, Mahmoud Reza Shah (reign: 1941-1979), his Western oriented policies and what was generally regarded as a corrupt government. Women started to wear the *chador* in the street in 'quiet' protest against the shah. But this protest later became more vocal and visual. For many women the wearing of the *chador* represented a mixture of political and religious reasons and beliefs, but mostly it stood as a protest against the shah (fig. 152).

When the revolution reached its climax in February 1979 the wearing of the veil was seen by many as a symbol of solidarity and militancy. Members of political parties to the left regarded the wearing of the *chador* as a sign of rebellion against Western ideas and imperialistic culture (Tabari and Yeganeh 1982:17; Brooks 1995:24). On the other hand, members of religious parties, especially those which may be regarded as traditionalist, regarded the sight of so many women wearing the *chador* at the time of the revolution as a sign that women wanted a return to Islamic conventions (figs 153 and 154). In a speech by Ayatollah Taleghani given at the beginning of 1979, he said:

"No one forced women to come with hijab on demonstrations ... But they themselves felt an Islamic responsibility to make this dress one of their Islamic and Iranian slogans, to show their genuine feelings and to show it to the world" (Tabari and Yeganeh 1982:107).

Another view of the introduction of *hijab* was noted by C. Mosteshar in her autobiography:

"When I first met Nahid the revolution was a year old, and her veil-wearing, prayer-saying model of the traditional Muslim wife was still a novelty to the circles in which I moved. My great-grandmother's generation had been the last in our family to have worn the veil. During my childhood the only people who wore the *chador* were servants. In those days the

chador was not this black crow-like outfit, but a beautiful, bright-coloured garment. Our cook used hers as a shield against dust rather than against lust, draping it over the back of her head and then wrapping it round her ample belly; this was a cultural outfit, not a sexual cloak" (Mosteshar 1995:244).

For many Iranian women the return to the *chador* was equated with a return to traditional moral and social values, including purity and dignity. However, an important point made at the time was that the wearing of the *chador* was a question of choice rather than compulsion. So there was considerable unrest when, at the beginning of March 1979, when Ayatollah Khomeini announced that all working women (namely women who did not stay at home), had to wear the chador when outside the house (fig. 155; Tabori and Yeganeh 1982:103-7). The decision led to the first of several demonstration. As a result of the unrest the role of women was clearly defined along strict Islamic principles and those stepping over the boundaries faced severe judicial punishment, which included death in some cases.

Another aspect of the enforcement of *hijab* was that women who were not wearing either the long *chador* or a long coat (*montoe*, *manteau*, or *rapoosh*; Goodwin 1995:106) plus a large headscarf (*roosarie*) could be subject to violent personal attacks in the street. M. Momen noted in his introduction to Shi'i Islam that: "There was also a drive in the same month [July 1980] to get women to wear the veil. Unveiled women were attacked in the streets by Hizbu`llahis" (Momen 1985:294).

There are also accounts of women having their legs painted or acid thrown at their faces. Later a special, 'morality' police called the *pasdar* was established. One of the functions of these police was to check that the correct form of clothing was worn. It would seem that in most cases, women were the targets of the *pasdar*. Male *pasdar* were officially meant to deal with men, while a special squad of female *pasdar* stop women:

"Four bearded men in the olive drab uniform of the *pasdar* leapt from the Nissan. One of them grabbed Moody as the others levelled their rifles. Simultaneously, four lady *pasdar*, in their uniforms of black chadors, assailed me, screaming in my face" (Mahmoody and Dunchod 1991:165)

During the summer of 1992 attacks on women increased. In this case it was for *bad hejabi* or improper veiling (Ramazani 1993:421). These attacks were carried out by zealots attempting to "uphold virtue and combat vice". Bad *hejabi* was a term which was gradually been taken up at this time as women started to wear brighter colours, patterned stockings and even lipstick. A number of women were also replacing the *maghneh*, a black head covering, with brightly coloured headscarves.

Figure 153.
A modern Iranian postcard depicting a peaceful revolutionary group at work in the fields (private collection).

Figure 154.
A modern Iranian postcard depicting a rally in support of the Islamic revolution (private collection).

149

During 1992 there was also an increasing number of demands by conservatives to suppress the growing attractiveness of women's outdoor dress. Public figures such as Mohammad Musavi Kho'iniha denounced *bad hejabi*, while the former prosector general, Sayyed Hosain Musavi Tabrizi, said: "Anyone who rejects the principle of the hejab is an apostate" (quoted by Ramazani 1993:422).

Although some conservative zealots advocated and carried out the beating of women for *bad hejabi*, others including Khamenehi called for words to be used to persuade women to wear correct *hijab*.

Although there was and still is considerable unhappiness at being forced to wear the chador, Iranian women are seen to have more 'freedom' than some other national groups. Iranian women are allowed to attend a number of university courses, especially those which relate to the health and eduction of the nation, for example, teaching, nursing, medicine. In addition, in order to defend the Iranian homeland are allowed to join military organisations and learn how to use firearms, as well as ride around on the motorbike with their black *chadors* fluttering in the wind (Ramazani 1993). In contrast Saudi Arabian urban women are still prohibited from even driving a car (see page 141) and may be subjected to arrest if seen outside of the house with too much of their face or hair uncovered.

Iran and Afghanistan

Finally, the political influence of Iran upon Afghanistan can also be seen in respect to the use of veiling. Women in the larger cities of Afghanistan traditionally wore the *chadri* (see page 73) which is made up of a skull-cap with circular cloak. The woman's face is totally concealed when wearing this garment. Several factors effected the discarding of the veil in Afghanistan's urban areas (Moghadam 1993:218). During the 1920's a comparative large number of unveiled women, especially Turkish women, were living in Kabul. Their presence added an impetus to the Afghan women in the city to remove their veils. More importantly, in late 1927 Amanullah, the ruler of Afghanistan, and his wife visited several countries in the Middle East and Europe. On their return an edict was proclaimed which stated that all women in Kabul should go unveiled (Hiro 1995:230). By October 1928, some 100 Afghan women, led by Queen Soraya, had publically discarded the veil. Nevertheless, following the overthrow of Amanullah one year later the edict was rescinded.

During the summer of 1959 the government further encouraged women to discard the veil in all towns in Afghanistan. In August 1959 the queen and wives of officials were seen in public unveiled during the visit to Kabul of Prime Minister Nehru of India (Wilber 1962:200). At the same time the police were given instructions to protect unveiled women, rather than arrest them. The new 'uniform' of women consisted of a scarf, dark sunglasses, heavy coats, gloves, and cotton stockings. Gradually, various elements of the uniform vanished, notably the coats, gloves and thick stockings.

Inevitably, there was a reaction against both of these attempts to remove the veil. Traditional religious leaders in Kabul and elsewhere protested and riots ensued. However, the Russian invasion of Afghanistan in 1979 meant that a speedily return to veiling took place. This movement was seen by many as a means of protecting the honour of women, and thus the family, and as a statement of Islamic/Afghan solidarity.

Many of the refugees who fled Afghanistan to Pakistan also readopted and indeed strengthened the use of veiling and especially *purdah* in order to keep some form of control in their insecure lives and to install a sense of continuation (Moghadam 1993:242-247). Kathleen Howard-Merriam suggested that:

> "the Mujahideen leaders recognize women's importance to the *jihad* (or holy war) with their exhortations to preserve women's honor through the continued practice of seclusion. The reinforcement of this tradition, most Westerners have failed to notice, serves to strengthen the men's will to resist ... *purdah* provides the opportunity for preserving one's own identity and a certain stability in the face of external pressures ... Westerners who have been quick to impose their own ethnocentric perceptions should note the value of this seemingly anachronistic custom for a people under siege whose very survival is at state" (Howard-Merriam 1987:104, 114).

In a United Nations report about the Afghan refugees in Pakistan, Hanne Christensen wrote that because of the overcrowded nature of the refugee compounds many women "are enveloped in veils day and night, even in sleep" (Christensen 1984:46). One of the main results of the reinstatement of *purdah* is that many women have become very isolated, and that this has resulted in severe mental and physical health problems.

Notes:

69 The following section is based on Hiro 1995:61-64.

70 Quoted by Hiro 1995:62; from *Nation*, 28th June 1986:883.

71 Yaukacheva 1959:76; Sanasarian 1985:91.

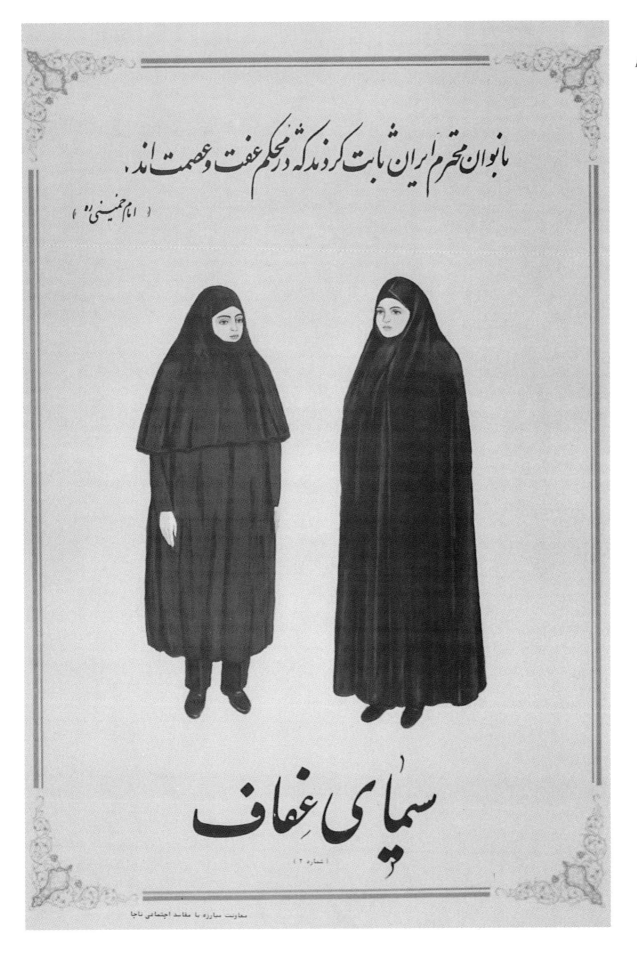

Figure 155.
*Modern Iranian
poster showing how
respectable women
are meant to be
dressed in public
(courtesy of the
Stichting Textile
Research Centre,
Leiden).*

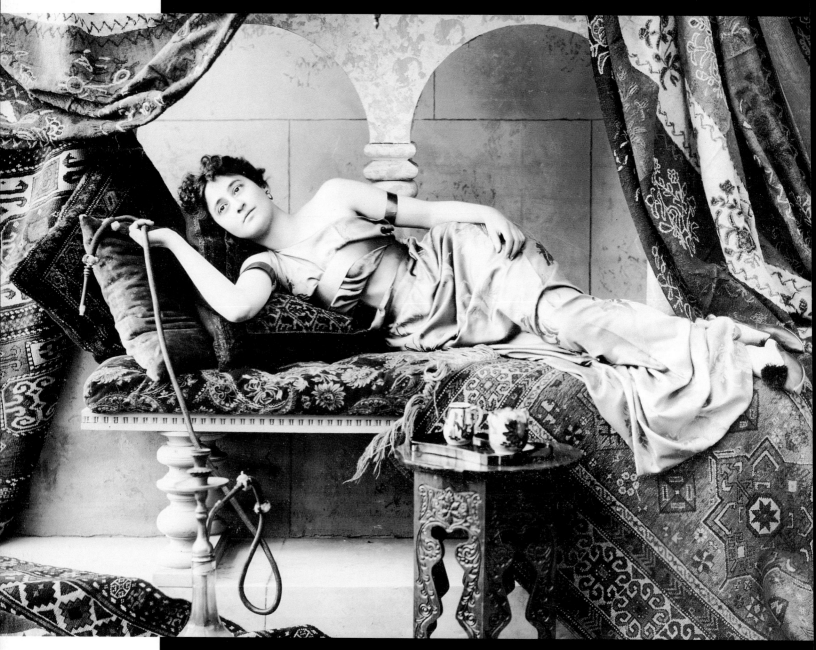

*Photograph of a mock harem scene entitled
"Hookah" by James Arthur, c. 1900.*

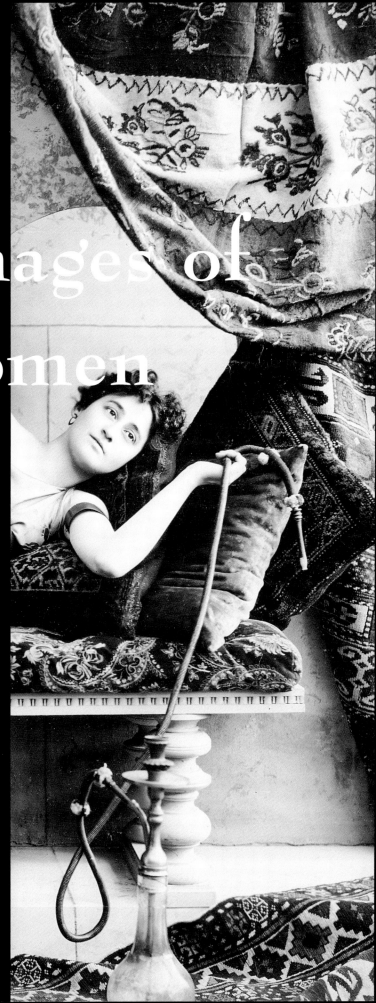

Visual images of
veiled women

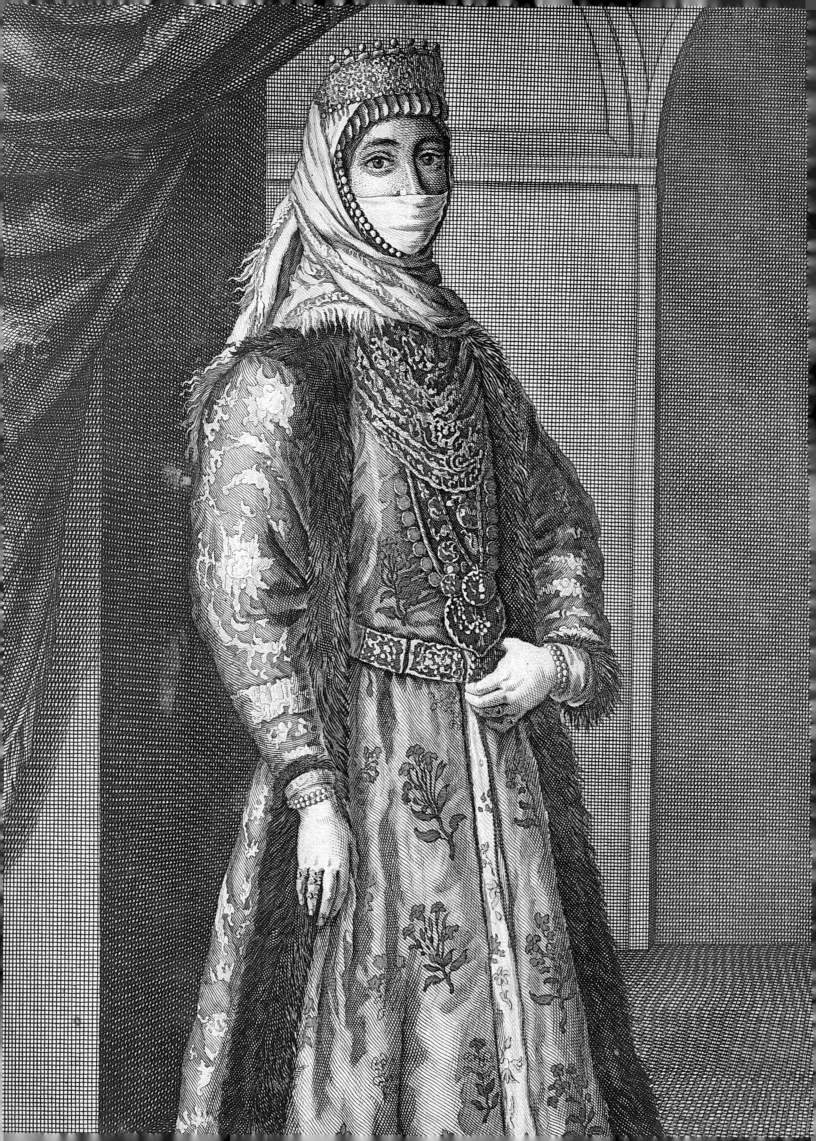

Chapter 13

Images of veiled women

The West has long been fascinated by the 'mysterious East' and many ideas and theories have been put forward to explain this attraction. One of the most quoted phrases about the East-West relationships comes from a poem by the English writer, Rudyard Kipling:

"Oh East is East and West is West,
and never the twine shall meet
till earth and sky stand presently
At God's great judgement seat."[72]

A general term, 'Orientalism', has been developed over the centuries in order to describe the West's interest in and curiosity about the East. The term now has a number of meanings relating to the study of eastern languages, literature, religion, philosophy, art, as well as social life. In addition, it has been used since the nineteenth century to describe a genre of painting with predominantly North African and Near Eastern subjects. In fact, 'Orientalism' has been used to describe anything inspired by the East and includes Islamic, Indian, Chinese, Indonesian, as well as Japanese sources. For the purposes of this chapter, the general nature of orientalism is being looked at, while at the same time attention is being focused on the written and visual depictions of women from the Near East and North Africa.

There have been numerous books in recent years about the general concept of Orientalism. One of the most well-known works is E. Said's *Orientalism* (1978). However, this book is extremely biased towards a negative concept of Orientalism and its function in colonialism and imperialism. A more sympathetic approach to the subject can be found in J. MacKenzie's, *Orientalism: History, Theory and the Arts* (1995). Two different views about the portrayal of women can be seen in S. Graham-Brown's, *Images of Women: The Portrayal of Women in Photography of the Middle East 1860-1950* (1988; this book follows Said), and A. L. Croutier's, *Harem: The World Behind the Veil* (1989). In Croutier's book, she is trying to understand the world in which her Turkish grandmother, mother and aunts grew up.

As may be expected, the way in which veiled women have been portrayed during the few centuries has varied considerably according to the viewer, when they were looking, what they were looking at and, perhaps most importantly, why. At different times in the past various aspects were selected. Sometimes it was for the exotic nature of the clothing worn by the subjects. On other occasions it was the erotic nature of the clothing and the way it was worn which was being highlighted.

In this chapter two aspects of 'Orientalism' will be looked at. Firstly, the role which literature and painting has played in the image people have of the Eastern woman. Secondly, the continuing and developing role played by photography and in particular, postcards. In the following chapter there will be a discussion about the role of music, dance and Hollywood, and some of these

Figure 159.
A Persian lady
c. 1700 (private
collection).

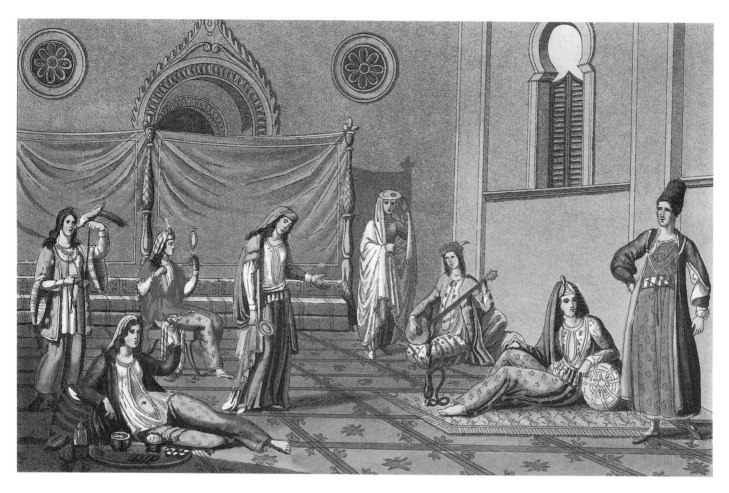

Figure 160. An 19th century print depicting a harem scene. The print was used to show the costumes worn by women from different regions of the Near East (private collection).

influences on modern day preconceptions about the Oriental woman.

Illustrations and paintings

After the Crusades an increasing number of travellers went to the Near East and wrote about their travels and the peoples they had met. These travellers included men such as P. Belon du Mans, who wrote *Les Observations des Plusieurs Singularités et Chose Mémorables Trouvées en Grèce, Asie, Judée, Redigées en Trois Livres* (1553); Joanna Helffrich (*Kurtzer und Warhafter Bericht von de Reiss aus Venedig nach Hierusalem* (Leipzig 1578) and Anthony Shereley (1565-1635; *His Relations of His Travels into Persia*). In addition to such travellers, merchants began to send artists to places such as Turkey specifically in order to obtain new ideas. One such artist was Pieter Coeche van Aelst (1502-1550) who was sent to Istanbul in 1533 by the Brussel's tapestry producer, Van Der Moyen, in order to create a series of 'Turkish' tapestry designs.

Some of the information provided by the various travelogues was included in costume books, notably those by Christoph Weiditz, *Das Trachtenbuch des Christoph Weiditz von seinen Reisen nach Spanien und den Niederlanden, 1529-32*, and Cesare Vecellio, *Habiti antichi, et moderni di tutto il mondo* (1598). Later works such as the *Codex Vindobonensis* (late 16th c.; Austrian National Library, Vienna), provide considerable information about

contemporary costume, in this case sixteenth century clothing worn in the Topkapi Palace, Istanbul.

In Vecellio's work there are numerous examples of veiled women from Europe (including Spain, Italy and Sicily), as well as Turkey, Persia and Egypt (fig. 156a-b). In general, those garments labelled as European or Near Eastern (Western Asia) are reasonably accurate. On the other hand, the costumes from remoter areas such as Russia, Eastern Asia, China and America should be regarded with suspicion.

Some of the problems of using early paintings and costume books as a source of information about women's clothing can be seen when looking at a painting by Gentile and Giovanni Bellini, *St. Mark Preaching in Alexandria*, Milan (started 1492, finished about 1510; fig. 157). In this painting there is a group of Egyptian women in the centre of the picture dressed in the "Mamluk mode" (Raby 1982:41). The standing figure to the left of the group appears to be the source of the *Donna del Cairo* (Lady of Cairo) in Vecellio's costume book mentioned above (rather than the other way around, as might be expected; fig. 158). So even by the late sixteenth century her style of costume had already been transported from Alexandria to Cairo.

Bellini's veiled figure was also used by artists and writers including Belliniano (*The Martyrdom of St. Mark*, Accademia, Venice); Breydenbach (*Peregrinationes*),

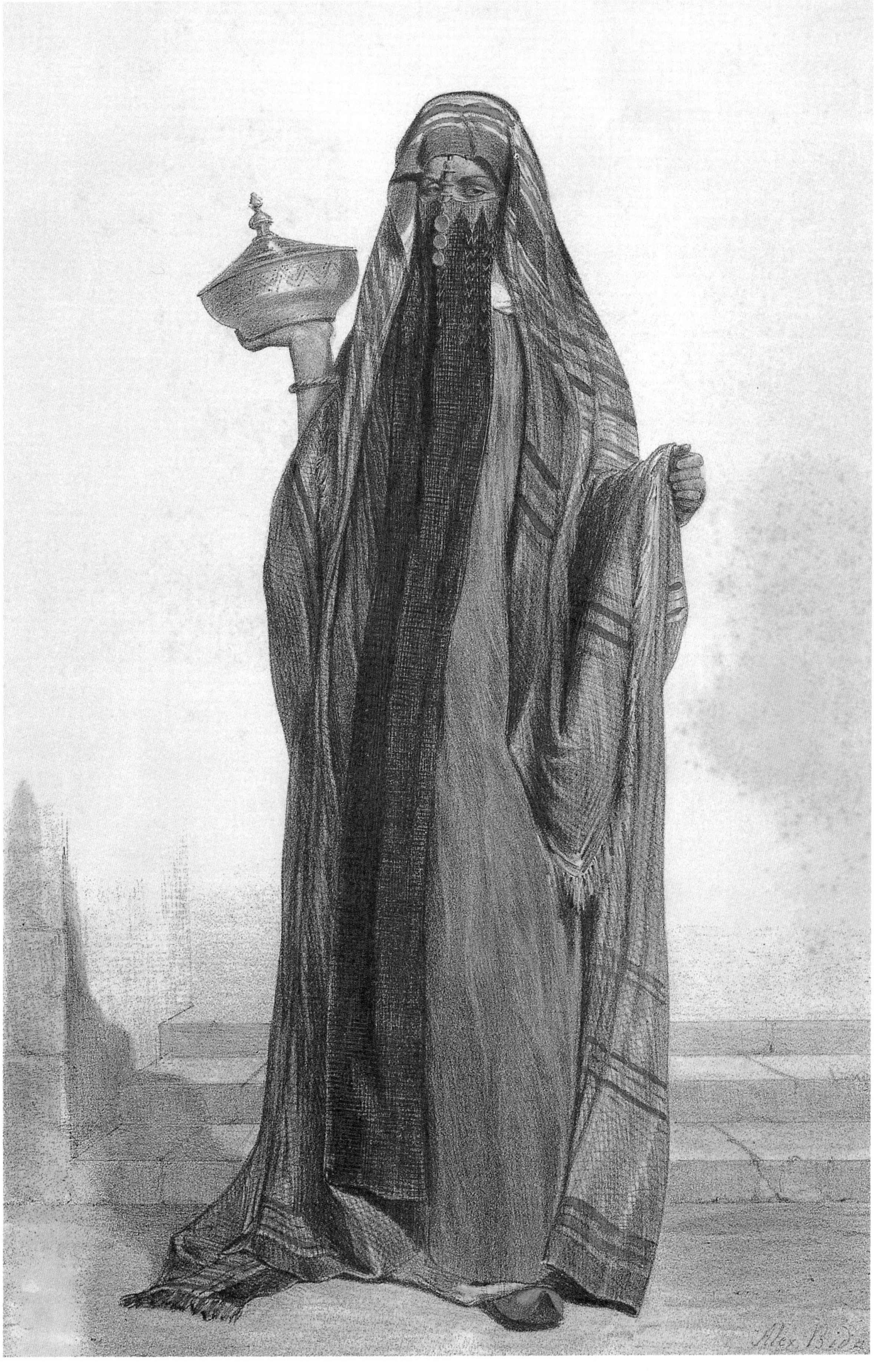

Figure 161.
*A print by A. Bida,
entitled "Woman of
Cairo" (no date).*

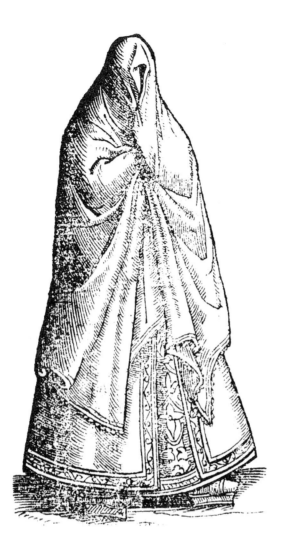

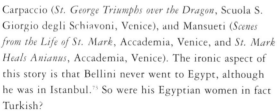

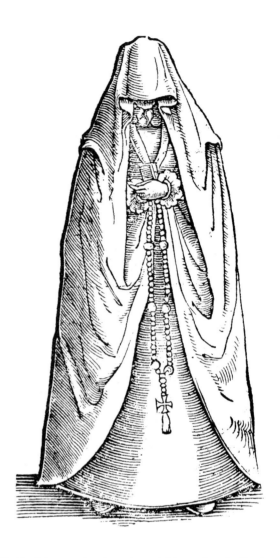

Carpaccio (*St. George Triumphs over the Dragon*, Scuola S. Giorgio degli Schiavoni, Venice), and Mansueti (*Scenes from the Life of St. Mark*, Accademia, Venice, and *St. Mark Heals Anianus*, Accademia, Venice). The ironic aspect of this story is that Bellini never went to Egypt, although he was in Istanbul.[73] So were his Egyptian women in fact Turkish?

During the seventeenth and eighteenth centuries there was a dramatic increase in the number of factual and fiction books about the Near East as the number of people travelling there increased sharply. Among the more serious works are books by people such as Thomas Herbert (1606-1682); Cornelis De Bruin (1652-1726/7) and Karsten Niebuhr (1733-1815).

From 1674 onwards, De Bruin, for instance, travelled through Syria, Iran and other countries. His journal was published in 1698 under the title: *Reizen Van Cornelis de Bruyn door de Vermaardste Deelen van Klein Asia, De Eylanden Scio, Rhodus, Cyprus, Metelino, Stanchio, etc Mitsgaders de Voornaamste Steden van Aegypten, Syrien en Palestina, Verrijkt met Meer als 200 Kopere Konstplaaten, Vertoonende de beroemdste Landschappen, Steden, etd. Alles door den Autheur Selfs na het Leven Afgetekend.* Later there were English (1702) and French (1704) editions of the book.

De Bruin's second major trip took him to Russia, Persia and India: *Reizen over Moskovie, door Persie en Indie: Verrykt met Driehondert Konstplaten, Vertoonende De Beroemdste Lantschappen en Steden, ook de Byzondere Dragten, Beesten, Gewassen en Planten, die Daer Gevonden Worden: Voor al derzelver Oudheden En wel voornamentlijk heel uitvoerig die van het Heerlyke en van Oudts de Geheele Werrelt door Befaemde Hof van Persepolis, By de Persianen Tchilminar genaemt* (1711). Again there were English and French editions.

The De Bruin books contain numerous depictions of people wearing traditional and local clothing (fig. 159). Because he was a skilled artist and he was working from his own sketches the representations in these two books appear to be accurate.

During the nineteenth century one of the most influential writers about Egypt was E. W. Lane. He was a student of Arabic and published numerous works on the subject. In addition, in 1836 he published *The Manners and Customs of the Modern Egyptians* (this book is still available), which was intended to be a serious, methodical study of lives of Egyptian men and women. Lane also provided considerable information about the garments worn by both men and women from various social levels (see figs. 67, 68 and 84).

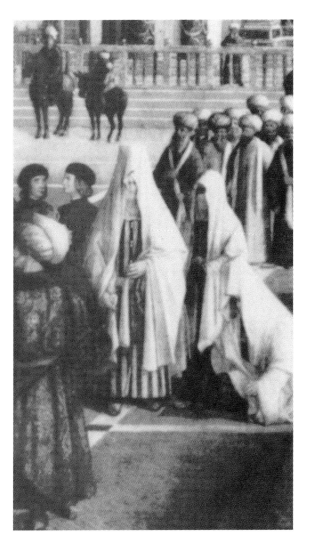

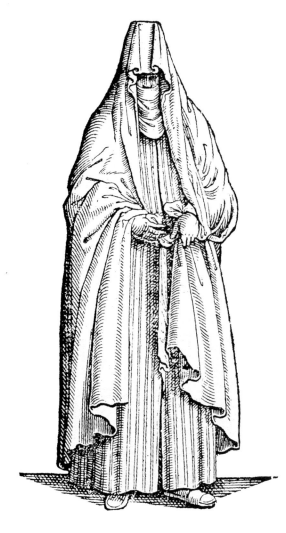

Figure 157. *A detail from G. Bellini's painting* St. Mark Preaching in Alexandria, *showing a group of women wearing 'Egyptian' style costume, c. 1500.*

Figure 158. *Vecellio's "Donna del Cairo" (after Vecellio,* Habiti antichi, et moderni di tuto il Mondo, *1598).*

With respect to information about Near Eastern women and how they lived, one of the most important female traveller's was Lady Mary Wortley Montague, who left London on the 1st August 1716, to accompany her husband to Turkey. Her husband had been appointed "Ambassador Extraordinary to the Court of Turkey". Her travels resulted in numerous letters which have since been published on various occasions, including by R. Halsband, *The Complete Letters of Lady Mary Wortley Montague* (1965, 3 vols). The letters of Lady Mary were followed by travellers such as those by Lady Lucie Duff Gordon, who went to Egypt in the mid-nineteenth century (*Letters from Egypt*, 1865).

Throughout the late nineteenth and early twentieth centuries there were numerous, albeit less serious (yet often well-meant), travel books about the Near East. These works include E. de Lorey and D. Sladen's, *Queer Things about Persia* (1907); M. E. Hume-Griffith's, *Behind the Veil in Persia and Turkish Arabia: An Account of an Englishwoman's Eight Years Residence Amongst the Women of the East* (1909) and J. Foster Fraser's, *The Land of Veiled Woman: Some Wondering in Algeria, Tunisia and Morocco* (1911).

As may be expected, however, there was an even greater number of works of fiction based around the Oriental theme. One of the earliest and most influential was the translation of Antoine Galland's *Arabian Nights' Entertainments* in the early eighteenth century (French ed. 1704; unauthorised English ed. 1704/5), which led to a fashionable taste for "Eastern" or "Persian" architecture, fashion and decorative arts. Some of the earliest stories in this genre include John Hawkesworth's *Almoran and Mahet* (1761); Clare Reeve's *History of Charoba, Queen of Egypt* (1785) and Maria Edgeworth, *Murad the Unlucky* (1804). On a more 'erotic' level the Oriental mode led to sexual fantasy worlds as described in the anonymous novels *The Lustful Turk* (1828) or *One Night in a Moorish Harem* (no date). But perhaps some of the more influential works were the two fictional autobiographies by Pierre Loti called *Aziyadé* (1877) about his love for a Circassian woman, and the later story *Les Désenchantées* (1906) concerning life in a Turkish harem.

In addition to writers visiting North Africa and the Near East, there were numerous artists (fig. 160). Painters who travelled in the region or were directly influenced by Orientalism, included artists such as Mouradja d'Ohsson (for example, *Tableau général de l'Empire Otoman*, 1789);

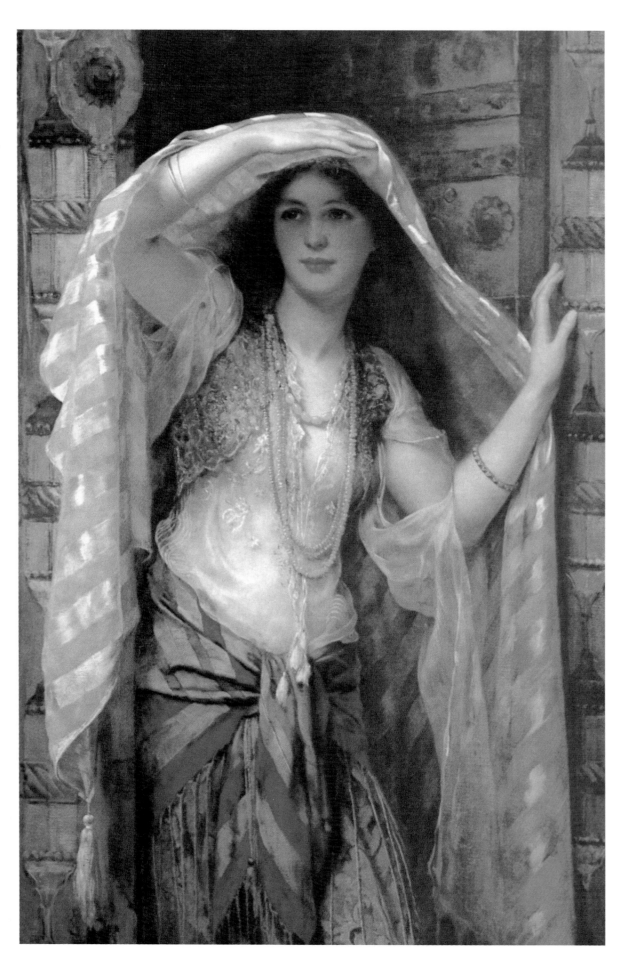

Figure 162. *The original title of this painting by W.C. Wonter is "Safie, One of the Three Ladies of Baghdad" (1900). In this Egyptian print of the painting the scene is called: "Luscious Safie with her transparent blouse".*

Dalvimart (*Turkish Cengi with Brass Finger Cymbals*, 1802, Victoria and Albert Museum, London) and Mayer (*Celebration at Ned Sili*, 1801, *Dancers with Tribal Tattoos*, 1801, Victoria and Albert Museum, London).

An upsurge in interest in all things Egyptian came following Napoleon's reconnaissance of the country at the end of the eighteenth century. There was a systematic survey of the country and much of the information was published with numerous illustrations in works such as V. Denon's, *Voyage dans la basse et la haute Égypte, pendant les campagnes du Général Bonaparte* (3 vols, 1802). These works led to the Egyptomania which swamped much of Northern Europe during much of the nineteenth century.

By the end of the nineteenth century increased affluence and ease of travelling meant that the number of both professional and amateur artists rose considerably. Many of these artists seem to have been fascinated by the apparently hidden lives of women. As a result, this 'world' was frequently deduced, fabricated and depicted.

There seem to be two main types of representations within the Western genre. On the one hand there are those depictions based on first hand experiences and accounts which were depicted by artists who were attempting to be as accurate as possible (fig. 161). Artists of this school who visited the Near East and North Africa, included Ludwig Deutsch (1855-1935). His works *At Prayer* and *The Scribe* are typical of this type, while the artist David Roberts (1796-1864) became famous for his mixture of ancient architecture with small, 'modern' figures. More gentler forms of architecture can be seen in paintings by Arthur Melville (1855-1904), such as his work *Arab Interior*.

On the other hand, there were many more artists and writers, who were attempting to produce a sensational and sensual image of the places they depicted (fig. 162). For many of these painters the more secluded and erotic the scene the better (fig. 145). Artists in this genre of Orientalism include Rudolf Ernst (for example, *The Manicure*); Jan-Baptist Huysmans (*The Beauty Spot*); Paul-Désiré Trouillebert (*The Harem Servant*, 1874); Eugène Delacroix (*Femmes d'Alger dans leur appartement*, 1834), Jean-Jules-Antoine Lecomte de Nouy (*The White Slave*, 1888), and John Frederick Lewis (*An Intercepted Correspondence*, 1869 and *The Siesta*, 1876).

It is also worth noting that a number of painters made extensive use of photographs (see below). William Holman Hunt, for instance, is known to have used the works of G. Lékégian, H. Béchard and the Bonfils family. One of Hunt's most famous works, The *Scapegoat* (1854-5), is distinguished for having actually been painted on the shores of the Dead Sea. Yet it would appear that he spent only a short time there making sketches, while the background and even the goat was photographed for future reference. Other 'Near Eastern' artists who made extensive use of photography include Rudolf Weisee; Gustav Bauernfeind and Ludwig Deutsch.

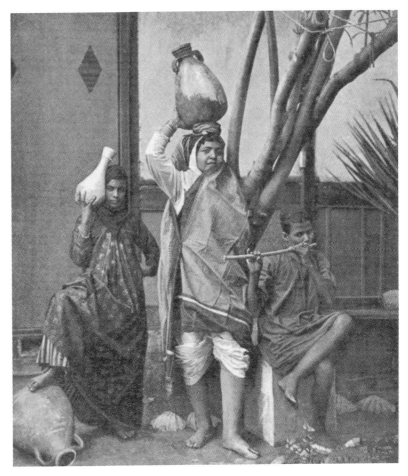

At the beginning of the twentieth century there was a new rage for the oriental image. This was partly due to the publication of the unexpurgated version of *The Thousand and One Nights*, edited by the Arabist R. Burton (1885), and the later French translations by J.-C. Mardrus (16 vols, 1899-1904). The impact of these works upon fashion, ballet, theatre and illustrations were considerable. The Western images of the Eastern woman, for instance, can be found in book illustrations in works such as E. Dulac's *The Rubaiyat of Omar Khayyam* (1909) and *The Thousand and One Nights* (1907). Another version of the *Thousand and One Nights* was illustrated by L. Carré (1929). In all of these works the heroines are beautiful, delicate, slender and scantily dressed.

Finally, the stereotype veiled woman seems to have come to rest in the cartoon world, where a simple piece of cloth across the face of a woman makes her instantly into an 'Arabian Princess' or 'Turkish harem lady'.

Photography

More information about the lives of women, their appearance and the use of veiling came with the advent of photography in 1839. Indeed the influence of photographs and studio tablaux was to play an important role in modern concepts of 'Orientalism' and images of the veil. But it should be stressed that although photographs now became available it does not necessary mean that the information provided is any more reliable.

Figure 163.
A theatrical set for a postcard (c. 1900; courtesy of the Stichting Textile Research Centre, Leiden).

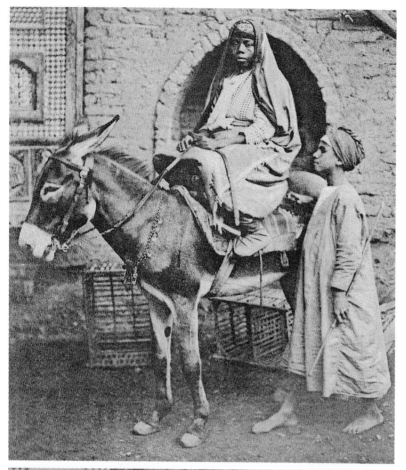

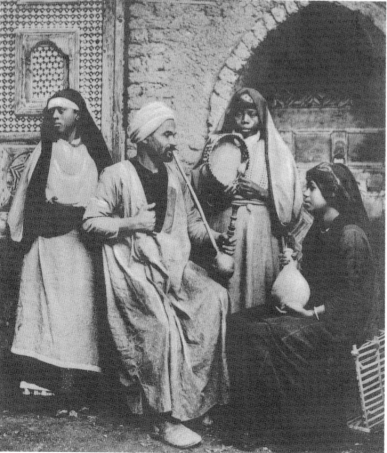

Early photography

The beginning of photography in the Near East coincides with the start of photography itself. In 1839 a new method of producing permanent images was announced. This discovery was called the daguerreotype system after its inventor Louis Jacques Mandé Daguerre. At the announcement of the invention in January 1839 at the French Academy of Sciences, François Arago suggested that the new daguerreotype system should be used to copy Egyptian monuments. As a result of this and other suggestions photographers went to the Near East almost immediately after the technique became available.

Another important development at the time included that by William Henry Fox Talbot, who announced a new system of making positive negatives called the calotype (1840). And in 1850 Louis Désiré Blanquart-Evrard introduced a new system of printing using albumen, which became a standard process for much of the nineteenth century. The following year (1851), Frederick Scott Archer perfected the wet collodion negative process, which replaced both the daguerreotype and the calotype systems.

Perhaps one of the most influential forms of photography, following the introduction of photography itself, was the widespread introduction in the 1890's of the Eastman's Kodak cameras. These cameras meant that literally anyone could take a relatively small and light camera while travelling. The era of the tourist snapshots had arrived.

The professional photographers

Following the introduction of the daguerreotype a large number of European photographers travelled to the Near East and North Africa and a number opened their own commercial firms. Some of the first to arrive in the Near East were Frédéric Goupil-Fesquet, Charles Marie Bouton and Horace Vernet. Most of these early photographers were French, followed by the British, Germans, Italians, Greeks and Americans. In addition there were a small number of Dutch, Poles and Russians. As a generalisation, the French and British were known for producing commercial photographs and those for military use; the Germans seem to have been especially active with respect to archaeological work. The Americans on the other hand, were initially mainly interested in photographing the Holy Land.

In addition to European and American photographers there were also a small number of Muslim photographers. These included Mohammed Sadic Bey from Egypt, and Suleiman Hakim who was working in Damascus.

Photographs, albums and postcards

Various forms of photographs taken during the nineteenth century and early twentieth centuries, were intended for both domestic and commercial purposes. These forms included simple photographs taken by tourists for themselves as well as more complex studio photographs.

Another form of commercial photography which developed at this period was the Album. Scenes and peoples with specific themes were collected together and then sold in Europe and America. The first album of photographs showing Near Eastern scenes was commercially published by N.-M. Lerebours of Paris between 1841 and 1844 (*Excursions Daguerriennes: Vues et Monuments les plus remarquables du Globe*). This was followed by albums such as de Pragey's views of Italy, Egypt, Palestine, Syria and Greece (1842) and Teynard's album of Egypt and Palestine (1849-50). In 1866 Lallemand published an album entitled *La Syrie; Costumes, Voyages, Paysages*, which was one of the first albums specifically to include costume as part of the country's exotic nature.

During the 1860's photography became an important medium for 'capturing' glimpses of life, both in Europe and elsewhere. In Europe studios were often used to make portraits of clients, as well as for the creation of specific tablauxs. Most commercial (European) studios in the Near East, however, seem to have relatively little portrait work, while the production of 'scenes', especially for the tourist trade, was much more important. Studios were set up in various cities including Istanbul, Beirut, Damascus, Jerusalem, Cairo, Alexandria and Port Said.

One of the most prolific of the studios in the Near East was the famous Maison Bonfils (Beirut, 1867-1918). Other lesser known firms include Laroche (Egypt; c. 1870's), Cateby and Marsha (Ramallah; c. 1880's); Levy and Lepage (Algeria and Paris, c. 1875) and the Zangaki Brothers (Port Said, c. 1870-1900). There was also the firm of Boesinger and Co., of Baghdad, who were working at the beginning of twentieth century in Iraq.

Setting the scene

Postcards were available in the Near East from the late nineteenth century onwards. These cards can be used as a source of information about the garments worn by women at the time. However, it is necessary to be aware that these cards were made to satisfy a particular market, namely, the tourists' desire to tell home where they were and what they had seen. Such postcards also tended to reinforce certain stereotype images.

Generally, early postcards depict scenes which were often simply made to look like theatrical sets. All too often, these cards use studio props borrowed from the world of Orientalist paintings including the water pipe (*narghileh*), a few palm trees, the laying figure evoking the lounging pose of an 'odalisque' (young, female servant), and a semi-lit room richly decorated with luxurious textiles (fig. 163). In addition, the unnamed people in these postcards were often later 'identified' in the captions and this information was used to stress their identification on the basis of racial or tribal origins, religion, and, sometimes, class.

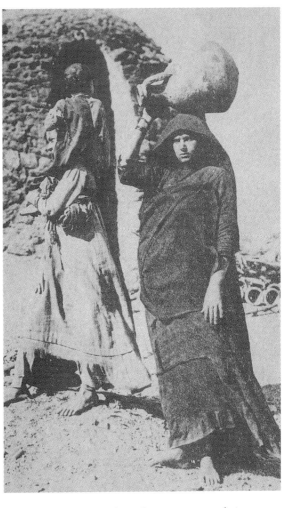

Figure 165. Two women and a child from Egypt, c. 1900 (courtesy of the Stichting Textile Research Centre, Leiden)

It is also apparent that when women were being portrayed the emphasis was usually placed on the face, and especially the eyes. As a result face veiling became an even more striking feature. Thus the erotic, forbidden and unobtainable nature of the 'Oriental' woman, which was so important in paintings, can again be seen in such photographs.

Real life and street scenes

At first glance, old photographs would appear to be a valuable aid to the understanding of how garments were worn. However, certain points need to be considered. With respect to early photographs, the length of time that early photographers needed in order to produce a negative meant that many of the so-called scenes of daily life were in fact carefully staged and posed.

Another problem which may be encountered is that of scenes which appear to be set out-of-doors and thus true to life, but which uses one specific location on several occasions. For example, there are various postcards probably initially produced by the Zangaki Brothers of Port Said, Egypt, at the turn of the century. By about 1905 the Cairo Postcard Trust, Cairo, and Lichtenstern and Harari, Cairo, were also using some of these photographs. In addition, the photographs were being used in fashionable French and English magazines.

Figure 164a-b. Two postcards with scenes using the same set and female model (c. 1900, courtesy of the Stichting Textile Research Centre, Leiden).

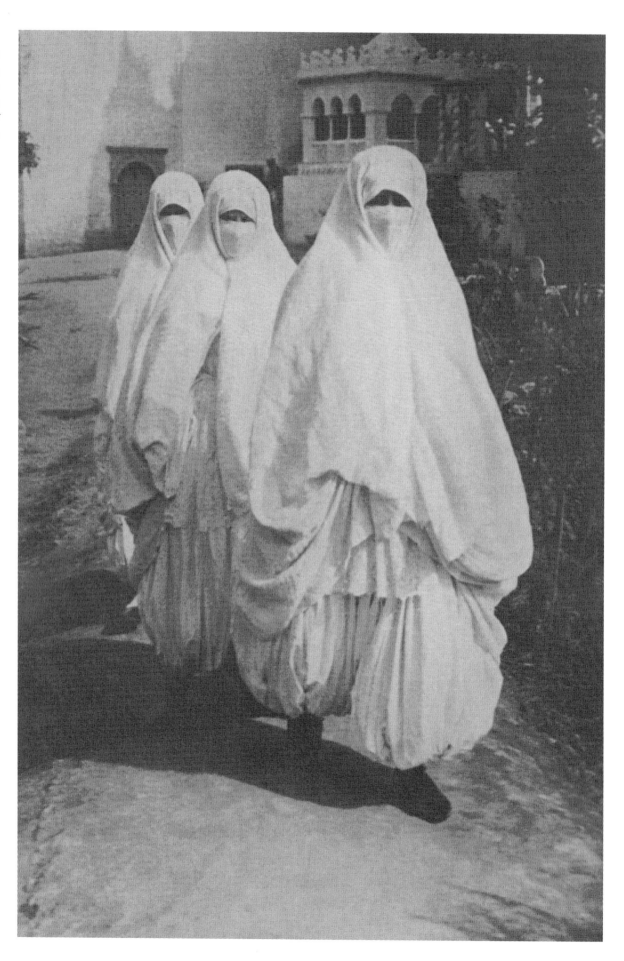

Figure 166a-c.
A group of postcards
from the beginning
of the 20th century
showing "Arab
women" (courtesy of
the Stichting Textile
Research Centre,
Leiden).

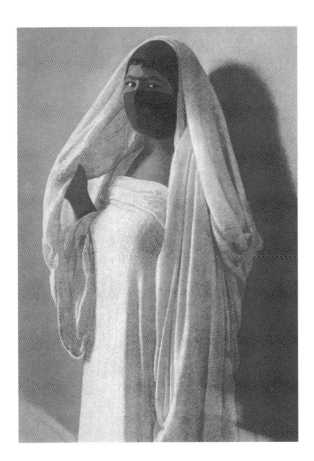
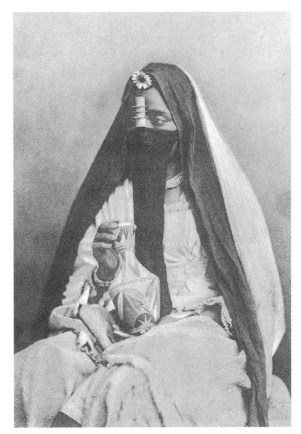

One of the outdoor sets frequently used by the Zangaki Brothers includes a mashriiyaa (latticed window), set close to the ground, with an archway and tree just to the right. The same scene has been used for a variety of themes including: the *Captive dans son palais*: (*Femina*, Paris, 1 Jan, 1906); *L'Amour egyptienne*; *Dame negresse sur Bouricos*, and *Famille Arabe* (fig. 164a-c). In the last two examples, the same model is riding on the donkey and holding the tambourine.

The use of one photograph by different publishing houses at different times, can make it very difficult to be certain where a particular photograph was taken, who the women represent and when the photograph was taken. These details are of importance when trying to understand regional clothing and variations.

Daily life scenes

One of the reoccurring themes when looking at postcards of peasant or fellahin women in the Near East is the water pot. It appears in many photographs, especially those from Algeria and Egypt. An example of such a photograph was published by M. Castro (Edit - Cairo - 84133; Platinoid Photo. Set. A N. 29) and dates from between 1905-1910. The photograph shows a married woman, with a younger girl who is carrying a child (fig. 165). There is part of a mud house in the background and a large number of pots drying in the sun. The married woman is carrying a water pot on her head. She is wearing a dark coloured *galabiyeh* with a *malayeh laff* wrapped around her upper body and then draped over her

head. The younger girl is wearing a light coloured *galabiyeh* probably with long under-trousers.

Some (stereo) types

Often a general title was given to a photograph which can make it difficult to be sure of the wearer's origin. Sometimes this was a deliberate 'deception' on the part of the postcard manufacturer, on other occasions it seems to be more a case of laziness.

"Femme Arabe"

All of the following three postcards have been given the title *Femme Arabe* (fig. 166a-c). The first two are by LTL, a company working in North Africa, especially Algeria. The first postcard shows a woman dressed in local clothing with a *lithma* type of veil which covers her nose and lower face. The second postcard shows a woman wearing the *lithma* of Tunisia which was bound around the upper forehead and around the lower part of her face, leaving only the eyes uncovered. Both are wearing a *huik* or large outer mantle. The third postcard depicts a young girl wearing the typical *burqa`* veil of northern Egypt, which has become especially associated cities such as Port Said, Cairo and Alexandria. In addition a daisy has been added to her hair and she carries the ubiquitous pot.

It could be argued that all of these woman are Arabs. However, when trying to understand clothing, it should be understood that there is a great deal of difference between the clothing worn by women in North Africa, Egypt and the Arabian Peninsular.

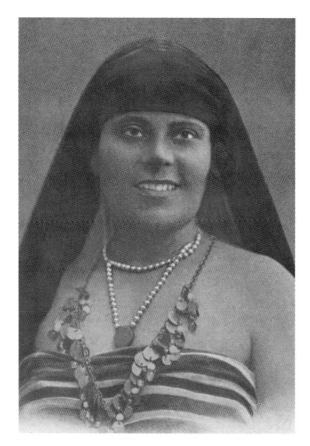

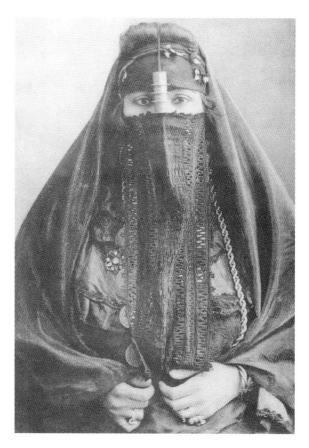

Figure 167. A pretty 'Egyptian' girl (courtesy of the Stichting Textile Research Centre, Leiden).

Figure 168. An Egyptian woman (courtesy of the Stichting Textile Research Centre, Leiden).

Egyptian Women

Above we briefly looked at the problems of recognising Arabic women. Now comes the problem of looking more closely at one particular nation, Egypt. Traditionally, there is a very wide range of clothing worn in this land. This variety is based on many factors, including social (urban versus nomad), economic (rich versus poor), as well as marital position (married or unmarried). In addition, there are differences according to the place of origin. These differences were often shown by photographers in so-called "Types and Scenes" series.

Various 'types' of women are depicted in the following postcards. In the first postcard (fig. 167) it is clear that the photographer had been instructed to photograph a pretty girl, add one or two accessories and call her Egyptian. The publisher of this postcard is not known, while the scene is simply, entitled "Femme Égyptienne".

In other postcards an effort was made to show a specific type, namely an Egyptian woman (fig. 168). Between 1895 and 1900, G. Lekegian and Co. of Cairo, produced a series of postcards which show young, presumably unmarried girls, as water carriers. The scenes have vague titles such as *Fille arabe portant Ballas* and *Le Caire, fille du Caire*. The models may be different, but their dresses look remarkably alike. The sensuality of these portraits makes it likely that these scenes were regarded as having an attractive face with soft pornography connotations rather than anything else

The untrustworthy nature of these postcards as direct evidence for the identification of garments can be illustrated by comparing the next two postcards. Both postcards date from about 1912 and were sent from Port Said. They are nos 93 and 94 in a series entitled *Edition Egyptienne*. It was produced by A. and M. B. Both cards depict the same two women in the same garments (fig. 169a-b). In no. 93 the veiled woman is seated holding a tambourine, while the young girl kneels by her side. In no. 94 the pose has been altered so that the girl is now standing with a pot in her hand. The veiled woman continues to sit with her tambourine. Scene no. 93 is entitled, *Deux femmes d'Alexandrie*, while no. 94 is *Deux filles de Damiette*. These two cities are several hundred kilometres apart, so their use as evidence for identifying particular, regional types of clothing should be regarded as none.

Turks?

When looking at photographs it is hard sometimes to tell whether the photographer was interested in producing a general series of Near Eastern types, or was interested in the various nationalities living in one particular country. For example, for several hundred years, up to the beginning of the First World War, the Turks were the official rulers of Egypt. As a result Turkish style clothing was adopted by many high-class Egyptian women. This led to a divergence in Turkish/Egyptian clothing, Firstly, there were the garments worn by women of Turkish descent and Turkish style garments worn by women of Egyptian descent.

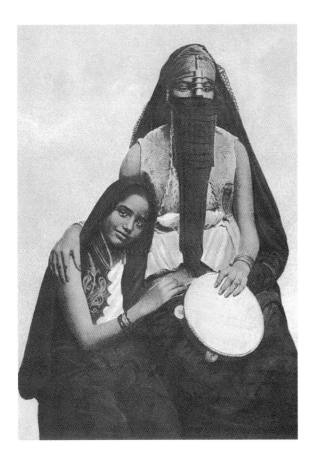

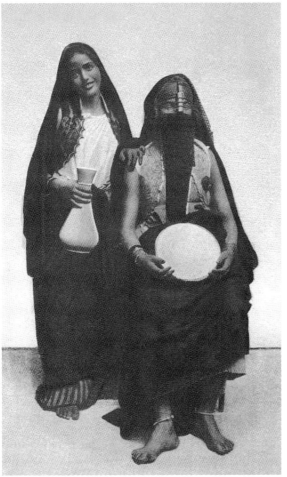

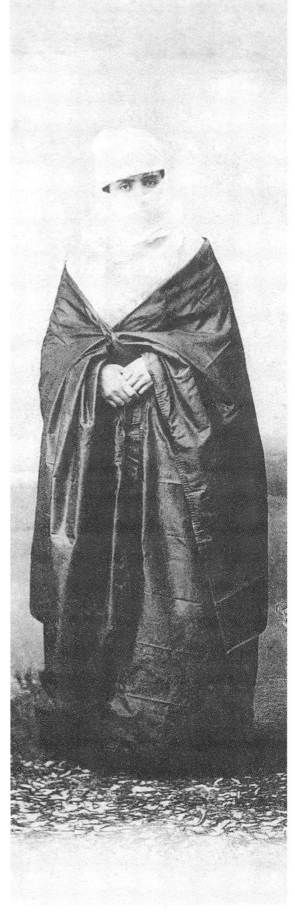

Figure 169a-b.
Two postcards
showing the same
models posing as
women from
Alexandria and
Damiette (courtesy
of the Stichting
Textile Research
Centre, Leiden).

Figure 170a. *Two*
postcards showing
'Turkish women' in
indoor and outdoor
costume (courtesy of
the Stichting Textile
Research Centre,
Leiden).

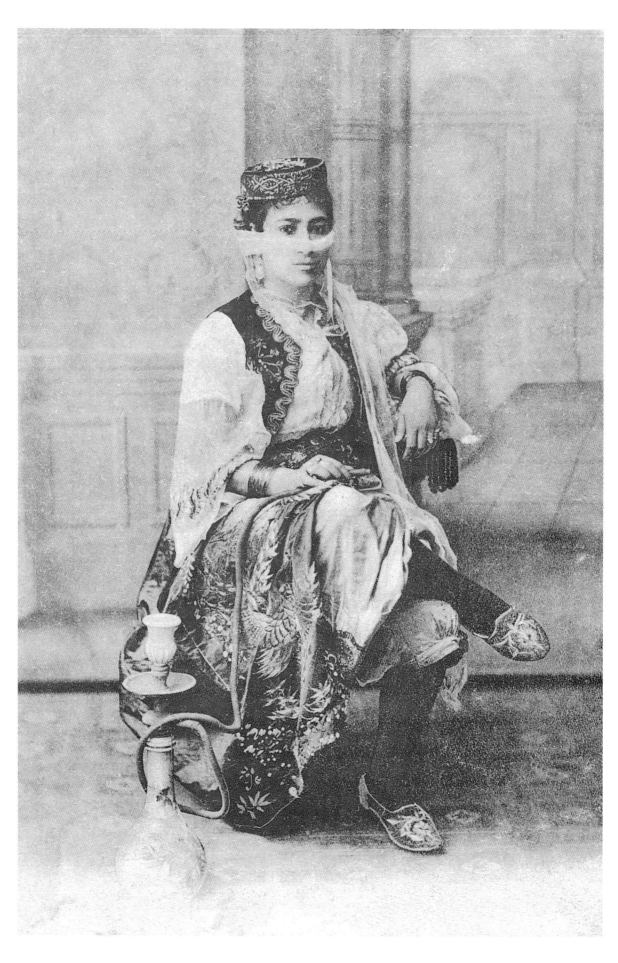

Figure 170b. Two postcards showing 'Turkish women' in indoor and outdoor costume (courtesy of the Stichting Textile Research Centre, Leiden).

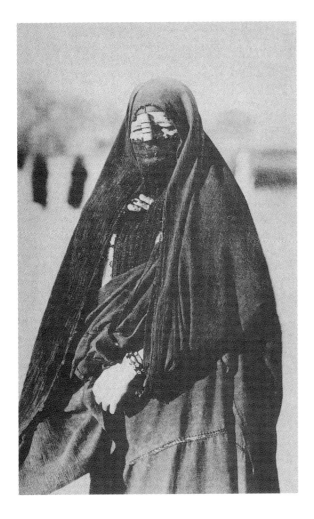

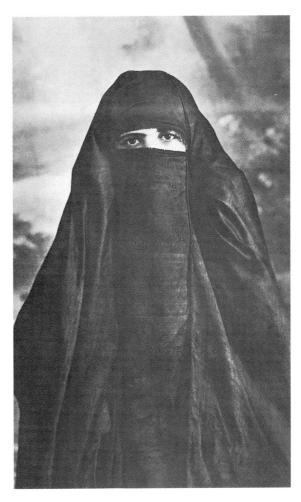

The situation is further complicated by the fact that the wearing of Turkish style garments (real or otherwise) was regarded as the prerogative of middle and higher class women. It is highly unlikely that such women would have posed for the following photographs. Where then did the garments come from? Where they simply part of the photographer's prop chest? This suspicion lingers as all of the following photographs were taken in various studios.

Two photographs show what preport to be Turkish women. Both postcards date to about 1895-1905 (fig. 170a-b). One of the postcards was produced by Lichtenstern and Harari (no. 357; Egyptian card). The second postcard is not signed although it was posted from Cairo in 1905 and has the no. 66 745 on the front. The first card shows a *Dame Turque* wearing outdoor clothing complete with a *ferangi* or out-of-doors coat and a *yashmak* style veil made from two strips of material, one of which covered the forehead. The second veil covered the lower part of the face (this should probably have come much higher up the shoulders). In the second card the woman is showing wearing an indoor version of a Turkish costume and is only wearing the lower half of the *yashmak*. The 'harem' background is emphasised by the fact that she is smoking a water pipe.

Reality versus sensuality

Words such as harem, mysterious, unapproachable, sensual, and lascivious give an impression of some of the images associated with the 'Oriental Woman'. In all of the images clothing, or the lack of it, plays an important role in showing the unobtainable. Certain props reoccur in these postcards, namely, water jars, pipes, servants and couches.

Perhaps the greatest contrast between a daily-life and a studio portrait can be seen by comparing the following two postcards. The first post card was produced by M. Castro Edit - Cairo (84189, Platinoid Photo. Set. A N. 35). It shows a more mature woman wearing a tradition urban veil (*burqa`* type) with brass amulet holder (fig. 171). She is also wearing a draped *miláyeh laff*. In the background there are vague shapes of other women. There is the feeling with this photograph that the manner in which the woman is wearing her garments represents reality.

In contrast, the second photograph is by Boesinger and Co., Baghdad (Iraq), and is part of a long series of postcards showing "Mohamedan Types". In this case "Mohamedan Typo [sic] of Baghdad" is being depicted (fig. 172). The scene behind the woman is obviously a set. More importantly, she is not wearing her clothes very well. They have the appearance of being thrown on with little care.

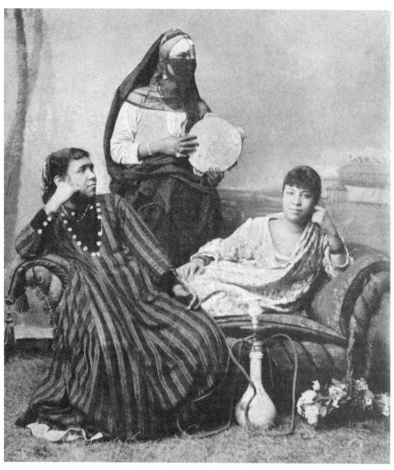

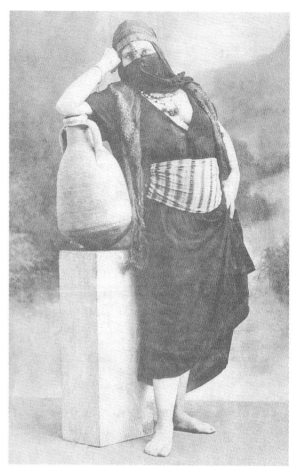

Boesinger is believed to have frequently used prostitutes as models for his postcards and it was said that he was more concerned with the sensual aspects of the image rather than depicting reality.[74]

One of the most 'obvious' examples of soft pornography can be seen in a postcard which was posted in either 1909 or 1919 and comes from the "collection artistique P. Custoulides, Alexandria, Egypt (fig. 174). The series is *Types d'Egyptiennes*, no 25. The woman is wearing a long black *galabayeh* which has been raised in her left hand to show her ankles. Around her waist is a wide cumberband. The top of the garment is wide open so that her breasts are clearly visible. Her urban style veil is 'casually tossed' over her left shoulder. She has a patterned shawl draped over her shoulders and head. Her right arm rests upon yet another water pot.

Curiously, it is the servant (this time with a tambourine rather than water pot) who is veiled in the following postcard produced by M. Handras of Port Said (no. 21). The card is entitled: *Deux dames arabes et la servante.* The servant is wearing an urban veil, a light-wight scarf with a dark *maleyah laff* (fig. 173). Her 'mistresses' are both lounging on a couch wearing indoor galabyehs one of which has been deliberately left open at the top.

A very bored looking lady is shown in another studio scene (fig. 175). The garments she is wearing are unusual in that she appears to be dressed in an European style day gown with a light coloured blouse and long light skirt. She would seem to be wearing a narrow belt around her waist. The post card was part of a series produced by 'B.B.' which has the captions in French on the back and English on the front. The card has the caption: *40 Egypt - Arab lady smoking her narghilet - B.B.*

Notes:

72 The poem however, then goes on to state:
    "But there is neither East nor West,
    Border or Breed or Birth
    When two strong men stand face to face,
    tho' they come from the ends of the earth."
73 Tietzes 1944:156-157; Raby 1982:41.
74 See comments by Graham-Brown 1988:67. Her figure 29 is another example of the "Mohamaden Typo" series.

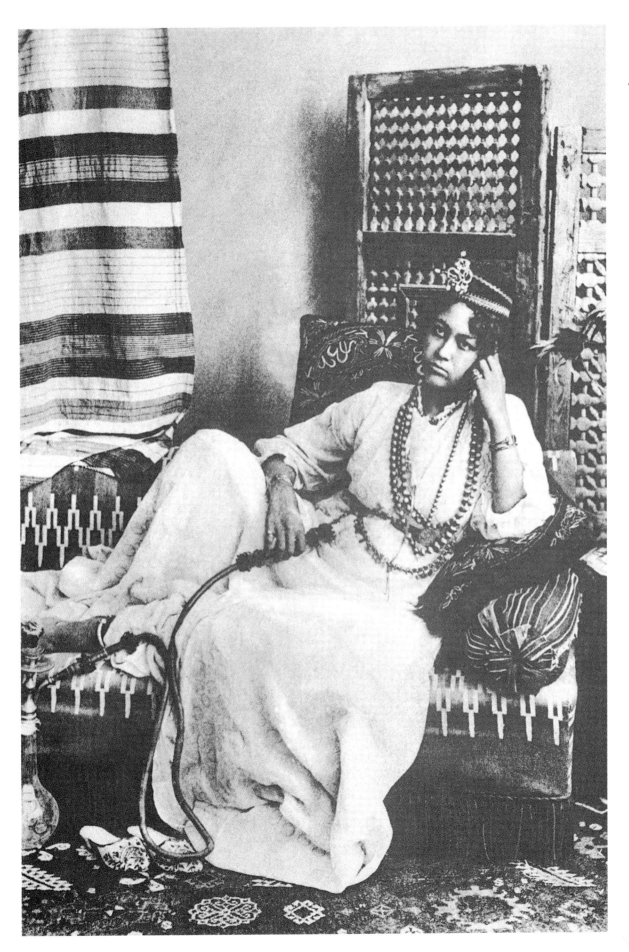

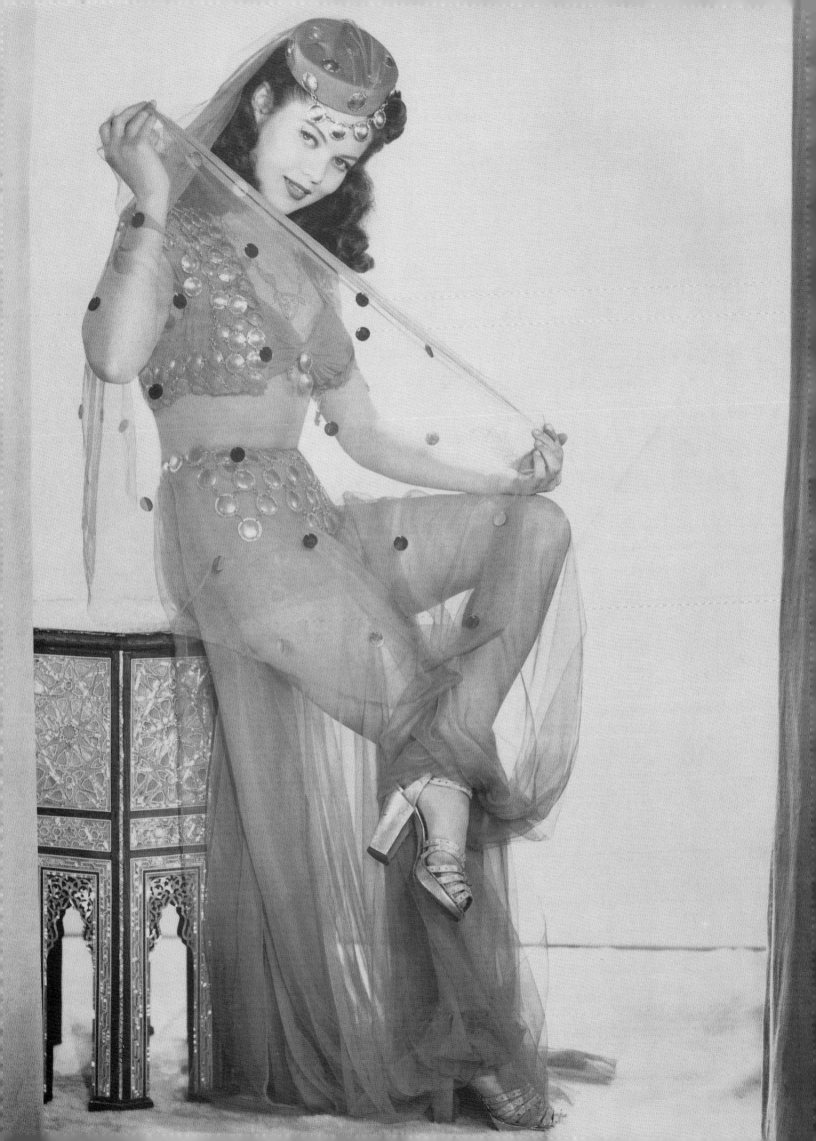

Chapter 14

Veiling, the theatre and Hollywood

I n the last chapter attention was paid to the role of painting and still photography in the development of this preconception of Middle Eastern women. In this chapter particular attention will be focused on the image of the so-called belly-dancers in cabaret and films. It will soon become apparent that the theatre, closely followed by Hollywood and movie films have played an important role in how people in the West see and regard the 'typical' woman of the Near East.

Baladi dancing

Baladi or traditional (peasant) dancing can be regarded as the traditional dancing of the Near East. There are special dances for men and for women. They are characterised by being separate, men do not normally dance with women. Sometimes women's *baladi* dancing was only performed at home by the women of the households on special occasions. But for various festivals or celebrations, there were also groups of professional dancers who could be hired (fig 176).

There are various forms of *baladi* dancing throughout the Near East. That found in Turkey, for example, is very different from the dances of Algeria. It would be impossible in this short study to refer to all the different forms of dancing, so attention will be focused on some professional *baladi* dancing in North Africa, and the development of traditional dancing into its cabaret form in Egypt.

The various names given to *baladi* dances by Western writers indicates a strong degree of confusion about the nature of this form of dance. It was called *danse du ventre* (veil dance), *belly dancing* (a corruption of baladi dancing), and even *hoochie koochie* (after the Kooch dancers of India). The actual origin of the dance was not important, what counted was the idea that the dance was Oriental.

During the nineteenth century two groups of professional dancers were well-known both locally and from the tales of European travellers. The first were the Oud Nial (Ouden Nail, Ouled Nail) of North Africa, whose women were famous as dancers. The second group were the *ghawazee*, a nomadic group from Egypt whose women earned a living as entertainers.

The Oud Nial lived in Northern Africa, especially in Algeria, and it was from there that they had an influence upon French 'oriental' dance styles. Similarly, at the beginning of the twentieth century, Egypt was a colonial outpost which had a strong cultural influence upon both Europe and America. Later, Egypt became the centre of the Middle Eastern entertainment industry and is now known for its development of the so-called Arab Cabaret form.

Traditionally, Oud Nial women learned to dance from infancy. When they were about twelve years old they left home and began a life in the oases. Here they entertained in the cafes, combining the profession of dancer with that of prostitute. When they had earned enough money for their dowry they stopped working and married. In North

Figure 180. Scene from the film "Road to Morocco" with Doris Lessing (courtesy of BFI Stills, Posters and Designs, London).

Figure 177.
A women from the
Oud Nail tribe of
North Africa
(c. 1900; courtesy
of the Stichting
Textile Research
Centre, Leiden).

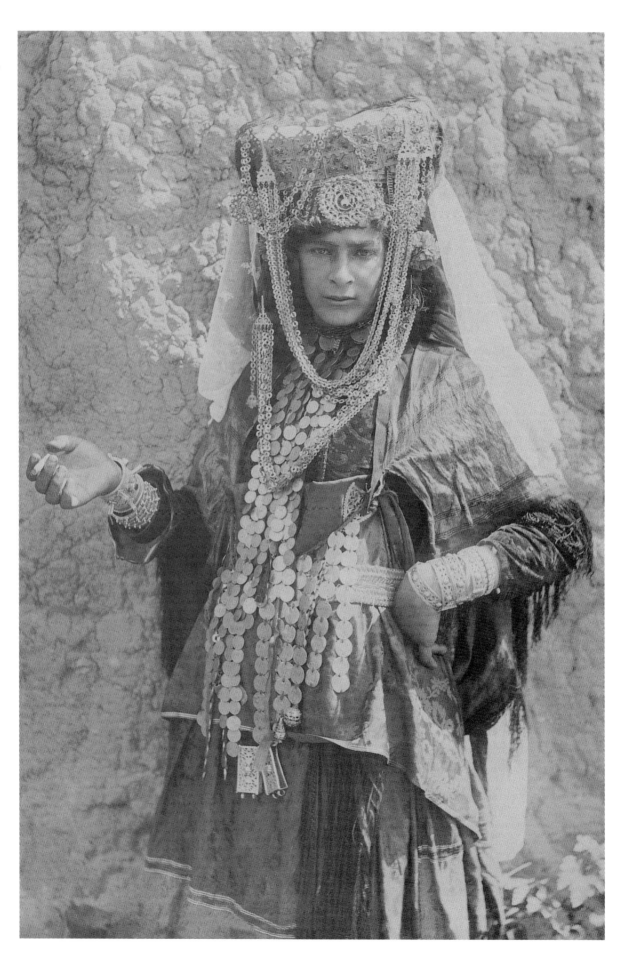

Africa, the term Oud Nail has come to mean dancers in general, no matter where they come from. One result in the region is the closely linked association of professional dancer with prostitute.

The dance of the Oud Nial has a rhythmic element and is closely related to black African dance forms. One American traveller, Ted Shawn, noted that:

"Unlike the Egyptian dancers, who specialize in soft, undulating, serpentine movements of the abdominal muscles, the Ouled Nail pride themselves in being able to make their belly pulsate violently and in syncopation to the music" (Shawn 1929:182).

Shawn went further in his description:

"It is not a suggestive dance, for the simple reasons that it leaves nothing to the imagination, and because of this unashamed animality, revolts the average white tourist to the point of being unable to admire the phenomenal mastery these women have of parts of the body over which we have no voluntary control at all" (Shawn 1929:182).

The costume of an Oul Nial consisted of an embroidered, smock dress worn one on top of the other, with open bell-like sleeves either left hanging or gathered in at the wrists (fig. 177). Over the dresses was worn a *haik* which was draped around the body and secured at the shoulder with a *bezima* or clap. In addition they wore vast amounts of large jewellery. Their long hair was braided with wool and twined around their ears. Some wore tiaras inlaid with coral, turquoise and enamel and huge earrings:

"Their costume while pursuing their craft is very wonderful indeed, they are so wrapped up, and overloaded with clothes, that it is difficult to get any idea of their figures, as one sees nothing but a tangled mass of long draperies and handkerchiefs and chains, which don't seem to belong anywhere in particular..."

"The body is draped, in the first place, in a long gown, that trails far behind, made usually of Manchester cotton print or some flimsy native stuff, which is joined at the shoulder by large silver pins, and doubled under the arms, as to leave the sides bare to the waist. To one of the silver pins is attached a loose banana handkerchief, used sometimes in the dance, and sometimes to mop the perspiring face of the beauty. Round the waist is an immense length of silken belt, wound round and round the body, and hanging in tassels to the feet. Their feet are encased in little embroidered slippers, or red morocco boots, over which fall the monstrous silver anklets, whose clanking gives notice of the approach of the fair one, and reminds the traveller of a prison yard. From the

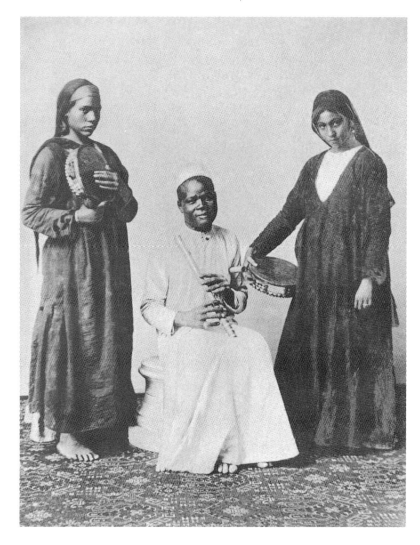

shoulders falls a cloak, dark and thick, and over that again is hung a white-striped cotton and silk sort of burnous, which sometimes trails in the mud, and is occasionally drawn over the head ... Under the chin is often tied a gauze veil of red or green, which is knotted about the neck, and covers the whole construction [hair decoration]. ... Their silken burnouses and gowns are almost hidden under the weight of ornament with which they are encumbered - yards of sliver chains about their necks and waists, on which are strung daggers and looking-glasses, and great boxes of talismans, all of solid silver" (Wingfield 1868:42-4).

At the beginning of the twentieth century there was some confusion in people's minds about the origins of various types of Near Eastern dancers. This can be seen in the following description of the costume worn by someone dancing in the 'Egyptian style'. At that time the dancer usually wore a body stocking (then called a fleshing) with veils and jewellery:

"A dancer in the nude always means something in the Egyptian style, and that entails a good ten pounds'

Figure 176.
Postcard showing Egyptian dancers and musicians wearing traditional clothing (c. 1900; courtesy of the Stichting Textile Research Centre, Leiden).

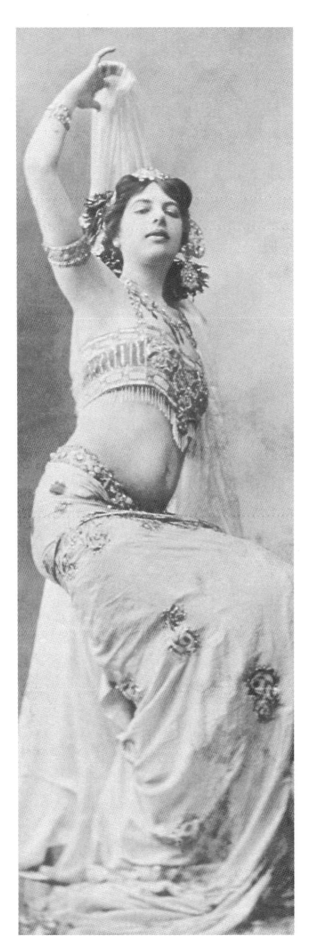

Figure 178. *Mata Hari wearing an oriental style dancing costume (Paris, c. 1905; courtesy of the Mata Hari Collection, The Fries Museum).*

Figure 179. *Scene from the film "Son of the Sheik" with Rudolf Valentino (courtesy of BFI Stills, Posters and Designs, London).*

weight of beaten metal straps and belts and ornaments, beaded latticework on the legs, necklaces from here to there and no end of veils" (Colette 1967:180).

In fact the amount of jewellery shows the influence of the Algerian dancers, the Oud Nial, described above rather, than that of Egypt. However, by this time Egypt had become associated with the Near East and Arabic society, just as China represented the Far East.

The second group of professional dancers were the *ghawazee* who lived in Cairo and travelled through the Delta region. At all times they lived on the fringes of society and were treated as such.

"The Ghawázee often perform in the court of a house, or in the street, before the door, on certain occasions of festivity in the hareem ... They are never admitted into a respectable hareem" (Lane 1895:373).

Despite people's attitudes towards them, the basic costume of the *ghawazee* was based on the everyday costume of middle and upper class urban Egyptians, rather than *baladi* clothing.[75] They tended to wear undershirts of transparent white muslin with long sleeves which reached to above the knees (*thaub*), a long, tightly fitting jacket (*yelek*), Turkish style pantaloons (*shintiyan*) gathered in at the ankle, and one or more shawls tied around the hips.[76] In addition they wore large quantities of ornaments (but not the heavy jewellery worn by the Oud Nial).

E.W. Lane gave a description of the *ghawazee* entertaining at a private party:

"their performances are yet more lascivious .... Some of them, when they exhibit before a private party of men, wear nothing but the shintiyán (or trousers) and a tób (or very full shirt or gown) of semi-transparent, coloured gauze, open nearly half-way down the front" (Lane 1895:373).

During the 1830's the *ghawazee* were banished from Cairo to Upper Egypt due to religious pressure and the notoriety of the dancer's lives. Ironically their place in Cairo was taken up by Khawals or boy dancers who originally came from Istanbul. Often these male dancers dressed up as women and danced more salaciously than the *ghawazee*. In 1860's the ban on the *ghawazee* was lifted and they returned to Cairo.

In general, Near Eastern women have usually refused to dance naked, especially in front of strangers. During the nineteenth and early twentieth centuries, one of the few dances which involved the removal of garments is the so-called "Bee Dance". In this dance the (professional) dancer pretends to have a bee loose in her clothing and she becomes desperate in trying to remove both the bee

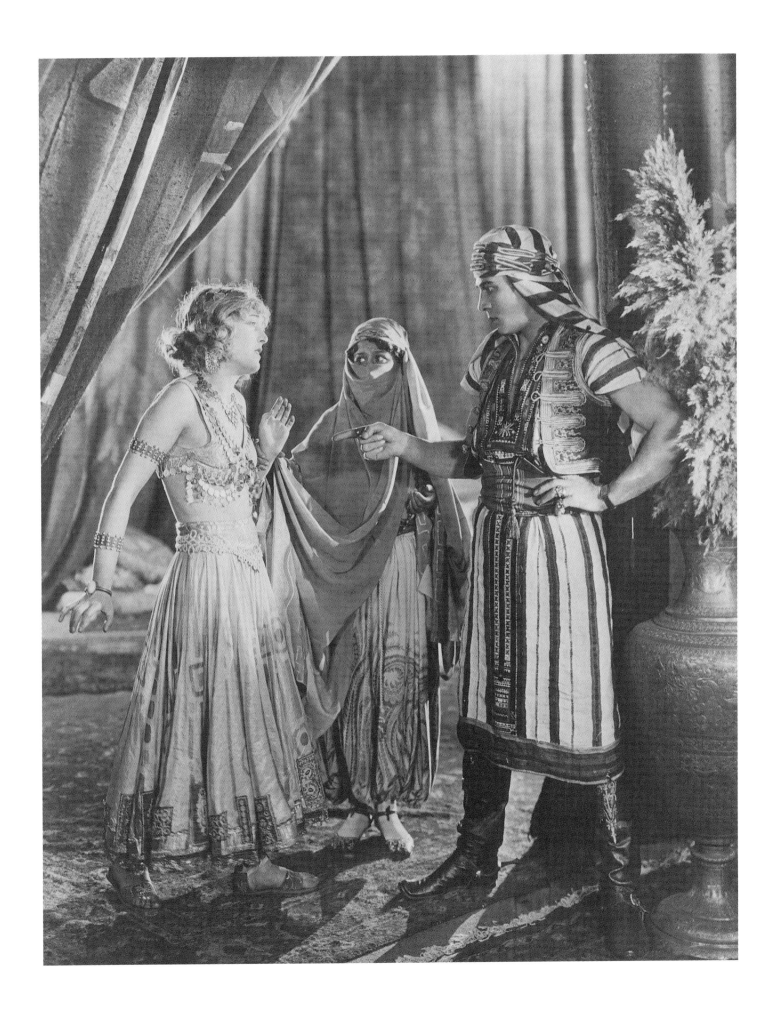

Figure 181. *James Bond from the harem scene in the film, "The Spy Who Loves Me" (the Museum of Modern Art/Film Stills Archive. Courtesy of United Artists).*

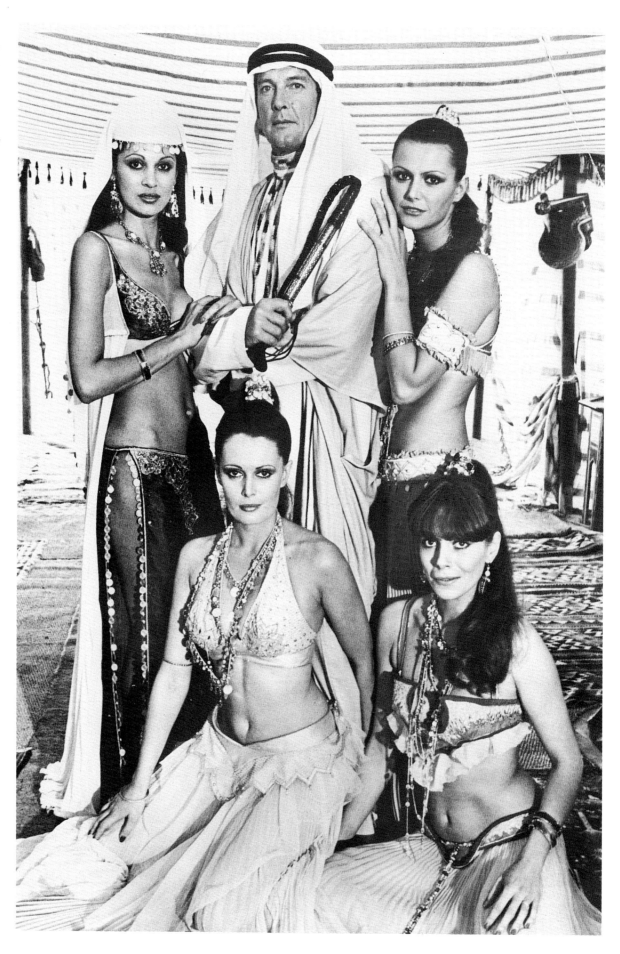

and her garments. There are several nineteenth century descriptions of this dance, but perhaps one of the clearest is given by H. de Vaujany in *Le Caire et ses environs*:

"One of the most popular is the dance of the bee (el-nahleh). The *ghawazi* [professional dancer] pretend to have been stung by a bee which they search for inside their costume, uttering little cries, trying to catch hold of the imaginary insect. Without stopping the dance, they quickly remove a first piece of their clothing, and throw it down; then they throw aside a second piece, calling 'nahleh, nahleh', with gestures which express by turn the fear of being stung and the hope of soon getting rid of the enemy. After much fruitless reaching, they end up with only one very light veil which they leave to float at the march of their movements. Little by little the dance becomes more lively, the figures animated and then, 'quite unintentionally' the last piece of the costume joins the others" (de Vaujany 1883:88-93).

Although there are still some *ghawazee*-style dancers in Egypt, their place has been taken by professional cabaret dancers (see below). Nevertheless, their presence is still felt both in the attitudes people have towards cabaret dancers, namely that the latter are not entirely respectable, and in their ability to change their costume and dance to current demands.

Western Cabaret or Belly Dancing

Written and pictorial descriptions of dancers began to filter through European life during the eighteenth and nineteenth centuries. In the early nineteenth century there was an explosion of Oriental themes in the theatre. Although most are based around Indian and Chinese themes, there were a few which were strongly influenced by the Near East. Some of the most influential productions in England were the *Earthquake or the Spectre of the Nile*, produced at the Adelphi Theatre in 1828 and 1829 (based on ancient Egypt and the then recent archaeological finds); *Hassan Pacha or the Arab's Leap* (Adelphi Theatre, 1838), which included a troupe of 'Bedouin Arab' dancers, and *The Desert* of 1847. The latter was a theatrical presentation of Félicien David's musical *Mélodies Orientales*, which were written following the composers visits to Turkey, Syria and Egypt. According to John Mackenzie, *The Desert* was: "a classic Orientalist performance, a European vision of vast geographical and meteorological effects, architectural grandeur, impressive ceremony and human and animal processions. It is essentially a circus vision" (Mackenzie 1995:192).

Perhaps one of the most important sources of 'information' were the great exhibitions held throughout Europe and America from the middle of the nineteenth century onwards. Here halls and even complete buildings were constructed in order to present different cultures.

People and cultural activities including dancing and music formed an essential part of the entertainment.

In Europe one of the most influential with respect to presenting the Near East and its music was the 1889 Paris Exposition Universelle. Dancers came from Africa, the Near East as well as Asia. Similarly, in 1893 the Great Columbia Exposition in Chicago included a Moorish palace, Turkish and Persian theatres and a Cairene street including indigenous entertainers (Buonaventura 1994:101). The Egyptian dancing was performed by Fahreda Mahza (originally from Syria), who proved to be the sensation of the fair.[77]

Ironically, one of the comments made about the dancers was that physically they were a disappointment:

"Their kinky hair, dirty butter complexions, bad features, stained teeth, and tendency to *embonpoint* are dreadfully disillusioning, their voices are of a timbre that would drive an American cat in disgrace from any well-regulated neighbourhood" (*The Illustrated American*, Chicago Nov. 1893).

By this date people's expectations of an oriental dancer had already been formed by Western art and literature. Oriental women, especially dancers, were meant to be mysterious, veiled beauties, rather than being plump with kinky hair and stained teeth.

From 1893 onwards the first so-called Oriental dancers began to appear in the various vaudeville and burlesque shows throughout America as well as salons and theatres of European cities. These dancers appeared under names as varied as Fatima, La Meri, Kishka and Poupik (English transliterations of Jewish words for the navel and other parts of the body; Buonaventura 1994:123).

Although one of the most renowned of these dancers was Colette (see below), one of the most famous was the Dutch 'dancer' Mata Hari (Margaretha Zelle), who was later executed at the end of the First World War by the French as a German spy. Facts about Mati Hari are difficult to come by as she was a compulsive liar (Waagenaar 1995). She pretended to be the daughter of a temple dancer and produced a style of Indian/Indonesian dancing. In addition she claimed to have been to Egypt and other Near Eastern lands to study *baladi* dancing. Although there is no evidence of such visits, several of her costumes certainly indicate a Near Eastern/Oriental feel, with their use of breast pads, veils, and low cut pantaloons (fig. 178).

Gradually, a more refined, Westernized Oriental dance took form. This dance combined upper torso movements, dramatic poses and ritual mime (Buonaventura 1994:118). The influence of Russian and French ballet was seen in the way the dancers used the complete area of the stage to dance. In addition, instead of emphasis being on the hips (explicit movements of the pelvis were forbidden in the West), it was moved

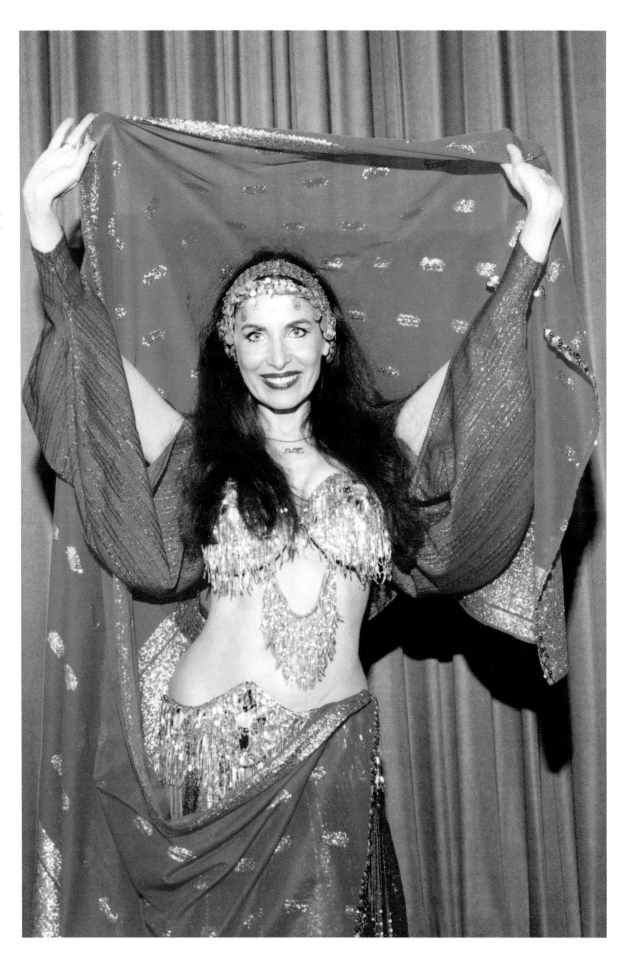

Figure 182.
Modern Oriental-style dancer, Yanina of Amsterdam (courtesy of the Oriental dancer, Yanina, Amsterdam).

Figure 184.
Modern baladi clothing suitable for dancing in (RMV 5826-2,6; photo. by B. Grishaaver).

upwards to the upper torso and the hands. The hands, for
example, were allowed to move in wide circles,
something which was not normal in *baladi* dancing

In her novel *The Vagabond*, "Colette" drew upon her
own experiences as a professional dancer to describe a
society party at which she was one of the attractions:

> "My hand trembling with stage fright, I wrap myself
> in the veil which constitutes almost may entire
> costume, a circular veil of blue and violet, measuring
> fifteen yards round. I began to writhe as my hands
> slowly loosen. Little by little the veil unwinds, fills,
> billows out and falls, revealing me to the eyes of the
> audience, who have stopped their frantic chatter to
> gaze at me ... I dance and dance. A beautiful serpent
> coils itself along the Persian carpet, an Egyptian
> amphora tilts forwards pouring forth a cascade of
> perfumed hair, a blue and stormy cloud rises and
> floats away, a feline beast springs forwards then
> recoils; a sphinx, the colour of pale sand, reclines at
> full length, propped on its elbows with hollowed
> back and staining breasts" (Colette 1964:38).

Perhaps one of the most famous 'oriental dances' in
Western culture is the so-called *Dance of the Seven Veils*.
This dance is associated with the story of Salome and the
death of John the Baptist (Matt. 14:3-11; Mark 6:17-28).
Yet in neither of the two New Testament accounts of the
Baptist's death is there a description of Salome's dance.
All that it says is that Salome danced: "For when
Herodias' daughter came in and danced, she pleased
Herod and his guests" (Mark 6:22).

In fact, the 'infamous' *Dance of the Seven Veils* only
dates back to the first decade of the twentieth century. In
1893 Oscar Wilde published a one act play in French
called *Salomé*. The lurid nature of the play meant that it
would have been automatically banned in England. In
1896, however, the play was produced in Paris and
starred the famous French actress Sarah Bernhardt. In
1905 Richard Strauss composed an opera based on the
Wilde play also called *Salome*, with lyrics by Florent
Schmitt and a ballet sequence for the dancer Loïe Fuller.
The "decadence and psychological intensity" of the music
meant that Salome caused a controversy (MacKenzie
1995:161). But perhaps one of the most famous elements
to come out of the opera was in the last act, the notorious
"Dance of the Seven Veils" in which the dancer slowly
removes most or all of her clothing.

As noted by Mackenzie, the influence of the Near East
and Orientalism was felt deeply throughout the theatre:

> "Clothed in such costumes, and set against flying
> drapes and exotic backdrops, the dancers created new
> moods; religious reverie, majestic display, unbridled
> sexuality or fabulous myth, conveyed by extremes of
> languor and muscular frenzy, slow unfolding patterns,
> twisting arabesques, sensual motions, themselves

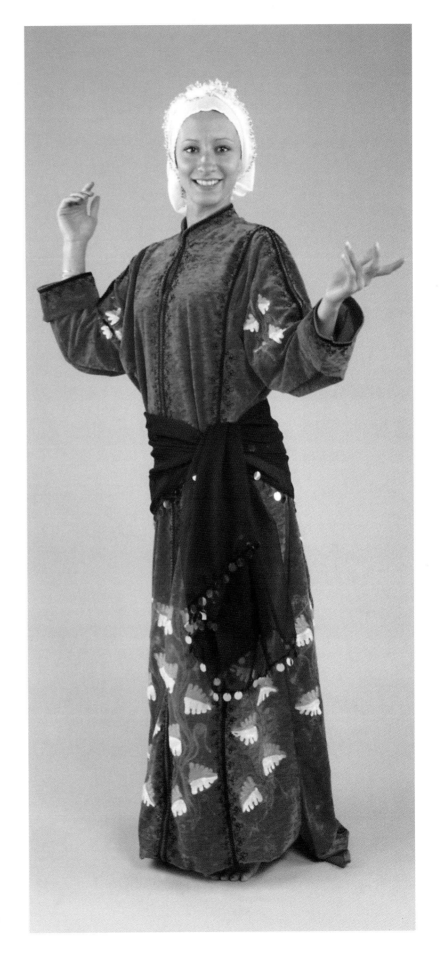

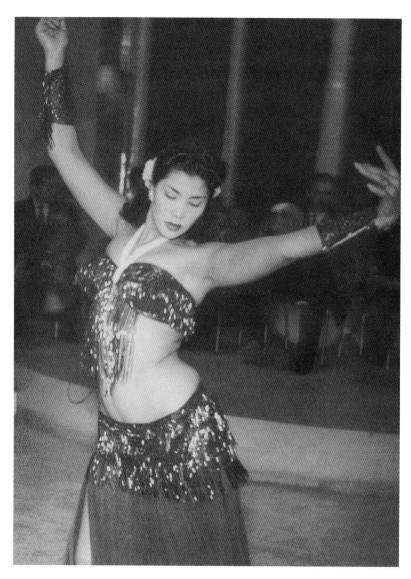

Figure 183. Egyptian cabaret costume (courtesy of the Stichting Textile Research Centre, Leiden).

emblematic of the non-linear, curved and mobile character of eastern design. The key point, however, is the Orientalist creations served to influence design, movement and production in the musical theatre generally, Those that ceased to have any connections at all to supposedly eastern themes still bore the mark of this revolution" (MacKenzie 1995:199).

With all of the various influences from the American and European stage, it is not surprising that by the 1900's Hollywood was already beginning to pick up the oriental style of dancing.

One of the first films of this genre would seem to be the *Danse du Ventre* (also called the *Passion Dance*) made in 1896 and featuring the American dancer Dolorita. It would appear that by this date the belly dancing costume had already developed as Dolorita was wearing a:

"voluminous low-slung pantaloons, her breasts barely concealed beneath a fine lawn chemise and a bodice bursting at the seams. Straddling the stage, she gyrates wildly, her body a mass of shaking, pulsating

flesh. With a smile of singular sweetness she sinks to her knees, thrusting her pelvis at the camera" (Buonaventura 1994:104).

Other films of this type were to follow. These included *Intolerance* by D.W. Griffith (1916), complete with troupe of Babylonian dancing girls; *Salome* (1918) with Theda Bara; *The Sheik* (1921; Rudolf Valentino); *The Son of the Sheik* (1926; Rudolf Valentino; fig. 162) and the *Thief of Baghad* (1924; Douglas Fairbanks jr),. Mae West also appeared in costumes based on the oriental mode as can be seen in the film, *I'm no Angel* (1933). Other Oriental style films include *Ali Baba Goes to Town* (1937, Edie Cantor), *The Mask of Demitrios* (1944, Zachary Scott), *Ali Baba and the Forty Thieves* (1944; Jon Hall), *Salome* (1953; Rita Hayworth), and *Road to Morocco* (1942; Bing Crosby, Bob Hope, Dorothy Lamour; fig. 180) and *Yankee Pasha* (1954; Jeff Chandler). Even James Bond has not been allowed to escape from a bevy of beauties dressed in virtually nothing (notably, the tent scene in *The Spy Who Loved Me*, 1977, Roger Moore; fig. 181).

Nowadays there are numerous single and groups of dancers still performing Oriental forms of *baladi* and belly dancing. Currently, one of the most famous dancers in The Netherlands is Yonina (working from Amsterdam), who wears the more discreet cabaret style dancing costume (fig. 182). In Germany, there is Salome (Regina Hentschker), who wears what can be classed as a traditional Western belly dancing costume, complete with navel jewellery and large veil, and Leila (Regina Adib) who wears even less clothing with more beads and sequins (see Askari 1993). On the other hand there are also German groups who are trying to get back to a more traditional form of dancing and actually wear *baladi* style clothing. El Kahina (Dorothea Prill), for instance, has a group called *Ouled As-Sahra* (Children of the Desert), all of whom wear a more traditional style of clothing.

The influence of films and various stage productions, and dance interpretations, especially those from the beginning of the twentieth century, gradually began to have an influence on Eastern professional dancers. In particular, they began to modify their dances in order to make them more acceptable to Western tourists. One of the more famous truly oriental dancers was the Armenian dancer, Armen Ohanian, who published an autobiography of her life as a dancer and her views of what was happening to her particular dance form (Ohanian 1922). Originally from Armenia she had lived and travelled extensively in Egypt as well as Europe. She was one of the first to note that Western concepts of Oriental dancing were beginning to have an effect upon the Eastern forms of the dance:

"In Cairo one evening I saw, with sick, incredulous eyes, one of our most sacred dances degraded into a horrible bestiality. It was our poem of the mystery and pain of motherhood. In olden Asia, which has kept the dance in its early purity, it represents maternity, the mysterious conception of life, the suffering and joy with which a new soul is brought into the world ... but the spirit of the West had touched this holy dance and it had become the *hoochie koochie*, the *danse du ventre*, the belly dance. I heard the lean Europeans chuckling, I even saw lascivious smiles upon the lips of Asiatics, and I fled (Ohanian 1922:246).

Not only was the dance beginning to change, but, as will be seen, the costume worn by the dancers was also significantly altered.

'Arab' cabaret dancing

The 'Arab' cabaret style developed in the nightspots of Algiers, Beirut and Cairo, which sprang up in the 1920's. These clubs were established, in the first instance, to satisfy the demands of a colonial audience. However, it was during this time that Egypt become established as the centre of a Near Eastern entertainment industry, and it was through this medium that the idea of the cabaret dancer was exported to the rest of the Arab world. Egyptian films were especially popular in the Near East, for their rags-to-riches plots in which dancers were often featured as heroines (notably Samia Gamal and Tahia Carioca). Cabaret dancing invariably featured in these films, even if only as a brief diversion from the main plot. Initially, Hollywood exerted a strong influence on Egyptian films and as a result American/European fantasies about Oriental dance filtered through to the Near East. All too often Arab dancers unconsciously parodied these fantasies in their desire to emulate Western behaviour and modes of fashion.

The first Egyptian cabaret, the Casion Opera, was opened in 1926 in Cairo by the Syrian actress-dancer, Badia Masabni (Bounaventura 1994:147ff). Initially, Masabni offered a varied all-round Arabic form of entertainment. However, with an eye on Western ideas, she decided to broaden the scope of Egyptian *baladi*. This discussion resulted in 'Arab cabaret'.

Until then, the upper torso and arms of a dancer had not played an important role in *baladi* dancing. Traditionally the arms were lifted and held in place. Dancers, however, now started using their arms in flowing, serpentine movements. Performers also began to use far more space, whereas previously they had performed more or less on the spot.

Another of Masabni's innovations was the introduction of veils. The use and manipulation of sheer veils was not a feature of *baladi* dancing. Instead, it was taken over from the repertoire of Western Oriental dancers. The form of cabaret dancing which developed at this time has been described by Wendy Buonaventura as follows:

"At one one end of the scale is an act which combines Arabic dance movements, Western notions of glamour and echoes of the Oriental dance of early Hollywood. At the other end is the sexy turn performed by women who know little or nothing about the dance, but who use it as a convenient money-spinner in which the only skill required is the ability to parade around in a revealing costume" (Buonaventura 1994:147)

Scantily dressed entertainers were often compelled, due to the demands of the commercial world, to highlight the more provocative elements of their dance (fig. 183). As a result they were not seen by many traditionalists as a good advertisement for Arab womanhood, which was to have severe repercussions on their traditional way of life (see below). Inevitably, at the lower end of the scale, dancers used the cabarets to advertise their charms to potential clients.

Baladi and cabaret costumes

An important difference between *baladi* and cabaret dancing is the clothing worn by the dancers. The traditional *baladi* costume is usually made up of the everyday clothing of the women, whether professional or amateur. It consisted of a long underdress, an overdress, kerchiefs and shawls around the head, and most importantly a shawl around the hips to emphasise this area of the body (fig. 184). This shawl is tightly wrapped around the hips and was not normally removed. In general, the quality of the material and overall appearance is one of more opulence and sparkle in the professional costumes. Variations on this costume are worn throughout the Near East and Northern Africa.

In contrast to the *baladi* costume, the outfit worn by cabaret 'artists' has more in common with the Western image of a 'belly dancer' or 'Oriental' dancer, rather than the Arabic original. The Egyptian cabaret costume seems to have appeared in the 1920's and is based on the Burlesque/Hollywood outfit. The costume was made up of a combination of "bra, low-slung gauzy skirt with side slits and bare midriff" (Buonaventura 1994:152). Traditionally, dancers were either barefooted or wore flat slippers. However, to show off their wealth and western influences, high heeled shoes were often worn by the cabaret dancers.

The early Arab cabaret dancers were not allowed to show their navels in public, so they used a long strip of material which went from the dancer's bra to the top of the skirt. In later cabarets, however, the 'navel veil' was sometimes discarded and replaced with a jewel in the navel.

Nowadays, the essential cabaret costume remains, in essence, the same since it was created in the twenties (fig. 184). The modern bra and hip-belts encrusted with rhinestones and sequins can be seen as a more "brassy version of the Hollywood's fantasy of an Oriental charmer" (Buonaventura 1994:152).

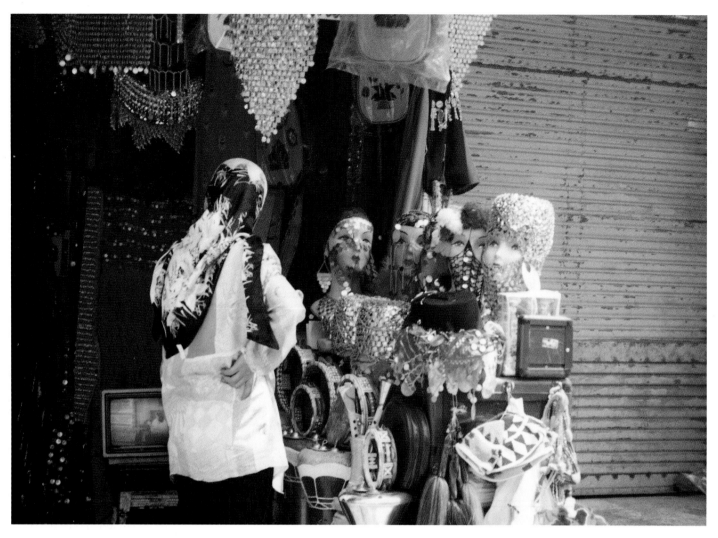

As noted above, another introduction into the Eastern cabaret dancer's clothing repertoire was the veil. This had already become one of the most important elements of the Western cabaret dancer's equipment. In the West veils were first used by the exotic dancers who began to appear at small parties and on the public stage at the end of the 1890's and beginning of the 1900's. Indeed, "society hostesses were among the many who pieced together an Oriental act consisting of theatrical poses, 'passionate writhings', angular mock pharaonic gestures and the discarding of veils in a graceful manner" (Buonaventura 1994:132).

In conclusion, the Near Eastern cabaret dancer's costume can be seen as a pastiche of the original, strongly influenced, if not created, by Western imagination fed on exotic images from literature, art and theatre.

Finally, something should be said about some of the current threats to the traditional art of *baladi* and Egyptian cabaret dancing. The two main problems currently encountered by Arab dancers are the number of professional dancers and even half-trained amateurs who are flooding the market. More importantly for this study, the clothing that these 'foreigners' wear while dancing is causing considerable concern amongst more traditional religious groups.

Egyptian cabaret dancers are currently coming under the threat of extinction because of religious pressures which are forcing dancers in Cairo to wear a one-piece costume that does not expose their midriffs. If the garment is considered to be too revealing then it is likely that the dancer would be visited by a special police group, known as the 'politeness police'. Certain dancers, such as Sahar Hamdi, have frequently been arrested for wearing garments which were considered to be too revealing, so the effectiveness of the police is in question. Nevertheless, the threat of imprisonment remains.

In addition, a number of Egyptian fundamentalists have tried to get cabaret dancing totally banned because dancing is regarded as indecent and immoral. However, the dancers are an important source of income for Egypt because they draw visitors from the Persian Gulf region. As a compromise the Egyptian government has stopped issuing permits to new performers, other than classical folk artists (*baladi* dancers), but they have not banned cabaret dancing outright

Another source of trouble lies in the influx of foreign dancers, especially those from Russia. The *Sunday Times* (30th July 1995) included an article, entitled "Cairo belly dancers feel the breeze", about these dancers:

"Ancient art of belly dancing is under threat in Egypt from foreign interlopers only too willing to work for low pay and to expose more flesh. This may well delight visiting Arabs from the Gulf states eager to savour the delights of western style shows, but veteran Cairo belly dancers are up in arms."

"The traditionalists reserve most of their barbs for hip-swivelling Russian dancers, who frequently are blonde and buxom."

Apparently many of the dancers were ballerinas in Russian companies. In addition there are now a number of 'Oriental dance academies' which specialise in teaching foreigners the art of belly-dancing. Among the foreign graduates from one school, were several Turks, a Russian, a Swede, an Ukrainian, and finally, a 'German', who turned out to be an Israeli (figs. 185 and 186).

A traditional dancer, Boosie, commented in the *Sunday Times* article that the danger to belly dancing did not apply to dancers from this generation, but that of the next who were not receiving the training and work necessary to continue the traditions. In addition, she noted that the European dancers were too skinny, although being a blond was a considerable plus point. Boosie then went on to say that:

"They [the night club owners] would let a Russian dance in a bikini ... If the vice squad saw an Egyptian dressed like that, they'd make a real fuss. We're eastern women - they want to protect us."

As noted previously, Egypt is the centre of the Middle Eastern film and cabaret world. Stars such as Soheir el-Babli, Fifi Abdou, and Suhair Zaki are well-known figures and in some cases, considerable box-office successes. Yet in recent years there have been a number of Egyptian artists who have suddenly renounced show business for good and who have adopted *hijab* clothing. With respect to Cairo's belly dancers these resignations date back to the late 1980's when dozens of singers and actresses were "hanging up their spangles, wiping off their makeup, donning *hijab* and haranguing their former audiences about the evils of the artist's world" (Brooks 1995:213).

Shortly later a joke began to circulate in Cairo in which a more cynical attitude to the renunciations of the dancers is presented:

"Who are the second-best-paid women in Egypt? The belly dancers, of course, because the Saudi tourists throw hundred-dollar bills beneath their feet when they dance. Who are the best paid? The dancers who've retired for Allah, of course, because the Saudi sheiks throw thousand-dollars bills into their bank accounts when they stop dancing" (Brooks 1995:214).

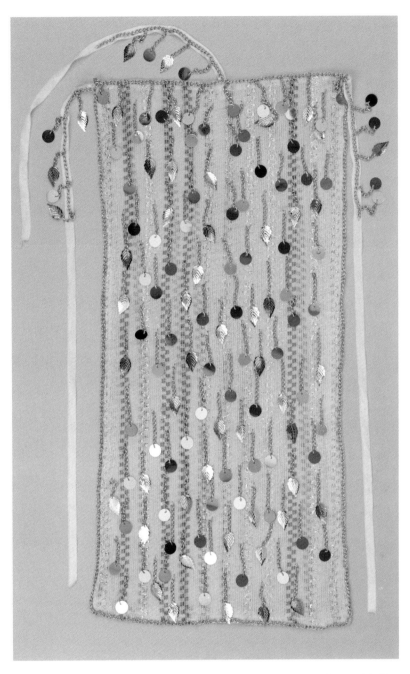

The Egyptian feminist writer, Nawal Saadawi pointed out that many of the women were past their prime as actresses or dancers anyway: "They know they're soon going to have to retire, so why not go out in a blaze of publicity" (Brooks 1995:214).

Figure 186. Face veil made for the tourist market (Cairo, Egypt; photo. by B. Grishaaver).

Notes:

75 Such garments are portrayed in John Frederick Lewis' paintings: "Lilium Auratum, (1871) and "Indoor Gossip" (1873).
76 Lane 1895:49-50; Scarce 1987:127.
77 Other dancers at the fair included Zareefa, a bedouin dancer, Jamelee from Syria and Rosa from Turkey (Buonaventura 1994:123).

Bibliography

ABADAB-UNAT, N., 1981. *Women in Turkish Society*, Leiden.

ABU-LUGHOD, L., 1988. *Veiled Sentiments: Honor and Poetry in a Bedouin Society*, Berkeley and Los Angeles.

ACHJADI, J., 1976, *Indonesian Women's Costumes*, Jakarta.

ADRIANI, A., 1948. *Testimonianze e Momenti di Scultura Alexandrina*, Rome.

AELST, P. C van., 1553. *Moeurs et Façons de Faire les Turez*, Antwerp.

AHMAD, A. al-Raziq, 1973. *La Femme au Temps des Mamlouks en Égypte*, Cairo.

AHMED A.S. 1980, *Pakhtun Economy and Society*, London.

AHMED, L., 1991. "Early Islam and the position of women: The problem of interpretation", N.K. Keddie and B. Baron (eds), *Women in Middle Eastern History*, New Haven, 58-73.

AKKENT, M. and FRANGER, G., *Das Kopftuch/Baörtü*, Frankfurt, 1987.

AKURGAL, E., 1961. *Die Kunst Anatoliens*, Berlin.

AL'AZZI, M. 1990. *The Battulah: Origin and Development* (English abstract), The Gulf States Folklore Centre, Dohar, nos. 13 (1989), 16-39; no. 20 (1990), 17-26.

ALBENDA, P., 1983. "Western Asiatic women in the Iron Age: Their image revealed", *Biblical Archaeologist*, 46 (1983): 82-8.

AMNESTY INTERNATIONAL, 1995. *Vrouwen Rechten zijn Mensen Rechten*, Amsterdam.

ANATI, E., 1968. *Rock-Art in Central Arabia*, Louvain.

ANDERSON, R.M., 1942. "Pleated headdresses of Castilla and Leon (12th and 13th centuries)", *Notes Hispanic*, (1942), 41-79.

ANON. 1986. *Historical Costumes of Turkish Women*, Istanbul.

ANON. 1993. "Omani fashion parade", *PDO News*, 2:30-35.

ARIÉ, R., 1965. "Quelques remarques sur le costume des Muselmans d'Espagne au temps des Nasrides", *Arabica*, 12 (1965), 244-261.

ARIÉ, R., 1965. "Le costume des Musulmans de Castille au XIIIe siècle d'après les miniatures du Libro del Ajedrez", *Mélanges de la Casa de Velazquez*, Paris.

ARIÉ, R., 1969. *Miniatures hispano-musulmanes*, Leiden.

ARIÉ, R., 1973. *L'Espagne musulumane au temps des Nasrides*, Paris.

ARIÉ, R. 1968. "Notes sur le costume en Egypte dans la 1ere moitié du XIXè siècle", *Revue des Etudes Islamiques*, II (1968), 211-12.

ARRIBAS, A., nd. *The Iberians*, London.

ASKARI, U., 1993. *Bauchtanz - Ein Trend mit Folgen?*, Berlin.

AZARI, F. (ed)., 1983. Women of Iran: *The Conflict with Fundamentalist Iran*, London.

BAMBAD, G. OL-MOLUK, 1977. *From Darkness into Light: Women's Emancipation in Iran*, (trans. F.R.C. Bagley), Hicksville.

BARTHES, R., 1957. "Histoire et sociologie du vêtement", *Annales: Economies-Sociétés-Civilisations*, 3 (1957), 430-441.

BATTO, B.F., 1974. *Studies on Women at Mari*, Baltimore.

BEAUMIER, A., 1860. *Roudh el-Kartes: Historie des Souverains du Maghreb*, Paris.

BEESTON, A.F.L., JOHNSTONE, T.M., SARJEANT, R.B. and SMITH, G.R., 1983. *Arabic Literature to the End of the Umayyad Period*, Cambridge.

BERANIS MADRAZO, C., 1956. *Indumentaria Medieval Espanola 700-1500*, Madrid.

BERNIS MADRAZO, C., 1962. *Indumentaria Espanola en tiempos de Carlo V, 1500-1600*, Madrid.

BERESNEVA, L., 1976. *The Decorative and Applied Art of Turkmenia*, Leningrad.

BESANCENOT, J., 1942. *Costumes du Maroc*, Paris.

BETTERIDGE, A., 1986. "To veil or not to veil: A matter of protest:, in: G. Nashat (ed), *Women and Revolution in Iran*, 109-128.

BEURDEN, L. van, 1994. *Over Mode en Mensen*, Nijmeagen.

BJÖRKMAN, W., 1986. "Litham", *Encyclopedia of Islam*, Leiden, vol. 5, 769-770.

DE BRÉVES, F. Savary. 1630. *Relations des Voyages - Hierusalem, Terre-Sainte, Constantinople, Aegypte, Afrique,* Paris.

BRIGGS, L.C., 1960. *Tribes of the Sahara,* Cambridge Mass.

BROADMAN, J., 1985. *Greek Art,* London.

BROOKS, G., 1995. *Nine Parts of Desire: The Hidden World of Islamic Women,* London.

BROUGHTON, J.C.H., 1855. *Travels in Albania and Other Provinces of Turkey,* London, 2 vols.

BOARDMAN, J., 1989. *Greek Art,* London.

v. BRUCK, G., 1987. "Re-defining identity: Women in Sana", in: Daum, W. (ed), *Yemen,* Innsbruk.

BUITTELAAR, M., 1993. "Veiled virgins, beautiful brides", in: P. Faber, *et al., Dreaming of Paradise,* 1993, Rotterdam, 151-168.

BUONAVENTURA, W., 1994. *Serpent of the Nile: Women and Dance in the Arab World,* London.

BURNS, A.R. 1971. *The Pelican History of Greece,* Harmondsworth.

BURTON, R.F., 1853. *Personal Narrative of a Pilgrimage to Al-Madinah and Meccah,* London (Dover ed. 1964; 2 vols).

CARRETERO, C.H., 1988. *Museo de Telas Medievales: Monasterio de Santa María la Real de Huelgas,* Madrid.

CASAJUS, D., 1985. "Why do the Tuareg veil their faces?", in: R.H. Barnes, D. de Coppet and R.J. Parkin, *Context and Levels: Anthropological Essays on Hierarchy,* Oxford, 68-77.

CASTLE, W.T.F., 1942. *Grand Turk,* London.

CHANDRA, M., 1973. *Costumes, Textiles, Cosmetics and Coiffure in Ancient and Medieval India,* Delhi.

CHARDIN, J., 1720. *The Travels of Sir John Chardin,* London (ed. N.M. Penzer, London 1927).

CHARLES, R.H., 1913. *The Apocrypha and Pseudepigrapha of the Old Testament in English,* Oxford.

CHRISTENSEN, H., 1984. *Afghan Refugees in Pakistan: From Emergency Towards Self-Reliance,* Geneva.

CLAVIJO, R. G. de, 1859. *Narrative of the Embassy of Ruy Gonzalez de Clavijo to the Court of Timour at Samarcand A.D. 1403-6,* London (Hakluyt Society ed. 1859, vol. V).

COLETTE, 1960. *The Vagabond,* Harmondsworth.

COLETTE, 1967. *My Apprenticeships and Music Hall Sidelights,* Harmondsworth.

COOPER, E., 1915. *The Harim and the Purdah: Studies of Oriental Women,* London.

CROUTIER, A.L., 1989. *Harem: The World Behind the Veil,* London.

CROWFOOT, E., 1977. "The clothing of a fourteenth-century Nubian bishop", in: V. Gervers (ed), *Studies in Textile History,* Toronto, 43-51.

CUNNINGHAM, P. and LUCAS, C., 1972. *Costumes for Births, Marriages and Deaths,* Oxford.

CUYPERS, J-B., 1994. *Touareg,* Tervuren.

DAR, S.N., 1969. *Costume of India and Pakistan,* Bombay.

DAVIES, E.W.L., 1858. *Algiers in 1857: Its Accessibility, Climate and Resources Described with Especial Reference to English Invalids,* London.

DENYAR, S., 1987. *African Tribal Architecture,* London.

DJÉBAR, A., 1960. *Vrowen van de Islam,* Utrecht.

DORSKY, S.J., 1986. *Women of `Amran: A Middle Eastern Ethnographic Study,* Salt Lake City.

DE JONGHE, M.C., 1976. *Marrying in White: Two Centuries of Bridal Apparel, 1765-1976,* The Hague.

DICKSON, H.R.P., 1949. *The Arab of the Desert,* London.

DJURA, 1994. *De Zusters van Scheherazade: Moderne Vrouwen en de Islamistische Traditie,* Baarn.

DUPREE, L., 1973. *Afghanistan,* Princeton.

DOUBLEDAY, V., 1988. *Three Women of Herat,* London.

DOZY, R.P.A., 1845. *Dictionnaire Détaillé des Noms des Vêtements chez les Arabes,* Amsterdam.

DRIVER, G.R. and MILES, J.C., 1935. *The Assyrian Laws,* Oxford.

EARLY E.A., 1993. *Baladi Women of Cairo: Playing with an Egg and a Stone,* Cairo.

EASTWOOD, G.M., 1983. "A medieval face-veil from Egypt", *Costume* 17:33-38.

EBERHARDT, I., 1992. *The Passionate Nomad: The Dairy of Isabelle Eberhardt,* London.

EICHER, J.B., 1995. "Introduction: Dress as expression of ethnic identity, in: J.B. Eicher (ed), *Dress and Ethnicity,* Oxford, 1-5.

EICHER, J.B. and ROACH-HIGGINS, M.E., 1992. "Definition and classification of dress: Implications for analysis of gender roles", in Barnes, R. and Eicher, J.B. (eds), *Dress and Gender,* Oxford, 8-28.

EPH`AL, I., 1974. ""Arabs" in Babylonia in the 8th century BC", *Journal of the American Oriental Society,* 94 (1974), 108-15.

FABER, P., HUYGENS, C., ROS, F. and RULLMAN, M., (eds.), 1993. *Dreaming of Paradise,* Gent.

FARMAIAN, S. F., 1982. Daughter of Persia, London.

FATHI, A., 1985. *Women and the Family in Iran,* Leiden.

FAIRSERVICE, W.A., 1971. *Costume of the East,* London.

FERDINAND, K., 1993. *Bedouin of Qatar,* London.

FERDOWS, A.K., 1983. "Women and the Islamic revolution", *International Journal of Middle East Studies* 15 (1983), 283-298.

FERNEA, E.W., 1969. *Guests of the Sheik: An Ethnology of an Iraqi Village,* New York.

FISKE, P., 1987-9. *Palms and Pomegrantes: Traditional Dress of Saudi Arabia,* New York.

TUGAY, E. FOAT, 1963. *Three Centuries Family Chronicles of Turkey and Egypt,* London.

FOGG, W.P., nd. *Travels and Adventures in Egypt, Arabia, and Persia, or the Land of "The Arabian Nights",* London.

FROBENIUS, L. and OBERMAIER, H., 1925. *Hadschra Mektuba,* Munich.

FUENTES, M.A., 1866. *Lima. Sketches of the Capital of Peru, Historical, Statistical, Administrative, Commercial and Moral,* Paris.

GALT, C.M., 1931. "Veiled ladies", *American Journal of Archaeology,* 35 (1931), 373-93.

GRACIÁ Y BELLIDO, A., 1971. *Iberische Kunst in Spanien*, Mainz.

GARNETT, L., 1890-1. *The Women of Turkey and their Folklore*, London (2 vols.).

GHERING VAN IERLAND, M.A. and WEYTS-RAMONDT, A., 1987. *Mode in de Zuidelijke Nederlanden 1490-1530*, Bergen op Zoom.

GHERING VAN IERLAND, M.A., 1988. *Mode in Prent (1550-1914)*, Den Haag.

GLOUDEMANS, F., 1975. *Arabische wereld*, Amsterdam.

GRAHAM-BROWN, S., 1988. *Images of Women: The Portrayal of Women in Photography of the Middle East 1860-1950*, London.

GOETZ, H., 1939. *The History of Persian Costume"*, in: ed. A. Pope and P. Ackerman, *A Survey of Persian Art*, London.

GOLDMAN, B., 1994. "Graeco-Roman dress in Syro-Mesopotamia", J. L. Sebesta and L. Bonfante (eds), *The World of Roman Costume*, Wisconsin, 163-181.

GOLDSCHMIDT, L., 1930. *Der Baylonische Talmud*, Berlin, vol. 1.

GOODWIN, J., 1994. *Price of Honour*, London.

GRIEBEWEGEN-FRANKFORT, H.A., 1951. *Arrest and Movement*, London.

EL-GUINDI, F., 1981. "Veiling infitah with Muslim ethic", *Social Problems*, 28 (1981), 465-486.

GUNAY, S., 1986. *Historical Costumes of Turkish Women*, Istanbul.

HALSBAND, R., 1965. *The Complete Letters of Lady Mary Wortley Montague*, (3 vols.), London.

HOWARD-MERRIAM, K., "Afghan women and their struggle for survival", in Farr, G. and Merrian, J. (eds), *Afghan Resistance The Politics of Survival*, Boulder 1987, 103-105.

HIGGINS, R., ND. *Tanagra and the Figurines*, London.

HIGGINS, R., 1967. *Greek Terracottas*, London.

HALLIDAY, W.R., 1928. *The Greek Questions of Plutarch*, Oxford.

HAMPE, Th., 1927. *Das Trachtenbuch des Christoph Weiditz, Vorwort und Einleitung*, Berlin.

HELLER, E. and MOSBAHI, H., *Hinter den Schleiern des Islam*, München, 1993.

HIRO, D. 1995. *Between Marx and Muhammad*, London.

HOLMGREN, V.C., nd. *Liberation à la Limena*.

HOLTON, P., 1991. *Mother Without a Mask*, London.

HOUIN, J., 1936. "Documents sur le costume des Musulmanes d'Espagne", *Revue Africaine*, 75 (1936), 43-46.

JASTROW, M., 1921. "Veiling in ancient Assyria" *Revue Archéologique*, 14 (1921), 209-38.

JEFFREY, P., 1979. *Frogs in a Well*, London.

JESSUP, H.H., 1873. *The women of the Arabs*, London.

JOHNSON, P. D., 1993. *Equal in Monastic Profession: Religious Women in Medieval France*, Chicago.

JOSHI, O.P., 1992. "Continuity and change in Hindu Women's Dress", in: R. Barnes and J. B. Eicher (eds), *Dress and Gender: Making and Meaning*, New York and Oxford, 214-231.

JOUIN, J., 1936. "Le costume de la femme israélite au Maroc", *Journal de la Société des Africanistes*, 6 (1936), 167-186.

JUYNBOLL, Th. W., 1930. *Handleiding tot de Kennis van De Mohammedaansche Wet*, Leiden.

KALTER, J. 1984. *The Arts and Crafts of Turkestan*, London.

KALTER, J. 1992. *The Arts and Crafts of Syria*, London.

KANAFANI, A., 1983. *Aesthetics and Ritual in the United Arab Emrites: The Anthropology of Food and Personal Adornment among Arabian Women*, Syracuse.

KEDDIE, N.R. and BARON, B., 1991. *Women in Middle Eastern History*, New Haven and London.

KEENAN, J.H., 1974. "The Tuareg veil", *Revue de l'Occident Musulman*, 17 (1974), 107-118.

KING, H., 1983. "Bound to bleed: Artemis and Greek women", in: eds. A. Cameron and A. Kuhrt, *Images of Women in Antiquity*, London, 109-127.

KIRAY, M., 1965. "The women of small towns", in: E. Lytle (ed), *Women in Turkish Society*, Leiden, 259-278.

KRAELING, C., 1956. *The Synagogue, The Excavations of Dura-Europos, Final Report 8.1*, New Haven.

KUPER, H., 1973. "Costume and identity", *Comparative Studies in Society and History*, 15 (1973), 348-67.

LA FOLLETTE, L., 1994. "The costume of the Roman bride", in: Sebesta, J.L. and Bonfante, L. (eds), *The World of Roman Costume*, 54-63.

LACEY, W.K., 1980. *The Family in Classical Greece*, Auckland (2nd ed).

LANE, E.W., 1895. *Manners and Customs of the Modern Egyptian*, London.

LAVER, J., 1995. *Costume and Fashion*, London.

LENCZOWSKI, G. (ed)., 1978. *Iran under the Pahlavis*, Stanford.

LERNER, G., 1986. *The Creation of Patriarchy*, Oxford.

LEON, L.C., 1981. *Traditional Dress of Peru*, Lima.

LESOURDE, M., 1954. "Le voile de la honte", *Bulletin de Liaison Saharienne*, XVI (1954), 27-4.

LEVY, R., 1935. "Notes on costume from Arabic sources", *Journal of the Royal Asiatic Society*, (1935), 319-338.

LEYENAAR-PLAISIER, P.G., 1986. *Griekse Terracotta's*, The Hague.

LEWIS, B., 1968. *The Emergence of Modern Turkey*, Oxford.

LISSENBERG, E., 1991. "Kleding in de gevangenis", *Textielhistorische Bijdragen*, 31 (1991), 114-129.

LLOYD S., 1967. *Early Highland Peoples of Anatolia*, London.

DE LOREY, E. and SLADEN, D., 1907. *The Moon of the Fourteenth Night: Being the Private Life of an Unmarried Diplomat in Persia during the Revolution*, London.

LYALL, C.J., 1918. *The Mufaddaliyat*, Oxford (2 vols).

MACARTNEY, Lady C., 1985. *An English Lady in Chinese Turkestan*, Oxford, 1985 (original version, 1931).

MACLEAN, F., 1985. *Eastern Approaches*, London.

McCRACKEN, G., 1995. "Clothing as language: an object lesson in the study of the expressive properties of material culture", in: B. Reynolds and M.A. Stott, *Material Anthropology: Contemporary Approaches to Material Culture*, Lanham, New York, London, 103-128.

MACKENZIE, J.M., 1995. *Orientalism: History, Theory and the Arts*, Manchester.

MACLEOD, A.E., 1992. *Accommodating Protest: Working Women, the New Veiling and Change in Cairo*, Cairo.

MABRO, J., 1930. *Veiled Half-Truths: Western Travellers' Perceptions of Middle Eastern Women*, New York, 1991.

MAHMOODY, B., 1989. *Not Without My Daughter*, London.

MAHMOODY, B., 1992. *For the Love of a Child*, New York.

MAKHLOUF, C., 1979. *Changing Veils: Women and Modernisation in North Yemen*, London.

MARÇAIS, G., 1930. *Le Costume Musulman d'Alger*, Paris.

MARMORSTEIN, E., 1954. "The veil in Judaism and Islam", *The Journal of Jewish Studies*, V:1 (1954), 1-11.

ACLA MAUDUDI, A., 1979. *Purdah and the Status of Woman in Islam*, Lahore.

MAY, F.L., 1957. *Silk Textiles of Spain: Eighth to Fifteenth Century*, New York.

MAYER, L.A., 1943. "Costumes of Mamluk women", *Islamic Culture*, XVII (1943), 293-303.

MAYER, L.A., 1952. *Mamluk Costume*, Genève.

EL-MESSIRI, S., 1978. "Self-image of traditional urban women in Cairo", in: L. Beck and N. Keddie eds., *Women in the Muslim World*, Cambridge Mass., 522-540.

MEYERS, C., 1978. "The roots of restriction: women in early Israel", *Biblical Archaeologist*, 41 (1978), 91-103.

MICKLEWRIGHT, N., 1987. "Tracing the transformations in women's dress in nineteenth-century Istanbul", *Dress*, 13 (1987), 33-43.

MINORSKY, V. (trans.), 1937. *Hudad al-Alam (The Regions of the World)*, London.

MOGHADAM, V.M., 1993. *Modernizing Women: Gender and Social Change in the Middle East*, London.

MOLLARD-BESQUES, S., 1963. *Catalogue Raisonné des Figurines et Reliefs en Terre-cuite Grecs et Romains Myrina*, Paris.

MOMEN, M., 1985. *An Introduction to Shi`i Islam*, Oxford.

MONTAGUE, M. W., 1708-1720. *The Complete Letters*, London (London, 1925 ed).

MOOSTERSHAR, C., 1995. *Unveiled: Love and Death among the Ayatollahs*, London.

MORIOKA, M. and RATHBUN, W.J. 1993. "Kasuri, Shiborizone and Koshi Patterns" in: Rathbun, W.J. *Beyond the Tanabata Bridge: Traditional Japanese Textiles*, 129-168.

MUHSEN, Z., 1994. *Sold*, London.

MÜLLER-LANCET, 1976. *The Jews of Yemen*, Chicago.

MUNDY, M., 1983. "San`a dress 1920-1975", in: R. B. Sarjeant and R. Lewcock (eds), *Sana: An Arabic Islamic City*, London, 529-40.

MUSIL, A., 1928. *Manner and Customs of the Rwala Bedouins*, London.

MURPHY, R., 1961. "Social distance and the veil", *American Anthropologist*, 66 (1961), 1257-74.

NAIPUL, V.S., 1982. *Among the Believers: An Islamic Journey*, New York.

NICHOLAISEN, J., 1963. *Ecology and Culture of the Pastoral Tuareg*, Copenhagen.

NIZAMI, 1881. *Iskandarnameh. Nizami, Sikander Nama e Bora*, (trans. H. Wilberforce Clarke), London.

OHANIAN, A., 1922. *The Dancer of Shamakha*, London.

ONNE, E., 1980. *Photographic Heritage of the Holy Land 1839-1914*, Manchester.

PAPANEK, H., 1973. "Purdah: Separate worlds and symbolic shelter", *Comparative Studies in Society and History*, 15 (1973), 289-525.

PERDRIZET, P., 1921. *Les Terres cuites grècques d'Egypte de la collection Fouquet*, Nancy, Paris, Strasbourg.

PEREZ, N.N., 1988. *Focus East: Early Photography in the Near East 1839-1885*, New York.

PETRIE, W.M.F. 1931. *Seventy Years in Archaeology*, London.

PHILIPPI, T., 1978. "Feminism and national politics in Egypt", in: L. Beck and N. Keddie (eds), *Women in the Muslim World*, Cambridge Mass., 277-294.

POSTGATE, J.N., 1979. "On some Assyrian ladies", *Iraq*, 41 (1979), 89-103.

QUESADA, A.M. 1968. *Lima, Ciudad de los Reyes*, Lima.

RABY, J., 1982. *Venice, Dürer and the Oriental Mode*, London, 1982.

RACKOW, E., 1958. *Beiträge zur Kenntnis der materiellen Kultur Norwest-Marokkos*, Wiesbaden.

RAJAB, J., 1989. *Palestinian Costume*, London.

RAMAZANI, N., 1983. "The veil - piety or protest?", *Journal of South Asian and Middle Eastern Studies*, 7 (1983), 20-36.

RAMAZANI, N., 1993. "Women in Iran: The revolutionary ebb and flow", *Middle Eastern Journal*, 47 (1993), 409-428.

RATTRAY, J., 1849. *The Costumes of the Various Tribes, Portraits of Ladies of Rank, Celebrated Princes and Chiefs, Views of the Principal Fortresses, and Interior of the Cities and Temples of Afghanistan*, London.

RICE, C. Coluver, 1923. *Persian Women and their Ways*, London.

RICHTER, G.M.A., *Handbook of Greek Art*, London.

ROSENTHAL, F., 1971. "A note on the mandil", *Four Essays on Art and Literature in Islam*, 1971, 63-100, Leiden (Brill).

ROSS, H.C., 1981. *The Art of Arabian Costume*, Switzerland.

ROTH, M.T., 1987. "Age at marriage and the household: a study of Neo-Babylonian and Neo-Assyrian forms", *Comparative Studies in Society and History*, 29 (1987), 715-747.

RUBENS, A., 1967. *History of Jewish Costume*, New York.

DE Sacy, S., 1826. *Chrestomathie arabe*, vol. 1, Paris.

RUDENKO, S.I., 1970. *Frozen Tombs of Siberia*, London.

RUGH, A.B., 1987. *Reveal and Conceal: Dress in Contemporary Egypt*, Cairo.

SANASARIAN, E., 1985. "Characteristics of women's movements in Iran", in: A. Fathi (ed), *Women and the Family in Iran*, Leiden, 86-106.

SAPORETTI, C., 1979. *The Status of Women in the Middle Assyrian Period*, Malibu.

SASSON, J., 1993. *Princess*, London.

SASSON, J., 1994. *Daughters of Arabia*, London.

SCARCE, J., 1975. "The development of women's veils in Persia and Afghanistan", *Costume*, 9 (1975), 4-14.

SCARCE, J., 1981. *Middle Eastern Costume from the Tribes and Cities of Iran and Turkey*, Edinburgh.

SCARCE, J., 1987. *Women's Costume of the Near and Middle East*, London.

SCHULMAN, A.R., 1979. "Diplomatic marriage in the Egyptian New Kingdom", *Journal of Near Eastern Studies*, 38 (1979), 177-193.

SENG, Y.K. and WASS B., 1995. "Traditional Palestinian wedding dress as a symbol of nationalism", in: J.B. Eicher (ed), *Dress and Ethnicity: Change Across Space and Time*, Oxford and Washington, 227-54.

SEYRIG, H., 1934, "Antiquités Syriennes", *Syria*, 15 (1934), 155-86.

SHAWN, T., 1929. *Gods Who Dance*, New York.

SHAY, A., 1982. "Traditional clothing in Iran", *Ornament*, 6 (1982), 2-9.

SPELLBERG, D.A., 1991. "Political action and public example: A'isha and the Battle of the Camel", in: N.R. Keddie and B. Baron (eds), *Women in Middle Eastern History*, New Haven, 45-57.

STILLMAN, Y.K., 1972. *Female Attire of Medieval Egypt: According to the Trousseau Lists and Cognate Material from the Cairo Geniza*, (Ph.D. thesis).

STILLMAN, Y.K., 1981. "Costume", in: Topman, J., *Traditional Crafts of Saudi Arabia*, London.

STILLMAN, Y.K., 1986. "Libas", *Encyclopedia of Islam*, 2nd ed,. vol. 5, 732-750.

STILLMAN, Y.K., "Jewish costume and textile studies: The state of the art", *Jewish Folklore and Ethnology Review*, 10 (1988), 5-9.

STILLMAN, Y.K. and MICKLEWRIGHT, N., 1992. "Costume in the Middle East", *Middle East Studies Association Bulletin*, 26, no. 1 (1992), 13-38.

STOL, M., 1995. "Women in Mesopotamia", *Journal of Economic and Social History of the Orient*, 38 (1995), 123-144.

STUKI, A., 1978. "Horses and women", *Afghanistan Journal*, 5 (1978), 140-9.

TABARI, A. and YEGANEH, N., 1982. *In the Shadow of Islam: The Women's Movement in Iran*, London.

THIENEN, F. van, 1930. *Das Kostüm der Blütezeit Hollands, 1600-1660*, Berlin.

THIENEN, F. van and DUYVETTER, F., 1968. *Traditional Dutch Costumes*, Amsterdam.

TIETZES, H. and TIETZE-CONRAT, E., 1944. *The Drawings of the Venetian Painters*, New York.

THOMPSON, D.B., 1950. "A bronze dancer from Alexandria", *American Journal of Archaeology*, 54 (1950), 371-85.

THOMPSON, D.B., 1963. *Troy: Supplementary Monograph 3*, Princeton.

THORNTON, L., 1994. *Woman as Portrayed in Orientalist Painting*, Paris.

TOPMAN, J., 1981. *Traditional Crafts of Saudi Arabia*, London.

TROFIMOVA, A.G., 1979. "The garments of the present-day Azerbaidzhan population", in: J. Cordwell and R. Schwarz (ed), *The Fabrics of Culture*, The Hague, 405-14.

TSEVAT, M., 1975. "The husband veils a wife: Hittie Laws nos. 197-8", *Journal of Cuneiform Studies*, 27 (1975), 235-240.

TUGLACI, P., 1984. *Women of Istanbul in Ottoman times*, Istanbul.

ULMER, R., 1918. "Südpalälstinensische Kopfbedeckungen", *Zeitschrift des deutschen Palästina-Vereins*, 41 (1918), 35-53.

VATANDOUST, G.-R., 1985. "The status of Iranian women during the Phalavi Regime", in: A. Fathi (ed), *Women and the Family in Iran*, Leiden, 107-130.

DE VAUJANY, H. de., 1883. *Le Caire et ses environs: caractères, moeurs, costumes des Égyptiens modernes*, Paris.

VAUX, R. de., 1967. "Sur le voile des femmes dans L'ORIENT ancien", *Bible et Orient*, (1967), 397-412.

VECELLIO, C., (1598) *Habiti antichi, et moderni di tutto il Mondo*, Paris (1859 ed).

VENEMA, B. and BAKKER, J. (eds), 1994. *Vrouwen van de Midden Atlas: Vrij of Vroom?*, Utrecht.

VÖLGER, G., v. WELCK, K and HACKSTEIN, K., 1987. *Pracht und Geheimnis: Kleidung und Schmuck aus Palästina und Jordanien*, Cologne.

VOGELSANG-EASTWOOD, G.M., 1983. "A medieval face-veil from Egypt", *Costume*, 17 (1983), 33-38.

VOGELSANG-EASTWOOD, G.M., *Textiles and Clothing from the Tomb of Tutankhamun*, (forthcoming).

WAAGENAAR, S., 1995. Mata Hari: *Geslepen Spionne of Onschuldige Schoonheid*, Baarn.

WALTHER, W., 1981. *Die Frau im Islam*, Leipzig.

WALKER S., 1993. "Women and housing in Classical Greece: the archaeological evidence", in: Cameron, A., and Kuhrt, A. (eds), *Images of Women in Antiquity*, London, 81-91.

WEIDNER, E.F., 1954-6. "Hof- und Harems-Erlasse assyrischer Könige aus dem 2.Jahrtausend v. Chr", *Archiv für Orientforschung*, 17 (1954-6), 257-93.

WEIDITZ, C, (1529-32). *Das Trachtenbuch des Christoph Weidtiz von seinen Reisen nach Spanien und den Niederlanden, 1529-32*, Nuremburg (1927, ed. T. Hampe).

WEIR, S., 1989. *Palestinian Costume*, London.

WIKAN, U., 1982. *Behind the Veil in Arabia: Women in Oman*, Chicago.

WILBER, D.N., 1962. *Afghanistan*, New Haven.

WILBER, D.N., 1975. *Riza Shah Pahlavi: The Resurrection and Reconstruction of Iran*, New York.

WILLS, C.J., 1891. *In the Land of the Lion and Sun or Modern Persia, Being Experiences of Life in Persia from 1866 to 1881*, London.

WINGFIELD, L., 1868. *Under the Palms of Algeria and Tunis, London*, vol. II.

YARWOOD, D., 1988. *The Encyclopedia of World Costume*, London.

YAUKACHEVA, G.-R., 1959. "The feminst movement in Persia", *Central Asia Review*, 7 (1959), 74-83.

ZENO, C., 1873. *Travels in Persia*, London.